Preventing

Is there any evidence that we can reduce the incidence of mental ill-health? Is it possible to prevent recurrence of mental ill-health?

Aspirations to achieve both these goals have featured in mental health policy and practice for over 100 years. This comprehensive and accessible book draws on research on the development and persistence of behavioural problems in childhood, adult depression and schizophrenia. The association between social disadvantage and mental ill-health, as well as the need for preventive care to start from conception and the crucial importance of maternal mental health, is discussed.

A variety of prominent programmes which have good evidence of efficacy are described. These include:

- targeted approaches with individuals and families;
- macro policies affecting housing and employment;
- lifestyle contributions such as diet and exercise.

However, some attempts to achieve preventive benefits have not succeeded, and reflecting on these problems is an important feature of this review.

Jennifer Newton has written extensively on these issues for over 20 years, and her careful examination of the research literature provides a succinct overview of the state of current knowledge which will benefit mental health professionals, and students of health psychology and public health. It also takes a life course perspective, and considers how, when and why vulnerability persists through childhood into adult life, so it will interest those whose work focuses on child well-being.

Jennifer Newton co-ordinates post-graduate programmes in the Faculty of Social Sciences and Humanities at London Metropolitan University, and also teaches and undertakes research in mental health, social work and management. Previous research posts led to books including *Preventing Mental Illness*.

Preventing Mental Ill-Health

Informing public health planning and
mental health practice

Jennifer Newton

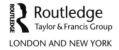

Routledge
Taylor & Francis Group

LONDON AND NEW YORK

First published 2013
by Routledge
2 Park Square, Milton Park, Abingdon, Oxon OX14 4RN

Simultaneously published in the USA and Canada
by Routledge
711 Third Avenue, New York, NY 10017

Routledge is an imprint of the Taylor & Francis Group, an informa business

British Library Cataloguing in Publication Data
A catalogue record for this book is available from the British Library

Library of Congress Cataloging in Publication Data
  Newton, Jennifer, 1953-
  Preventing mental ill-health: Informing public health planning and
  mental health practice / Jennifer Newton.
    p. cm.
  Includes bibliographical references and index.
  ISBN 978-0-415-45540-4 (hardback) — ISBN 978-0-415-45541-1
  (pbk.)   1. Mental illness—Prevention.   I. Title.
  RA790.N44 2012
  362.19689—dc23
                                                    2012012462

ISBN: 978–0–415–45540–4 (hbk)
ISBN: 978–0–415–45541–1 (pbk)
ISBN: 978–0–203–08564–6 (ebk)

Typeset in Times New Roman
by RefineCatch Limited, Bungay, Suffolk

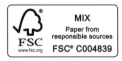

MIX
Paper from
responsible sources
FSC   FSC® C004839
www.fsc.org

Printed and bound by CPI Group (UK) Ltd, Croydon, CR0 4YY

Contents

Preface and acknowledgements

The reader might speculate on the hugely over-optimistic nature of the writer of this text, as few would be so foolhardy as to set out on such an enterprise. One might have thought that, having completed a similar enterprise in the 1980s and produced *Preventing Mental Illness* and *Preventing Mental Illness in Practice*, both commissioned by National MIND, I could have made a better guess at how extensive the literature had become in the intervening 24 years. But as discussed here later, optimists often do well in life because they persist long after others would give up, to achieve the unrealistic goals they can set themselves. My patient family will attest to the latter, and I must thank my husband Les for his unlimited tolerance and support of my long hours in front of the computer; also my patient son George. My daughters Josephine and Roxanne Newton tried to ensure I eventually met the fifth deadline set by taking on some of the bibliography checking themselves – thank you both.

An apology is offered to all the experts in each of the disciplines covered here for the simplification of complex ideas in your field. I have done my best to check that I have understood their essence correctly by sending each chapter to those who understand some of the specific areas better than I do. For this I must thank the kind friends and colleagues who helped along the way by reading sections or discussing them with me: George Brown, Tirril Harris, Tom Craig, Alan Rushton, Richard Skues, Liz Davies, Simon Brewer, and Mike Mills. Most also commented on the size of the challenge I set myself, and may not be convinced I have met it!

Much complex research is reviewed, with the aim of distilling the main points relevant to prevention with the minimum use of jargon or technical language. The approach has been to examine the evidence about what ought to work before turning to what has been tried. That is, what do we know about cause and course, what do we know about people who are resilient, what does it suggest we should be doing? The story develops then by exploring what has been tried, and whether it worked, and asking where we go next given the larger than expected gap between these two – important insights often seem not to translate to practice.

This is not a systematic review. It is more like a detective story. Find an informed recent review of the state of the evidence relating to part of the story of interest, and use this to direct me to other important sources. These sources have also sometimes redirected my investigations to cover other areas of evidence that had not been foreseen. In this particular detective story there are far too many suspects to investigate with as much rigour as a reader might wish. Some have been explored far less than others, but with the aim of at least arriving at some tentative conclusions about the significance of the role played by each one.

To locate the initial sources, I usually started with use of a library database, most frequently Academic Search Complete and PsycINFO. A database lists papers with most recently published papers first, and the discovery of a few helpful recent papers would in turn lead me to research considered particularly important by these experts. Although systematic reviews and meta-analyses are assumed to be the best evidence, it did not always seem to be so, as they were sometimes conducted without a strong theoretical rationale. Hence what was included and what was drawn out of these were sometimes less helpful than reviews that were less wide ranging but more analytic. And a review of a large number of weak studies that point in the same direction does not add up to a strong conclusion, though no doubt I fell into this trap occasionally too. Important studies are summarized from their original papers, not from reviews by others.

I have stayed with a wide focus, and will expect criticism from biological psychiatry for entertaining ideas that positive thinking, humiliating experience, or social status might be important, and from those in positive psychology who will dislike the engagement with diagnosed disorder and genetic evidence. In mental health, differing perspectives are often held with passion, and competing perspectives too readily dismissed. It can make criticism dangerous, though I have entered all houses of these new religions as an agnostic, and hope to take a reader through the arguments with as much critical intelligence as I am able to do given my limited history with each.

1   Introduction

To focus a book on prevention suggests there might indeed be some magic pill, a fish oil capsule perhaps, or other chemical or a psycho-social equivalent, that we could take or administer to others to immunize us against the often miserable, sometimes frightening, sometimes confused, occasionally exciting feelings we call mental illness. In a sense there is – we need to inherit the right genes, be kept safe from accidental damage and traumatic experience, feel the love and protection of a parent or parent figure throughout childhood, learn the life skills to keep us safe, and find our own place in society alongside people or at least one person who cares about us. Easy. But how important is each one of these, and how far can strength in one compensate for vulnerability in another?

The following 11 chapters tell this story, including the magic pill and the fish oil detour, but starting by questioning the words and assumptions behind the concept of prevention, and the reasons for our interest in this. Discussion of the possibilities requires engaging with hugely contested and controversial issues and ideas, not least of which is the choice of words to describe mental ill-health and whether it matters. Chapters 2 and 4 take these two areas of controversy in turn, setting out the basis of enquiry for subsequent chapters. In this first chapter, these difficulties will be side-stepped, to explore the increasing interest in prevention in policy, to provide a brief account of early progress, and to explain how this informs the structure of this book.

Why so much interest in prevention now?

To a large extent, the answer is – money. First and foremost, the realization that the increasing wealth of the Western world is not reflected in increasing happiness (Layard, 2006a). Second, that unhappy people, as well as those with diagnosed mental illness, are more likely to be found in poorer districts within a society, or to live in relatively poor material circumstances, these differences becoming ever more visible in wealthier countries (Wilkinson, 1996). Third, that those with poor mental health cost the economy a great deal.

The numbers of books appearing in the past few years on happiness, and on inequalities in health, attest to our renewed fascination with what is now popularly referred to as 'wellbeing'. Many question why, with all the wealth of the developed world, their peoples are not happier. Various estimates of population happiness do not show a greater proportion of happy people as GDP rises; in fact, in some cases changes can go in the opposite direction (Wilkinson, 1996; Layard, 2006a). Richard Easterlin was one of the first to describe the paradox that at any one point in time, happiness and income levels are correlated, and over the short term income and happiness continue to go together – happiness falls in an economic downturn, and rises during an expansion – but over a period of 10 years or more, happiness does not rise with rising GDP, a finding confirmed by drawing on data from developing countries and Eastern European countries as well as those in the West (Easterlin et al., 2010). Those exploring the differences between countries are emphasizing social factors such as trust, equality, full employment, crime, and willingness to help one another as likely to account for much of the difference (e.g. Putnam, 2000), and see a link between these societal characteristics not only with subjective happiness, but with mental and physical ill-health and with life expectancy (Marmot Review, 2010).

But the concern with cost is also linked to population change, and the increasing challenge for governments of funding welfare services to support people who are out of the labour market. This concern pre-dates the banking crisis that has shaken governments in the Western world over recent years, and policy has been shifting the priority from treatment and care towards prevention and public health for many years, as exemplified by an opening statement of the Report of the Surgeon General in the US (1999: 3):

> The report was prepared against a backdrop of growing awareness in the United States and throughout the world of the immense burden of disability associated with mental illnesses. In the United States, mental disorders collectively account for more than 15 percent of the overall burden of disease from *all* causes and slightly more than the burden associated with all forms of cancer (Murray & Lopez, 1996). These data underscore the importance and urgency of treating and preventing mental disorders and of promoting mental health in our society.
>
> (emphasis in original)

The Murray and Lopez reference is to the major study sponsored by WHO and the World Bank and based at Harvard University known as the Global Burden of Disease study, which calculated the health effects of more than 100 diseases and injuries in eight regions of the world, starting in 1990, and updated in 2004. It provided a comprehensive and internally consistent estimate of mortality and morbidity by age, gender and region, using a new measure of 'disease burden' – a calculation of years of life lived with disability of a defined level of severity, or years of life lost through premature death (together described as the disability adjusted life years or DALYs). As a proportion of total DALYs, cardiovascular diseases as a group were top of the list of days lost (18.6%) in established market economies in 1990, but 'all mental illness' came in second place with 15.4%, slightly ahead of cancers at 15%. Days lost to alcohol use and respiratory conditions, the next largest problems, fall a long way short of these figures, both just under 5%. Separating the cardiovascular and mental illness categories into specific disorders shows that unipolar major depression is the mental illness diagnosis contributing to the most DALYs, and in 'global burden' this is second only to ischaemic heart disease (Murray and Lopez, 1996).

The various costs associated with mental ill-health are not simply the costs to governments of treatment (including expenditure on services and drugs), or of state benefits to sustain those not working, but also the cost to industry of lost productivity through absence from work or from people working below full capacity, and the human costs to individuals and their families of reduced quality of life and often reduced income. About 7% of the UK population are without work and receiving incapacity benefit due to long-term health conditions or disabilities (Black, 2008); the average UK employee takes 6.4 days of sick leave, and over a third of short periods of sick leave (under a week) and about half of longer periods are due to mental health related problems (CBI, 2010). Numbers who are less productive than usual, perhaps reflected in impaired concentration or energy, are unknown, but thought to be substantial – a problem described as 'presenteeism' (SCMH, 2007), and bringing more attention now to preventive strategies in the workplace.

Government spending around the world on mental health varies greatly, with 28% of countries not having any allocated budget, and a further 36% allocating only 1% or less of public health funds to mental health (WHO, 2001). A study commissioned by the Alberta Mental Health Board (Canada) compared spending by a selected eight other developed countries with its own, finding the UK government to spend the largest proportion of the health budget on mental health (12%), more than twice the proportion allocated by Canada (5.4%) (Lim et al., 2008), though it is noted that these comparisons are not wholly reliable given the difficulty in ensuring comparable budget scope. The UK's *New Horizons* policy for mental health from 2010 quoted a more recent figure of 14% of NHS funds spent on mental health, and taking government, industry and individual and family cost together, estimates the total as £77 billion for 2003 (calculations by SCMH, 2007), a cost it suggests may double within 20 years. This presumably reflects the fact that by 2009, mental ill-health had overtaken cardiovascular diseases as having the highest total burden in the UK, with 26% of DALYs lost due to mental ill-health, and expected to rise to 31% by 2030 (DH, 2009b).

Funding associated costs is the worry – the challenge faced by public services that rely to a large extent on funds from a shrinking working population. Across the world, life expectancy is increasing, and the dependency ratio with it. For instance, the proportion of the population over the age of 65 in the UK is projected to rise from 16% in 2008 to 23% in 2033, meaning that there were 3.2 people of working age for each person of state pensionable age in 2008, but this will only be 2.8 by 2033 *after* taking account of increases in retirement ages planned during this period (ONS, 2009a). Given the correlations between dementia and age, many dramatic statistics have been published in recent years about the 'global epidemic' of Alzheimer's disease (e.g. Brookmeyer et al., 2007). Recent UK calculations are that spending on dementia will rise from 66% of all mental health service costs to 73% by 2026, and total spending on mental health will rise by over 40% (McCrone et al., 2008). Public policy in the UK and elsewhere has been responding to this challenge by looking for all kinds of cost savings, as public service arrangements come under strain. Keeping people of all ages out of the most expensive care options – hospitals and nursing homes – has been top of the list for many years already.

Not surprisingly, options that may prevent ill-health and disability are currently gaining much greater prominence, as are policies that bring people who may hitherto have considered themselves, or been considered by others, as disabled back into the work force (DH, 2009a). This change is one that many will welcome, along with a major shift in emphasis from a treatment focus to prevention towards inclusion and recovery (as defined by the service user), and towards social care and support deriving from communities, other people with similar problems, the individual themselves, and families, rather than the state, and for which the case is clearly laid out by the government (DH, 2008).

What have we tried in the past, and what did we learn?

The possibility of preventing mental illness has been a focus of policy and practice for at least 100 years, most notably among philanthropists and reformers; sociologists, psychotherapists and social psychiatrists; and psychiatrists attached to the military services.

Reformists and philanthropists

Some of the early reformists of treatment services, such as Philippe Pinel (1745–1820, whose grandson Samuel was the first to describe it as *le traitement moral* (Tuke, 1813)), believed mental ill-health had psycho-social causes. Pinel emphasized the importance of individual sentiments and their social context, such as being held in esteem, being treated with respect, retaining dignity (Gerard, 1997: 388), and the role of extreme experiences of frustration, disappointment and humiliation that he believed typically preceded an episode of 'mania or mental alienation' (Gerard, 1997: 389). The treatment he provided at the Bicêtre hospital in Paris also emphasized a healthy diet, firm management to ensure order, but through kindness, not force, and used recovering patients as attendants with important roles in creating a respectful therapeutic climate. In England William Tuke followed his example at the York Retreat (Tuke, 1813). Such therapy was far from typical of the time, when in fact 'manic' patients in many hospitals were still frequently restrained with chains, and patients in many hospitals for many decades after this experienced inhumane treatment, as Clifford Beers describes, documenting his own experiences in *A Mind that Found Itself* (published in 1908), hoping to stimulate public opinion against them.

An influential American psychiatrist, Adolph Meyer, became interested in Beers' writing, and persuaded Beers to work with him toward reform of the system, including public education and eventually the prevention of mental illness (Levine, 1981; Leighton, 1982). Meyer wished to integrate the best of the then declining tradition of moral treatment and the associated ideas for the role of the social environment with the more recent ideas on the biology of the brain. Together Meyer and Beers founded first the Connecticut Society for Mental Hygiene, and the following year (1909) in New York, the National Committee for Mental Hygiene.

A similar non-governmental organization, the National Council for Mental Hygiene, was formed in London in 1923, and Clifford Beers spoke at two of its meetings in the first year. As described by Newton (1988), it had six aims, of which the first two related to prevention:

1   The improvement of the Mental Health of the Community. This involves a closer and more critical study of the social habits, industrial life, and environments of the people, with a view to eradicating those factors that lead to mental ill-health and unhappiness and to educating the public in all matters that militate for and against good mental health.
2   To study the causes underlying congenital and acquired mental disease,[1] with a view to its prevention. To further this the Council will promote scientific investigation by competent workers.

Three subcommittees were formed, one to prepare reports on the prevention and early treatment of mental disorders, chaired by Sir Maurice Craig; the other two to work towards the other objectives, relating to the aftercare and treatment of the insane, and on mental deficiency and crime. Preventive proposals centred on child development: good antenatal care (diet, exercise, avoidance of infection), then regular checks on the child and early referral for signs of mental disorder (National Council for Mental Hygiene, 1927).

Both the British and the American mental hygiene organizations developed branches across the country to promote their ideals nationally, and, in line with the changing emphasis in psychiatry, renamed themselves associations for mental health. The hygiene and health movements had much in common, both being concerned with reforming mental hospitals, with community participation and with prevention. But the latter had anti-medical components that increased with time, and the rationale for moving away from institutional care became primarily social. From the 1960s, ideas relating to culture, social class, stress, social disorganization and unhealthy roles became prominent, and a new academic discipline came to the fore known as social psychiatry (Leighton, 1982; see Newton, 1988).

In the early days of the mental hygiene movement, however, child guidance centres were arguably the first preventive mental health service, numbers increasing rapidly to 617 separate agencies by 1935 in the US. The first child guidance clinic opened in London in 1927. Children with delinquent, difficult or neurotic behaviour could be seen by a psychiatrist, social worker or psychologist. The hope was that these services would lead to a better understanding of child development and psychological causes of difficulty, and by providing timely guidance would reduce current problems and help to prevent more serious problems later in life (Sampson, 1980). Their focus was soon extended to include educational problems, and their remit then greatly increased.

In the US, the origins of child guidance clinics were born from aspirations to prevent juvenile delinquency by the Commonwealth Fund, which funded a number of demonstration clinics in the US, and at first included a community outreach approach with a focus on the neighbourhood, school, family and home life. But this shifted quite rapidly towards a professional, institution-based service and a more medical ethos that located the problems in the child. According to Horn (1989), the psychotherapeutic focus and shift towards problems in middle class children were a consequence of this change in emphasis. She illustrates these points in her description of 179 cases seen in a Philadelphia clinic between 1925 and 1944, showing a shift from social to individual problems, from lower class to middle class families, and from referrals from schools to referrals from parents. Jones (1999) finds the same changes in her analysis of case records of the Boston Clinic. Horn notes that the increasing dominance of psychiatrists provided no improvement in positive outcomes compared to that achieved by the educators and social reformers who were early pioneers. Despite some critiques of the 'medicalization' of child difficulty (Horn, 1989) the description of the service in the south of England between 1984 and 1996 still showed the staffing to be psychologists, psychiatrists, nurses, social workers and psychotherapists, and to discuss their work in terms of treatment (Thompson et al., 2003). There was, however, during this period a shift in workload from doctors to nurses, and back towards a community outreach approach, which was beginning to be reflected in a higher proportion of working class service users, and engagement with the problems of very young children. The focus remained on the management of the young child's difficult behaviour and/or sleep problems, and often on the mother's parenting skills.

The American philanthropists behind the Commonwealth Fund also funded the first English child guidance centres, setting aside $68,000 in 1929 for the English programme (Stewart, 2006). In addition, the fund sponsored the first diploma for psychiatric social work at the London School of Economics in the same year, as it saw this role as central to its approach to supporting the family. In 1931, the fund contributed to one of the first successful child guidance centres in Scotland – conditional on the scheme adhering to its medical approach (led by a child psychiatrist, psychologist, and psychiatric social worker), despite being run by a Catholic nun, Sister Marie Hilda (Stewart, 2006). She combined her religious and therapeutic aspirations as:

> to socialise the neurotic and aggressive, encourage the dull and retarded, and redeem the delinquent, and thus to decrease the number of mental breakdowns and to lessen the number of prison inmates in later life. By its constructive methods, the (Notre Dame) Clinic hopes to build up integrated personalities capable of taking their place as members of the family, of the Church and of the State.
>
> (Sister Marie Hilda, in a 1950 pamphlet for the Catholic Truth Society entitled *Child Guidance*, cited by Stewart, 2006: 68)

The *Glasgow Catholic* newspaper heralded the opening of the centre with a slightly different summary of the target group: 'the study and treatment of children who, though given average home and school conditions, remain an enigma to their parents, and by their undisciplined behaviour form one of the chief difficulties of the classroom' (cited by Stewart, 2006: 61). The role of the psychiatric social worker was initially to help the mother to acquire better habits through simple advice and guidance, such as how to respond to temper tantrums (Horn, 1984). From 1931 onwards, their role appeared to be more supportive and encouraging and less directive, which Horn (1984) describes as due to the professional development of social work. As they became more professional, they became less moralistic.

But in the end, the effectiveness of the child guidance movement was judged to be very limited. Given the substantial numbers of children with behavioural, emotional and educational difficulties, these one-to-one methods could only hope to reach a very small proportion of them, and on this basis alone they could make little impact. Cartwright (1974) argued that one of the weaknesses of the clinics was their failure in many cases to establish collaborative relationships with families, resulting in children not attending for second or subsequent appointments. Sampson (1980) maintained that there was little evidence of their impact on delinquency rates, or in making adult neuroses more predictable. However, many lessons from their work (e.g. techniques using behaviour modification) have permeated lay understanding, featuring in child care manuals, radio programmes and popular journals, and they have contributed to thinking in remedial education and art therapy that has had wider application. In contributing to public knowledge on coping with problem behaviours in children, they can be argued to have played a valuable role in prevention.

Sociology, psychotherapy and social psychiatry

Gerald Caplan was one of many child psychiatrists who became disillusioned with the child guidance method. He had trained under John Bowlby in London, and set up a child guidance centre in Israel after the Second World War, aiming to build a programme of preventive child psychiatry (Caplan-Moskovitch, 1982). However, he realized that the childhood problems he saw could be traced back to mother–child relationships, and these in turn to the mother's childhood experience. A further disadvantage was the large number of highly trained professionals needed to help a small number of troubled individuals, and the aim of intervening at earlier and earlier stages in the development of disorder. Instead he proposed a method of helping large numbers of people to provide preventive support to troubled people of all ages, offering training to health workers of all kinds. He highlighted the role of life crises as the point at which those vulnerable to mental ill-health would be most likely to develop disorder, but when they would also be most receptive to outside efforts to help them. He saw potential in the work of Erich Lindemann, who was providing similar training to clergymen, teachers and others in a caring role in Boston, helping people to adjust to crises in their lives. Following his move to the Harvard School of Public Health in Boston, Caplan began to reconceptualize prevention along public health lines, defining primary, secondary and tertiary prevention. Coping with crisis became the focal point of his work, described in 1964 in his influential book *Principles of Preventive Psychiatry*.

Studying how people adapt to particular crises was expected to lead to the development of methods of anticipatory guidance and preventive intervention. These ideas were considered relevant to the newly emerging community mental health centres (CMHCs). The potential was that they could perhaps identify people facing stressful events and transitions and help them to improve their adaptive capability and resistance to mental disorder (primary prevention), or identify and offer help to those in early stages of mental ill-health (secondary prevention), and help to alleviate the disabling consequences of an established illness (tertiary prevention).

However, the CMHCs also failed to live up to expectations, as Leighton (1982) described. Only 500 of the projected 2000 were built in the US by the mid-1960s; there was disagreement on what was meant by mental health, and on the best ways to achieve it, and a growing realization about the feasibility and cost of helping the very large numbers of people with mental ill-health, more particularly the possibility of promoting 'positive mental health'. 'The goal of providing services for everyone with a psychological or social need began to seem more and more like trying to drink the ocean' (Leighton, 1982: 72).

Another early influential figure in the development of ideas in preventive mental health was Marie Jahoda, a distinguished social psychologist and researcher committed to social change and civil liberties. Arguably her most important contribution came from her analysis of the mental health effects of unemployment, based on a detailed descriptive study of the life of residents of Marienthal, Austria following closure of a local textile business (1928–30) where the majority of residents had worked. Most households were without a single member in paid work, and suffered great poverty as well as the psychological effects of worklessness. She described the apathy and resignation of the subjects – their reduced level of activity and demoralization, focus on the bare necessities, and loss of hope and future plans (Jahoda et al., 1933/1972; Eisenberg and Lazarsfeld, 1938). Some years later she was one of the first to conceptualize the differences between 'positive mental health' and health as the absence of illness, and saw unemployment as affecting the former rather than the latter. More than 20 years later, she published *Current Concepts of Positive Mental Health* in which she proposed six core elements of a state of positive mental health: having positive attitudes towards the self; self-development toward self-actualization; an integration of these two – positive attitudes with self-development; autonomy; a clear perception of reality; and environmental mastery. She suggested that for most people regular work is essential for positive mental health, because it provides a sense of identity and social contacts, and structures time.

These insights also informed the thinking of pioneering social psychiatrists such as Douglas Bennett in the UK in the 1950s, who developed vocational rehabilitation services for those treated in hospital for serious mental ill-health, and facilitated a much more optimistic view of recovery. This approach was supported also by sociologists such as Wolf Wolfensberger (1983) who was emphasizing the importance of a socially valued role in society for people with disabilities. Their perspectives have been more recently reflected in the 'recovery vision' of mental health service users, and in their aims to influence mental health services development (Anthony, 1993 and see Chapter 2).

Military psychiatry

The major world wars brought to prominence a differing perspective on the cost of mental ill-health, notably its role in the loss of military capacity, and the need to prevent this. About 118,000 men and women were discharged from the three British services for psychiatric reasons between September 1939 and June 1944, this being the most common reason for medical discharge during the Second World War (Ahrenfeldt, 1958; see Newton, 1988). Ahrenfeldt explains what was learned. Firstly, that high morale, maintained through skilled leadership, good discipline and adequate training, reduced psychiatric problems. (Shay (1994, 2002) makes a similar point in his account of his work with Vietnam veterans.) Even more important, however, was that the abilities and aptitudes of men were appropriately matched to the tasks demanded of them. A disproportionate number of men of limited intelligence fighting at the front as part of the infantry suffered a psychiatric breakdown, as did men of high intelligence assigned for general labouring duties in the Pioneer Corps. Part-way through the war psychiatrists were allowed to recommend for transfer to employment of a special nature men who were working in jobs for which they were temperamentally unsuitable. 'This procedure resulted in a great diminution of the numbers of cases admitted to hospital because of a psychiatric breakdown and was a notable achievement in vocational selection and psychiatric prophylaxis' (Ahrenfeldt, 1958: 19). By 1942 this led to procedures (selection tests) being set up to avoid such problems arising in the first place.

The duration of the time at the front was also, not surprisingly, found to determine the rate of breakdown. John Appel, who became the first chief of the newly created Preventive Psychiatry branch of the US Army Psychiatry Division during the Second World War, describes his role in identifying the point beyond which almost every man will break – '200 to 240 aggregate days of combat' – though he noted that British soldiers who had a four day rest away from the line every 12 days could last twice as long, 400 days. After this any man was ineffective, 'If he had not "cracked up," he was so jittery under shell fire and so overly cautious that in addition to being ineffective as a soldier, he demoralized the newer men' (Appel, 1999: 22). Along with Gilbert Beebe, a statistician in the Surgeon General's office, Appel set about analysing casualty rates in the Mediterranean fighting zone. They found that by 214 days all men who were not killed, injured or physically ill 'had broken down psychologically'. Appel's recommendation to the army Chief of Staff to limit all tours of duty for infantrymen to 180 days was accepted, becoming army policy that was applied in Europe and the Pacific, and in subsequent wars in Vietnam and Korea. While he was unable to report on the benefits of the policy, he argued that it provided a ray of hope to soldiers, a way to cope with the stress, knowing that providing they stayed alive, there was a known end point. Otherwise the only way out was death, injury or war's end.

At the end of the war, there were efforts to prevent psychiatric problems in returning military personnel through civil resettlement units (CRUs) offering rest and recuperation, specialist advice, and help to improve work skills and to find employment. The support and sense of gratitude extended towards returning British servicemen was not so evident, however, to the US veterans of Vietnam, nor to more recent veterans of unpopular wars. Vietnam veterans were often reviled, ostracized, seen as an embarrassment and given little help to reintegrate to civilian life, sometimes choosing not to seek it, preferring not to disclose their military past (Paulson et al., 2007). Daryl Paulson's review includes his own account of his service in Vietnam, and of the rejection and revulsion expressed of the war by civilian contacts after his return, and hence of his part in it, finding this to be as damaging to his mental health as any experience of the war itself (Paulson et al., 2007: xi). Suicide rates were reported to be very high (e.g. Salmon, 1985), although the numbers are disputed. Post-traumatic stress disorder (PTSD) was recorded in 15% of Vietnam veterans in the 1980s, and 10% of all veterans still had PTSD symptoms 30 years after their return from Vietnam (Koenen et al., 2008).

Shay's accounts of his work with those with PTSD (or a 'psychological war injury' as he would prefer to call it) devote particular attention to the difficulty faced by those soldiers who successfully build a 'warrior ethos' to perform well at war, and then struggle to adapt to the very different sets of values required for successful civilian life. Shay argues that governments need to invest in programmes to help returning soldiers to *unlearn* their ability to kill. He also advocates the institutionalization of some sort of communal purification ritual within the military, preferably alongside one's own unit (Shay, 1994, 2002).

Medical advances

One of the most important advances in the prevention of mental disorder has resulted from medical progress in treating physical disorder, particularly the discovery of antibiotics for the treatment of syphilis. As Shorter (1997) explains, an epidemic of venereal disease spread across Europe and North America in the nineteenth century, and the average time between infection and the appearance of psychiatric symptoms that would follow in many of those infected with syphilis was 10–15 years (Shorter, 1997). He calculates that 5–20% of the population would have contracted syphilis at some point in their lifetime, and about 6% of these would go on to develop neurosyphilis. Although most would die at home, die by suicide, or die in a private spa, a proportion would end their days in the asylums, contributing substantially to the apparent rise of mental illness and the numbers admitted to asylums.

Syphilis would at this time typically be spread through prostitution, and the sores or swelling would disappear after a relatively short time and no further

symptoms would be apparent for many years. But for those in whom the spiro-
chetes remained in the blood stream, symptoms affecting movement of the legs
and/or the functioning of the brain, depending on whether the infection lodged in
the spine or the brain, would start to surface a decade later (Shorter, 1997: 54).
The disease that reached this stage was invariably fatal, but its course would
usually include speech difficulty, mania, dementia, then paralysis. As Shorter
notes, it was frequently middle class, middle-aged men that were affected, and
admission rates to many hospitals, particularly the private wards, in the late 1800s
and early 1900s reflect this. Admissions for 'general paresis' or GPI (general
paralysis of the insane) in many hospitals exceeded those for mania and dementia
praecox (schizophrenia). However, from 1944, once mass production of penicillin
had begun, the effective treatment of people who contracted syphilis removed a
major source of inpatients.

Not all biological discoveries have yielded such important preventive gains,
however. The numerous autopsies of those who in life had been seriously affected
by mental illnesses did not take biological psychiatry forward very far in the
nineteenth century, despite the discovery at the end of this period by Arnold Pick
and Alois Alzheimer and others before them of deposits and atrophy in the brains
of those who had lived with dementia. Such clear physical difference was not
evident in other mental illness, hence the distinction now drawn between 'organic'
(Pick's disease, Alzheimer's disease) and 'functional' causes of mental ill-health
(those now labelled schizophrenia and manic depression for example). These
advances in understanding the dementias, however, have not produced indications
for prevention, as we do not yet know what causes the deposits or atrophy to
develop in one person more than another.

This section should not conclude without some comment on the discovery in
the 1950s and since of a range of psychotropic medication that has become the
mainstay of modern psychiatry, and can substantially reduce relapse rates from
recurrent disorder such as schizophrenia and bipolar disorder. These drugs
contributed greatly to the confidence of psychiatrists to discharge people from
long-stay hospitals, and for many people they facilitate some control over their
symptoms. However, the reader will need to look elsewhere for coverage of
issues related to use of medication and its potential for prevention, as the focus
here is on social, psychological and self-help factors that are open to change, and
related policy.

Conclusion, and focus of this book

As this short and highly selective review of past efforts indicates, there is a long-
established understanding that prevention can focus on: vulnerability established
in early childhood; the role of life events and difficulty in adult mental ill-health;
the importance of employment for positive mental health; the value of group
morale and an end in sight for people's ability to cope with extreme stress; the
need for traumatized people to unlearn behaviour that is maladaptive once traumatic experience is over; and the link between some mental health conditions and

some physical illnesses. The pressure to implement preventive measures derives in large part from the potential cost – financial, and emotional – to the individuals themselves, their families, employers, health and social services, and the military. However, there is great scope for well-intentioned action to cost more than it saves, hence the need to draw on good evidence that any action that is costly in human and financial terms will bring the desired benefits. As noted with the child guidance and crisis support developments (and discussed in an earlier review; Newton, 1988), a prevention strategy dependent entirely upon one-to-one support by expensive professional services cannot hope to support more than a small number of those likely to experience mental ill-health.

This review will take a path through this evidence. It starts with the clues thrown up by epidemiological studies (Chapter 3) and the research to date on the aetiology of two diagnosed disorders: the most common mental health condition seen in primary care – depression (Chapter 5), and the most common in secondary care services – schizophrenia (Chapter 6). The words used to describe them are discussed in the following chapter (Chapter 2), examining why we still need medical labels for certain purposes and the problems this can create for those so labelled.

The possibilities for action by individuals, communities, families and local services are a large part of the focus, but in the prevention of physical illness and disability it has often been population measures that have achieved most. Hence the differing approaches are discussed in Chapter 4, and inform the focus of many chapters to follow. The second half of the book looks at the evidence that is needed for intervention. What do we know about how to support adults through crises (Chapter 7), about childhood vulnerability and when intervention might be most successful (Chapter 9), and how the resilience of the young person might be strengthened (Chapter 10)? Links with physical ill-health are the subject of Chapter 8, and population strategies that of Chapter 11.

The conclusions drawn in Chapter 12 confirm much of what we know already about the need for a loving, safe childhood, and the importance of a sense of control over life difficulties, of close relationships, and of feeling valued. But they also highlight the difficulty of intervening effectively with those most at risk, and of demonstrating benefit. The challenges for policy are discussed, as the pursuit of individual choice and freedom does not always fit well with support for those starting life with many disadvantages. But this most difficult task – addressing early vulnerability – is clearly the most important.

Note

1 Later changed to 'defect and disorder'.

2 Labels, and why they matter

In a book about prevention, the reader might expect an early definition of what exactly is to be prevented. However, this is far from a straightforward undertaking. Mental ill-health – something linked to emotions and thinking, reflected in behaviour, in adults and children; something not as it should be. The *Diagnostic and Statistical Manual* (DSM) *IV* described mental disorder as:

> a clinically significant behavioural or psychological syndrome or pattern that occurs in an individual and that is associated with present distress (eg a painful symptom) or disability (ie impairment in one or more important areas of functioning) or with a significantly increased risk of suffering death, pain, disability, or an important loss of freedom.
>
> (APA, 1994)

It clarifies that this does not include culturally sanctioned responses to events such as bereavement, nor behaviour that is deviant in relation to one society's political, religious or sexual norms unless associated with 'a symptom of a dysfunction in the individual'. These two qualifications take the discussion immediately into dangerous territory, with great differences in views on what is culturally sanctioned, and what is deviant, and where society rather than the individual is the problem. Yet most of us have a clear view of what we mean by mental illness, and it is a state associated with distress, confusion, problems with mood or thinking that is interfering with our ability to enjoy life or carry out everyday tasks that were previously unproblematic: that is, more or less what the DSM says. The degree of distress, confusion or problems with thinking must be well beyond the 'normal' range, and must be more long lasting before it becomes something anyone would want to give a name to or to do something about.

So what's the problem? There are three – probably others could list many more. First, we now label many more conditions and many milder difficulties as mental illnesses than 50 or so years ago. Second, these labels have problems of reliability and validity. Third, the labels carry stigma that is associated in turn with negative consequences for individuals that are in some cases more problematic than the symptoms so labelled. This chapter reflects on how these issues should be addressed in a review of the prospects for prevention, and concludes that some categorization remains essential for many research, planning and treatment purposes, but that the use of labels by practitioners seeking to help those with symptoms of mental ill-health needs careful consideration, and problems associated with the stigma of mental ill-health should be a core component of a comprehensive prevention strategy.

Problems exist with the reliability, validity and use of differing labels and definitions for positive mental health and wellbeing too, of course, but the potential negative consequences for individuals are less worrisome. Jahoda's (1958) definition was focused on the individuals themselves, in line with a traditional concept of the word 'health', but others take a much wider view; for instance, Jourard and Landsman (1980) assumed that mental health has a moral dimension and an interpersonal focus, which include caring about the natural world and caring about other people.

Problems – reliability, validity, medicalization

Psychiatrists have spent many decades defining and redefining categories of mental illness on the basis of clusters of symptoms, adding (and occasionally subtracting) diagnoses in each refinement of the two most widely used diagnostic manuals: the DSM (*Diagnostic and Statistical Manual*, developed and used in the USA) and the ICD (*International Classification of Diseases*, developed through WHO (1992) in 39 countries around the world). According to John Cooper (1999: 306), the revisions leading to the 10th version of the ICD, and comparisons with the DSM, now demonstrate 'that a large measure of agreement has been reached between psychiatrists and other mental health professionals world-wide about which disorders they should be concerned with'. A diagnosis identifies a related cluster of signs and symptoms that are assumed to represent an underlying disorder, which can then be described in terms of its expected course or natural history, its causes, and should guide the clinician toward appropriate action. But as Mechanic (2003) explains, diagnoses are hypotheses; some have more evidence behind them than others.

The diagnoses have only moderate inter-rater reliability. Many would say this is an understatement (e.g. Kutchins and Kirk, 1997; Horwitz and Wakefield, 2007). In the 1960s American psychiatrists were much more likely to label people as suffering from schizophrenia than their British counterparts (who more often used other diagnoses), as confirmed through a study of those watching the same video interviews of patients (Cahn, 1999). Since then diagnostic practice and tools to guide it have greatly advanced, and their use also in research involves training raters to employ the same thresholds (see Chapter 3). But Cooper (1999) noted that in the latest versions of the diagnostic manuals, there remained a discrepancy between the two in how long symptoms must have lasted before schizophrenia could be diagnosed. A review of 92 studies comparing diagnostic practice by Jansson and Parnas (2007) suggested that concerns remain about the validity of the diagnosis of schizophrenia using these tools, even though reliability may have improved.

Reliability refers to the likelihood that two different raters (or the same rater at different times) will arrive at the same diagnosis for the same person rated, using the same assessment tool. Validity refers to whether the diagnosis arrived at appears to hold meaning and relevance; that is, it agrees with clinical judgements made by psychiatrists, and/or distinguishes people reliably according to a level of difficulty they experience over time as shown by other indicators (reports by relatives, difficulties retaining work, relationships, managing daily living tasks and so on), and/or accurately differentiates people likely to benefit from a particular type of treatment. What Jansson and Parnas suggested is that in trying to increase reliability, refinements to diagnostic tools have to some extent reduced the validity of the label; for instance, now limiting the label schizophrenia to people who have experienced severe and continuous psychotic symptoms for a long time. These are a subgroup of all those who might meaningfully be grouped together on grounds of experiencing similar difficulty and judged as having psychotic symptoms by a psychiatrist.

The diagnosis of mental illness remains as controversial today as it did in the time of Scheff (1966), who argued that such labels are what we give behaviour for which all other explanations fail. Kutchins and Kirk (1997) have brought together many of the criticisms in a provocative book, focusing in particular on the development of the DSM, which they argue contributes to an increasing tendency to describe all kinds of difficulties in medical terms (one of many they quote is 'disorder of written expression' – a developmental or learning difficulty where the student has a poor level of writing that cannot be explained by their age, intelligence or education). They also argue that the reliability of the DSM 'has been exaggerated . . . and its impact on social work practice and clients is rarely studied, but often deleterious' (Kutchins and Kirk, 1995: 154). Robert Spitzer led the revisions to the third edition of the DSM, and Kutchins and Kirk (1997: 5) argue that 'he has undoubtedly defined, or refashioned more new diagnoses than any other living person in the field of mental health'.

If their popular usage and familiarity now are any indication of their validity and usefulness, then some of the new diagnoses added during Spitzer's chairmanship pass the test (if also continuing to be contested) – anorexia nervosa, bulimia, post-traumatic stress disorder are categories currently widely used in the West. Spitzer also played a key role in removing homosexuality – listed as a mental illness in DSM II but dropped from DSM III. Two factors in particular have helped to establish the many new labels (DSM IV has no fewer than 297 separate conditions!). A DSM diagnosis is required by US medical insurance agencies before they will sanction reimbursement for treatment; hence practitioners who wish their bills to be paid have a strong incentive to label. Labels are also advantageous to the pharmaceutical industry, as it can develop new products for each new diagnosis.

Spitzer himself has been moved to question some of his assumptions in his foreword to a more recent critique of the DSM by Horwitz and Wakefield (2007). The latter authors argued that psychiatry has moved too many normal experiences into the domain of illness, this time focusing on sadness and depression, arguing that the diagnosis needs to take more account of the context of the individual so that those with 'normal' and understandable sadness due to recent major loss events should not be diagnosed with a clinical condition. Support for at least part of their argument comes from some surprising quarters. Shorter (1997: 319), for instance, whose historical account of developments in psychiatry takes a strongly biological focus, argues that in the latter part of the twentieth century 'psychiatry increasingly became a specialty oriented to the provision of medication' and pharmaceutical companies rapidly responded to this huge market potential, which distorted psychiatry further. 'A given disorder might have been scarcely noticed until a drug company claimed to have a remedy for it, after which it became epidemic' (Shorter, 1997: 319). He cites the 2.5 million American children, more often boys, prescribed 'ritalin' in the mid-1990s for attention deficit disorder and/ or hyperactivity, commenting further that 'the entire notion of giving patient-status to people because they are troublesome to others represented a pathologizing of essentially normal if irksome behaviour. Thus these diagnoses . . . dipped greatly the threshold at which individuals were said to be ill' (Shorter, 1997: 291). This concern resonates when one reads recent epidemiological enquiries such as the Comorbidity Survey Replication (see Kessler and Merikangas 2004 and Chapter 3), which included the diagnoses 'impulse control disorder', 'oppositional defiant disorder' and 'intermittent explosive disorder'. (Interestingly, Shorter (1997: 325) also provides a counter-view for the value of psychiatric drugs becoming popular, citing the example of Prozac (to treat depression or panic attacks, with a side-effect of weight loss which helped generate strong demand) as encouraging the view that mental ill-health is both common and easily treatable, thereby helping to reduce associated stigma.)

Increasingly, a view is gaining ground that symptoms of mental ill-health of all types follow a continuum, rather than representing distinct conditions that we either have or don't have, for which our cut point to label 'illness' is based on consensus judgements. Social factors are implicated in almost all of them, and may sometimes also underlie the 'irksome behaviour' to which Shorter refers. It is not the case that marked symptoms represent a biological condition that has no link with the social environment. As later chapters show, severe and mild types of mental ill-health, as well as a good deal of physical ill-health (e.g. herpes, abdominal pain, myocardial infarction), are associated with life events and stressful living circumstances (Brown and Harris, 1989; Martin, 1998; and see Chapter 8). Adverse childhood experience is similarly widely implicated in vulnerability.

The concerns about medicalization and the validity of diagnoses are in the main linked not to reservations as to their use in research, but to a belief that the labels are applied too widely to people who may not have considered they had a problem, and encouraging people to assume that the solution to a host of minor as well as marked psycho-social difficulties may also lie with medicine.

This is not the same as suggesting that medical treatment for symptoms associated with distress is unimportant. When people *are* seeking help, why would a practitioner not offer talking treatments or medication if it brings some short-term relief (Kendler, 2008)? Most of us will take a pill to reduce pain, but will also take action on the causes. If it enables people to function better, achieve more, and does not divert expensive medical resources needed elsewhere to trivial purposes, it must surely be appropriate to do so.

Problems – stigma and discrimination

Social psychiatrists leading the way in rehabilitation have for many decades expressed their own reservations about the effect of labelling. Those promoting social models of rehabilitation in London from the 1950s were clear that diagnosis was not always an important predictor of the outcome of their efforts, and helping people back to a full life was a task more suited to psychologists and social workers than psychiatrists (Birley, 1999). In Italy, Franco Basaglia, a radical psychiatrist leading the deinstitutionalization of both staff and patients in Trieste in the early 1970s, argued that the patient's diagnosis should be 'put in brackets', 'since that diagnostic label hung fixedly on the patient like a preformed value judgement', creating potentially disabling attitudes in the mind of both patient and those around them (Donelly, 1999).

These are two of the concerns arising from diagnosis for people with mental ill-health – it can lead other people to make judgements about them that are disadvantageous; it can lead them to internalize the negative stereotype, contributing to a lowered self-image. Together these can lead to a tendency to avoid some situations where they might meet prejudice. This is the meaning of stigma, a concept brought powerfully to our attention by Erving Goffman in his book on the subject in 1963, where he defined it simply as an 'attribute that is deeply discrediting' that reduces the bearer from 'a whole and usual person to a tainted, discounted one' (Goffman, 1963: 3). Writers more recently would substitute the word 'label' for 'attribute', to shift the identified centre of the 'problem' from the individual to those labelling the individual. In fact, Sayce (1998) argues that the use of the term 'stigma' is itself problematic given its history of association with individual attributes, rather than the discrimination associated with the diagnosis.

A powerful illustration of how a group that is 'tainted' can be negatively affected even in its ability to capitalize on equal opportunities offered has been provided by Hoff and Pandey (2004). They conducted experiments involving competitive card games with groups of boys who did not know each other, but were descendant from differing Indian castes. Although the caste system is long gone (since 1950), some discrimination and deferential behaviour continue. Those descending from the 'Untouchables' won as much money in the games as other boys as long as their caste was not known by anyone playing the game. But their winnings were reduced by 42% if their caste was revealed by providing their surname in introductions at the start. Of interest was that such knowledge did not benefit the higher caste boys as far as might be predicted, as their expectations were also affected – they did not think they needed to try so hard to win.

While not wishing to liken the label of 'mentally ill' to the status of a low-caste Indian boy, the general point is that a label that carries a negative stereotype will affect the performance of the person only if others know the label, and do so largely through the assumptions and expectations of the individuals themselves, and to a lesser extent, those of other people. It is to be hoped that the label of mental illness does not carry such a powerful negative stereotype in the minds of the general public today, but although attitudes in the UK may have improved for some diagnoses, in 1998 people with schizophrenia, drug addiction or alcoholism were still judged more negatively than they might be. An ONS survey of 1737 members of the general public, commissioned by the Royal College of Psychiatrists (Crisp et al., 2000), found that people with these diagnoses were considered unpredictable (by over three quarters of respondents) and dangerous (by over two thirds of respondents), and those with drug addiction or alcoholism as being to blame for their own ill-health (over half of respondents). Although a much smaller proportion, there were still 25% of respondents who believed that people with severe depression were dangerous. Analysing responses by age showed that young people were, if anything, more negative in their views than people over 65.

Negative perceptions related to trustworthiness and competence have been reflected in discrimination in employment, immigration, and in access to insurance or loans (Sayce, 2000). Equalities legislation should now be reducing such problems of course, as litigation is one of the most important weapons to counter discrimination. But it has meant that many people with a psychiatric diagnosis have been disinclined to apply for jobs for *fear of* unfair treatment, according to a survey by Baker and Read (1996), as well as due to experience of prejudice and unfair treatment. A more recent survey by the UK charity Rethink of 661 carers and 3038 service users in the UK (Time to Change, 2008) asked about the effects of diagnosis on their lives, in order to inform a proposed anti-stigma campaign. When asked if they had stopped doing things they used to do because of stigma or discrimination, or because of fear of stigma or discrimination, two out of three confirmed that one or both of these was the case.

The most common fear (over half of respondents) was of disclosing their mental health problems to others, and the most common experience of stigma or discrimination (almost half of respondents) was in the area of employment. Friendships and activities outside the home were also affected. Many felt unsure whether this might be partly their own anxiety and low motivation. Workshop discussions with over 100 service users indicated they were particularly concerned with the lowered expectations of their close family members (Time to Change, 2008).

There is no shortage of evidence that employers are cautious about taking on those with a history of mental ill-health. A survey for the UK Department of Work and Pensions (Bunt et al., 2001), of 1200 employers, included 32 in-depth interviews about their experiences of and views on new government pilots to support the employment of benefit claimants. They found that employers were more willing to make reasonable (small) adjustments and offer flexibility to accommodate lone parents and, to some extent, people who had been unemployed a long time, but were less inclined to be flexible about accommodating people with physical disabilities or mental health problems. UK Labour Force Survey data (DWP, 2011) shows that mental ill-health is more of an obstacle than physical disability, with half or more of those with long-term health conditions or disability in employment in 2011, compared to less than one in five with a 'mental illness, phobia, panic or nervous disorder' and not many more (25–31%) of those with 'depression, bad nerves or anxiety'.

The anti-stigma campaigns in the UK do seem to be shifting attitudes very gradually, however. The latest of a series of surveys by the National Statistics Office (NHS Information Centre, 2011) is able to compare answers to the same questions in 11 of the years between 1994 and 2011. Some attitudes are changing very little – tolerance, fearfulness, willingness to live alongside those with mental ill-health – and one in six continue to believe that a major cause is lack of self discipline or will-power. But the proportion agreeing they should not hold public office fell from 29% to 21%, and that they should not be given responsibility from 17% to 13%, and slightly more felt they could talk about it with friends, family or employers. There is also increasing recognition that everyone should have the same rights to work and live in any neighbourhood.

Widely held negative stereotypes inevitably mean that a person receiving a psychiatric diagnosis will worry that the stereotype must be an accurate description of themselves, despite previously viewing themselves as competent and trustworthy (Festinger, 1957). But Festinger and Carlsmith (1959) demonstrated that publicly explaining to others a view that is not the one you hold shifts your own view substantially towards the one you express to others, which may be one of the reasons that supporting people into employment aids recovery. If a person who has come to see themselves as unreliable and incompetent explains to an employer (who is unaware of the person's mental health history) why they are reliable and competent enough to be offered a paid position, it is likely to shift their view towards this belief, particularly if the employer is convinced.

The implication is that a psychiatric diagnosis would be less pernicious if it did not carry the stigma it does in the West. Contrasting the Western context with beliefs about psychosis in many developing countries, drawing from international comparisons by WHO and a number of anthropological and related studies, Warner (1994) shows that psychotic symptoms that present little trouble to the community may not be labelled, may be treated with curing rituals that engage rather than exclude, and are often associated with strongly positive assumptions about recovery. Crucially, he argues, people are assumed to be able to return to work and, particularly in rural economies, are more easily able to do so. Together, he argues, these factors largely explain why the recovery rates in the developing world appear to be so much better than in the West (see Chapter 6 and Warner, 1994).

Categories and cut-points – essential for research

Researchers need to distinguish one disorder from another, and the 'ill' from those with some symptoms of borderline significance, and these from the 'well', to advance their analysis of cause, course, treatment and recovery, to inform service planning, and to evaluate service delivery. This is essential too for an exploration of the evidence base for preventive intervention. There are some obvious similarities in broad terms in the aetiology of many differing diagnoses, with, for instance, life stress being implicated in most. But there are also important differences in detail, with life events involving humiliation more important to depression than to anxiety (see Chapter 5), and social support more important in preventing depression than preventing anxiety. Childhood conduct disorder is more likely to continue into adulthood than is childhood emotional disorder, and more can be discovered about conduct disorder if this is disaggregated into aggression and opposition-defiance, which show different gender profiles (see Chapter 9); complications in birth may play a role in vulnerability to psychosis (see Chapter 6). Genetic factors appear to play a greater role in the disorders diagnosed as psychoses than in the more common types of mental ill-health, and in anxiety and obsessive disorders more than in depression. Many other examples could be listed.

The same is true of course for the estimation of the incidence and prevalence of disorder, and particularly when researchers wish to compare findings in different populations. They need a fair degree of agreement in their methods of labelling people as having the condition, as having a borderline condition (some symptoms or symptoms for a short while that might if worse or more long lasting reach the clinical threshold), or as not having the condition. Only then can they judge the role played by social differences in the lives of people with comparable difficulty.

To improve upon the variable practice between clinicians, researchers have developed interview guides, including advice on how to judge the severity of the problems revealed (e.g. the SCAN, CIS and CIDI; see next chapter). However, the threshold chosen by those standardizing the tools has been arrived at from consensus judgements about the level at which the symptoms should be judged as a disorder, something that would now benefit from treatment. That is, it is a man-made judgement and not in nature. The situation for mental ill-health is no different from the majority of 'diseases', as epidemiologist Geoffrey Rose (1992: 45) reminds us – there are almost no diseases in medicine that you 'have' or 'have not'; 'you either have a little or a lot of' most of them.

These tools are considered to be able to produce sufficiently reliable assessments for most research needs, though remaining far from perfect, as discussed further in Chapter 3. They have enabled researchers to demonstrate, for instance, that recovery from schizophrenia is better in some countries than in others, that depression is more common in inner cities than in county towns, that conduct disorder in children is linked to social disadvantages that are also more common in inner cities. The convincing evidence for the role of social and cultural factors in mental ill-health has not come from the radical campaigners against psychiatry, but from careful epidemiological enquiry using psychiatric categories and standardized measures of numbers, severity, duration and date of onset of pre-defined conditions.

It has been essential that researchers have been able to convince sceptics that they are comparing like with like, to gain credibility for claims for the role of social factors. The oft-cited international study of schizophrenia commenced in nine countries by the World Health Organization in 1973 revealed a marked variation in recovery at two-year and five-year follow-ups of the samples (see Chapter 6), linked not with clinical treatment but with cultural context. To their surprise, recovery in India and Nigeria was much better than that in many developed countries with vastly more psychiatric services available.

A more carefully designed study was launched in the 1980s to check whether this could really be the case. Jablensky and Sartorius (2008) have recapped on their methods, including diagnostic processes, in order to answer the latest critics of these findings, which again revealed marked variations between societies. They argue that 'a strong case can be made for a real pervasive influence of a powerful factor which can be referred to as "culture,"'; and that the higher rate of 'chronic disability and dependency associated with schizophrenia in high-income countries, despite access to costly biomedical treatment, suggests that something essential to recovery is missing in the social fabric' (Jablensky and Sartorius, 2008: 254).

Harris (2000) also describes how essential it was for their findings on the social origins of depression in the 1970s (see Chapter 5) to resist criticism by biological psychiatry that what they were studying was not 'real' mental illness. They needed to be rigorous in their use of standardized tools, recognized diagnostic practice, methods for dating onset, and measures of social factors, in order to convince sceptics that depression is indeed largely caused by social rather than biological factors.

Some service user perspectives

Studies in the 1980s in which service users were interviewed about their view of psychiatric labels showed a mixed response, some people finding the label helpful, but frequently with some associated problems too, and others reporting only negative effects arising – 'many, if not most, patients feel some shame and believe that others will respond negatively to the fact of their hospitalisation' (Link et al., 1987: 1472). According to Link and colleagues, much evidence suggests that even if it were helpful privately, a person would prefer not to risk sharing the label publicly, shown for example by the finding that many US citizens forgo treatment through their medical insurance rather than have a note of psychiatric treatment on their record. Others say they would falsify their CV to hide any gaps due to treatment when applying for work, clearly believing that the label itself would be harmful however effectively they had performed at work since.

On the other hand, most surveys of people newly diagnosed with any worrying health problem show that close to the top of their priorities is information – about the prognosis, effective treatment, support available, what is known about its cause. This facilitates participation in decision making about the best course of action. Mental ill-health is no exception (Read, 1996). Many service user organizations have developed their own management support advice for others sharing their difficulties, often based on diagnosis (for example, Bipolar UK (2011) offers self-management training).

Knowing that other people share these problems, and that there are particular responses and/or treatments that help, can be beneficial in the short term. Chadwick (1997: 147), a university psychology lecturer who has been diagnosed with schizophrenia, maintains that 'it was helpful to regard myself as having had an illness' in that he then had a respect for adhering to medication, which he has reduced to a low dose that has maintained his good health. He concludes that the 'best strategy is to accept the illness label in the short term and face and accept one's (often temporary) fragility and vulnerability and then dispense with it as one gains strength' (p. 171). He describes the symptoms he experienced in a psychotic episode in 1979: the droplets on the hospital ceiling were the souls of people who had died because of him; his bandage sling had moulded itself into the Madonna; the clouds had taken the form of his dog and his housemate; tapping noises from the wall, orchestrated by 'the Organisation' confirmed that it was essential he kill himself. He comments simply that 'It is obvious to anyone with a shred of common sense that I was ill. Any characterization of my behaviour as merely "bizarre", such that an illness attribution would then be an act of social control (to empower the medical profession), is clearly utterly absurd' (p. 44).

Chadwick has evidently adapted his life to cope with remaining symptoms in the way those with physical disabilities are assumed to be able to do but, until recently, those with diagnosed severe mental illness were often assumed unable to do. Many service users have been arguing for several decades that mental health provision needed to give as much attention to their social and vocational engagement and to the social disadvantages they experience as it does to the amelioration of symptoms. The goal should be an ordinary life, or better, as Deegan (1988) put it: to 'live, work and love in a community in which one makes a significant contribution'.

There is a large literature by service users on their views of the ways they are treated, much less on labelling. A priority frequently expressed is for the person to be the centre of the discussion, rather than a focus on symptoms as if they can be considered independently. Anthony (1993: 15) describes recovery as 'a deeply personal, unique process of changing one's attitudes, values, feelings, goals, skills, and/or roles. It is a way of living a satisfying, hopeful, and contributing life even with limitations caused by illness.' While discussed in relation to treatment services, these issues are relevant too to prevention. Two priorities are identified: strengthening provision of personal support, and looking for triggers that might enable the person to find new meaning and purpose in life. Given that Anthony likens the experience of a severe mental illness to the experience of other devastating events in life, he similarly likens recovery to the process of adaptation to any crisis, for which a core resource is: someone to 'be there' for you, to trust, encourage, understand. Outcomes for services should be improvements to self-esteem, empowerment and self-determination. As the chapters to follow suggest, these issues are also a central part of the prevention story – close, supportive relationships, improvements to self-esteem, a reappraisal of attitudes and goals, recognizing that we have some choices in life, and the capacity to achieve them.

How might stigma and discrimination be reduced?

Stigma has several components (Link and Phelan, 2001: 367). First the difference is labelled, and the meaning of the label is appraised in terms of cultural beliefs. A negative stereotype will link the labelled person to undesirable characteristics; this places 'them' into a category with good separation from 'us' (essential if attributing very negative characteristics to 'them'). The label brings loss of status and discrimination, and those making judgements must have power to affect the opportunities of the stigmatized person based on their approval, rejection, exclusion or discrimination.

Hence effective anti-stigma work should attempt to change attitudes and beliefs about what people with a psychiatric label are like, reduce the gap between 'us' and 'them', and reduce the power of others to exercise prejudice through strong law. As someone with flu is one of 'us', so the message needs to convey that someone with a diagnosis of schizophrenia is too. This need not only be an effort to shift 'them' towards 'us', but also to shift 'us' toward 'them'. Gilbert (1999) describes how professionals can inadvertently collude in the social distancing of patients, citing managers of one regional health authority who argued that staff did not have 'emotional disorders' (Gilbert noted wryly that 'apparently only patients suffer from this').

Recent media campaigns in the UK (e.g. Time to Change. www.time-to-change. org.uk) have addressed the aspect related to status by using well-respected and well-known media figures who have acknowledged that they have a diagnosis of mental illness, but continue their high-profile and successful careers. They have openly commented on their symptoms and diagnosis, and are people with whom the television viewer can identify; that is, they are one of 'us', and crucially, they have not lost status by disclosing their diagnosis. Numerous actors, presenters, politicians and others note their pride in surviving serious mental ill-health, their appreciation of their difference, their commitment to challenge discriminatory attitudes. This seems a more promising strategy, than avoiding naming the condition, to see that it is what makes us human – it can sometimes serve a useful purpose; it should not be shameful. Their evaluations indicate they are having some success (see Time to Change website).

Legal remedies for discrimination can be used to challenge any institutional discrimination as well as that on an individual level. As Link and Phelan (2001: 381) conclude, 'one should choose interventions that either produce fundamental changes in attitudes and beliefs or change the power relations that underlie the ability of dominant groups to act on their attitudes and beliefs'.

The media has been part of the problem, and is increasingly now part of the solution. Both fictional accounts and factual coverage had been a concern since the 1980s, TV dramas frequently portraying those with mental ill-health as violent. Philo (1994) showed that selective coverage of factual events relating to mental ill-health in the British media included stories where there was a violent incident as compared to more sympathetic accounts at a rate of four to one. Warner and Mandiberg (2003) describe how campaigners have achieved considerable success in improving coverage, citing the inclusion of a character with a diagnosis of schizophrenia in two TV 'soaps' (*EastEnders* and *Home and Away*) in response to lobbying by the UK mental health charity SANE, and the success of a 'stigma-busting' strategy started in 1990 by the New York State Alliance for the Mentally Ill. This co-ordinated monitoring of media stories across the state identified examples of negative coverage, then mass lobbying followed, through letters, emails and phone calls explaining why the story was considered offensive. Warner and Mandiberg cite the success of two similar actions that changed the portrayal of a character in the *Superman* comic in 1992 before it went to publication so that it was not after all a cosmic lunatic killer escaped from an interplanetary asylum. A 13 episode TV series was also withdrawn after two episodes after mass complaints over the violent antics of patients in a drama set in a psychiatric unit. These actions were by the National Stigma Clearing House and the National Alliance for the Mentally Ill in the US (see Warner and Mandiberg, 2003).

Summary and implications for prevention

The view that too many problems that are troublesome to self or others have been added to the list of psychiatric diagnoses in the past 50 years, thereby inappropriately categorizing them as medical conditions, is widely shared. Equally, there are a large number of distressing or disabling behavioural or psychological conditions that need to be distinguished one from another for purposes of research and treatment, which have been defined clearly in the diagnostic manuals and are widely known and used. While there are some problems with their reliability and validity, this is not the same as saying they are not useful (Kendall and Jablensky, 2003). Researchers have gained important insights with the measures used so far, as even the sceptics acknowledge (Kutchins and Kirk, 1995: 155). In the review to follow, the labels used in the research reported will need to be used to avoid misrepresentation of those findings, but are also needed to explore the subtleties of the development of differing types of mental ill-health, and the implications for prevention. When specificity is not required, the term 'mental ill-health' will be used.

However, diagnostic labels, some more than others, can and do have negative effects for the person gaining the label, through lowering their expectations and the expectations of them by others who know their label, impairing their recovery and return to work. Fear of such labelling may create reluctance to seek help from others. The label is not a major problem when it can be shed easily with recovery, and where recovery is a widely held expectation. But too often the label endures even when symptoms are well controlled, resulting in expectations that opportunities are not available or realistic, and the person identifies – and is identified – as different, less competent, less trustworthy, not like 'us'.

Balancing these concerns with the benefits of early treatment for those with psychotic symptoms is discussed further in Chapter 6, where it is noted that a reluctance to stigmatize may in part contribute to significant delays in receipt of effective treatment for many young people, in many countries. A long period of untreated psychosis has negative consequences for recovery (see Chapter 6), leading to the development of various models of service designed to achieve early intervention in the least stigmatizing way possible.

Reducing stigma requires policy and practice that: encourages more optimistic expectations about recovery after a period of mental ill-health; reduces links in the media between mental ill-health and violence; reduces the distance of 'us' from 'them'; notes that there can be positive as well as negative aspects; and provides more recognition that people at all levels of society have experienced mental ill-health and that they can maintain the respect of others and their social status.

3 Prevalence and distribution of mental ill-health

In the search for clues about how it might be possible to prevent mental ill-health, an obvious place to start is with a profile of those who have experience of it, to see if there are any obvious social factors that appear to distinguish their lives or their circumstances. Following the concern that too many trivial problems may now be assumed to be medical conditions, it may also be instructive to examine the profile of disorders for which people consult a doctor, and which people and how many do so. What proportion of disorders clear up quickly, how many become long-term conditions, and what we know about the difference are also important to explore, given the much greater impact on home and work lives that follows from long-term conditions. Their greater cost to individuals, families, employers and society means these are arguably the more important public health focus.

Epidemiology is the key tool. It is the study of the distribution of defined disorder in the general population. But cross-sectional data collected at one point in time does not tell us enough about either the course of disorder or direction of effects. High rates may represent low recovery rates more than high incidence, for instance. Associations found can be two-way – divorce may cause ill-health; ill-health may cause divorce. What is needed for the next step is longitudinal data, following up the study sample with and without the suspected causal factor, over time. Then, as Robins (1978) explained:

> The final proof is that modifying that cause changes the rate of disorder. Of course, the probable causes identified may not always be amenable to manipulation by the researcher, or government policy, and so cannot be proved. However, it is the psychiatric epidemiologist's hope that he will discover some link in the causal chain that *can* be broken.
>
> (Robins, 1978: 697)

The paragraphs to follow will summarize the within-population data on the prevalence and distribution of mental ill-health, profile those most likely to receive treatment, and follow up two of the 'clues' to demonstrate the difficulties of drawing clear conclusions from cross-sectional data. As discussed in the previous chapter, all such research relies first and foremost on the ability of researchers to measure disorder reliably and identify those who have 'a lot' rather than 'a little'.

Measuring disorder

The latest assessment tools are designed to be used by dozens of different researchers interviewing people at the same time across the country and across countries. Considered the best current tools for large-scale use, and heralded as a major step forward in facilitating study of mental ill-health in society, are two interview schedules: the Composite International Diagnostic Interview, or CIDI (Robins et al., 1988), and the Clinical Interview Schedule – Revised, or CIS-r (Lewis et al., 1992). Both are fully structured, and designed to be used by trained interviewers who are not clinicians. Both have been widely used across the world in prevalence studies.

An adapted version of the CIDI was used in the major National Comorbidity Survey (NCS) in the US in 1990–2 and in the NCS replication in 2001–3 (Kessler and Merikangas, 2004), and is available as a computer-assisted questionnaire that will compute a diagnosis on the basis of answers given to the questions set, hence it is very reliable in the sense that a certain pattern of responses will always lead to the same diagnosis. The CIS-r has also been fully structured and made available in computerized form, and has been used in the UK National Psychiatric Morbidity Surveys in 1993, 2000 and 2007. It needs to be used alongside a psychosis screening questionnaire as it assesses only 'neurotic symptoms' (see Jenkins et al., 2003). A third type of interview – the SCAN (Schedule for Clinical Assessment in Neuropsychiatry; Wing et al., 1990) – is a semi-structured interview allowing interpretation of responses, designed for use by psychiatrists and others trained at the WHO SCAN centre to mimic the clinical interview with a psychiatrist, and is thought to be the 'gold standard' measure, and the most valid of the three given its close approximation to the judgements arrived at by psychiatrists in their everyday clinical practice. Given that it requires more specialist training, it cannot so easily be used on the large samples for which the CIDI and CIS-r were developed. However, it can be used to check on the reliability and validity of the other measures.

How reliable are the measures?

It seems that the reliability of the information obtained on those interviewed in the community who may or may not have sought treatment is not as strong as hoped. Brugha and his colleagues have examined the results of using both the CIS-r (Brugha et al., 1999) and the CIDI (Brugha et al., 2001) against those obtained by using the SCAN. They found that both CIS-r and SCAN ratings showed that 137 of a sample of 205 people did not have any diagnosis, and that 17 people did. However, the CIS-r identified another 33 people as having a disorder not so identified by SCAN, and SCAN identified 18 people with a disorder that CIS-r did not. Using the CIDI, there were 96 out of 172 also assessed using the SCAN who were considered on both measures to be 'well', and 33 rated as having a disorder of some kind. But the CIDI identified 33 others with a disorder that the SCAN did not, while the SCAN identified 11 people as having a disorder that the CIDI did not.

When the samples are drawn from those attending primary care centres, the agreement between differing measures improves somewhat. Using all three, Jordanova and colleagues (2004) found slightly less disappointing concordance rates, with the CIDI finding exactly the same prevalence of disorder in primary care as the SCAN (though 10 of the 105 people were not the same people – each measure identifying five the other did not). The CIS-r identified 25 fewer cases than the SCAN.

These differences overall suggest that prevalence statistics must be treated with some caution, and should ideally be adjusted after a sub-sample has been assessed using the SCAN. Otherwise, these studies indicate that there is a substantial group of people, about 25% of the population, about whom there is likely to be disagreement as to whether they do or do not fall over the threshold of having a 'clinical' level of disorder. They will all have some symptoms, but the measures place one third or two thirds of this 25% just over rather than just under the threshold, depending on the measure. Hence, although the data cited in this review is drawn from the most rigorous large-scale surveys available to date, it would be reasonable to assume that these are at best a fairly rough guide.

In addition, CIDI asks about disorder in the 12 months prior to interview, while the CIS-r focuses on the previous week, and up to a month before interview only (hence identifying fewer cases than the SCAN or the CIDI). Data from the Netherlands illustrates just how large the difference between a one month and a 12 month prevalence figure can be. While the difference in rates of enduring severe conditions like those diagnosed as schizophrenia are small, the overall figure for all disorder changes from 23% in the past 12 months to 16% if only the last month is considered (Bijl et al., 1998), which also suggests that a good deal of mental ill-health is short-lived.

The second essential ingredient of a prevalence study is to ensure that the sample is fully representative of the population to be studied. To assess differing rates of disorder in different countries with very different arrangements for treatment, the rate should not be based on numbers treated, but on a random sample of the general population whether in treatment or not, and from across the whole country. This means interviewers going door to door to a representative sample of households, including care homes, hospitals and hostels for homeless people. Very few studies have included all these latter types of setting in their data, but more claim to have a representative sample of the population living in private households, hence their data if anything will underestimate rates of ill-health, particularly the more severe problems (e.g. Bijl et al., 1998).

What do the surveys tell us about prevalence?

The first *nationally* representative household survey to examine mental health in any country was in the US – the National Comorbidity Survey (NCS; Kessler, 1994), with over 8000 participants, although this study was preceded by an even larger survey involving over 20,000 people in five areas in the US (so not therefore a *national* sample; Robins and Regier, 1991). The NCS was replicated and extended in 2001–3, which involved face-to-face interviews with a nationally representative sample of 9282 adults. The first National Psychiatric Morbidity survey in the UK was conducted in 1993, and a second in 2000, using postal districts as the sampling frame, to provide a representative sample of people living in private households. This was supplemented with a study of residents of care homes, hospitals and homeless people from across England, Scotland and Wales. They used the CIS-r as their measure of neurotic disorder, with additional measures for drug and alcohol dependence and psychosis. More recent data from 2007 was on England alone, and did not include interviews with those in institutions.

In 2007, they found an overall prevalence rate among the 7403 people interviewed of 23%, which is nearly a quarter of the population screened positive for at least one of the disorders studied (ONS, 2009b). Almost one in five of these people screened positive for more than one:

- 15.1% had neurotic symptoms above the CIR-r threshold in the past week, most commonly a mixture of anxiety and depression
- 3.4% has a drug dependence in the past year
- 0.4% had a psychosis (confirmed by using the SCAN) in the past year.

If the age range is reduced to exclude those 65 or over, in order that the figures can be compared to the large number of surveys limiting their range to those aged 16–64, then the rates become slightly higher – 17.6% having a CIS-r score above 12. This is because older people have lower levels of mental ill-health. Age variation is most marked in drug dependence. The overall rate of 3.4% masks very high rates in young people, particularly young men, in black young men, and those on the lowest incomes (ONS, 2009b). The overall rate doubled from 1993 to 2000, but remained similar from 2000 to 2007. The tendency to mature out of drug dependence is reflected in the rapid decline from 13.3% of men aged 16–24, then in the next three 10-year age bands dropping to 9%, then 2.9%, then 1.3% of 45–54 year olds. The most commonly used drug, and the most common dependency, is cannabis. The UK is not alone in this trend, the national survey in the Netherlands reporting 21% of 18–24 year olds dependent on either alcohol or illicit drugs (Bijl et al., 1998).

The National Comorbidity Surveys in the US found a rate of all disorder of 30% using the CIDI (Kessler et al., 2005), while the NEMESIS study in the Netherlands reported a comparable figure of 23% using the CIDI with 7076 adults aged 18–64 years in 1996 (Bijl et al., 1998). Shen et al. (2006) interviewed a random sample of 5201 people in metropolitan areas (so not representative of the whole country) in China (Beijing and Shanghai) and confirmed the widely understood picture of low rates of mental disorder in their country, finding only 7% of the population with any DSM disorder in the previous 12 months.

The most common diagnoses identified by these surveys are depression and alcohol dependence. Figures quoted by Kessler (1994) from the first US National Comorbidity survey (NCS) (face-to-face household interviews of 5388 people, 1990–2) show that in the 12 months before interview, the former was more common in women (12.9% as against 7.7% of men), the latter in men (10.7% as against 3.7% of women).

The most recent UK data shows a similar gender difference, with 3.3% of women alcohol-dependent over the past six months compared to 8.7% of men, and the most common category of common mental disorder – mixed anxiety and depression – in 6.9% of men and 11% of women in the past week (ONS, 2009b). Anxiety disorders were also very common in both US and UK data, and about twice as prevalent in women as in men. A European survey including a representative community sample of 21,425 adults in Belgium, France, Germany, Italy, the Netherlands and Spain interviewed between 2001 and 2003 using a revised version of the CIDI confirms the overall picture of high rates of mental ill-health, those with major depression being the largest group (ESEMeD, 2004). Women were more likely to have any mental ill-health, and more likely than men to be anxious or depressed, while men were more likely than women to have an alcohol disorder. People who were unemployed, on sick leave or disabled, and never married were more likely to have mental ill-health, and though a less strong difference, living in a city had an association with mental ill-health.

As in the UK, non-affective psychosis was rare in the US (0.3%) and in the Netherlands (0.2%), the lower figure in the latter survey likely to be an underestimate as it omitted people resident in institutions (Bijl et al., 1998). Bipolar disorder is only slightly more common, 12 month prevalence rates across Europe ranging from 0.5% to 1.1% (Pini et al., 2005).

So what's the answer? There is considerable consistency in the broad picture across populations and between studies in demonstrating that problems characterized as one of the psychoses are rare, with about 1 in 100 people in any year experiencing either a non-affective psychosis or a bipolar disorder. Adding together rates of problems broadly grouped under a heading of neuroses, alcohol dependence, and substance misuse, mental ill-health is very common. Somewhere between 1 in 6 and 1 in 4 of the population living in urban areas in the US and Europe in any 12 month period experience these, but many fewer in some Asian countries – possibly less than 1 in 14 in China.

Should anyone believe that all such ill-health requires medical intervention, then the resources required would be enough to worry any government. A cynic might suggest that this helps to explain the growing influence of service user led responses, and support for self-management, and is where advantages identified by pharmaceutical companies may increasingly be seen to be disadvantages for government if to be funded by the state. These high numbers have, of course, been used to argue for more resources for mental health, and will no doubt stimulate further debate on where the boundaries of medicine should lie. These numbers also have implications for the affordability of preventive intervention, and imply that expensive methods need to be directed carefully where they will achieve most.

Clues to aetiology: Comparing those with and without symptoms

A list of factors that correlate with disorder is supplied in all studies. Data from the UK National Morbidity Survey of 2000 (Singleton et al., 2001) illustrates the kinds of demographic profile usually found. It shows that people who are separated or divorced, or live alone, or are lone parents have higher rates of mental ill-health. So too do those who live with a longstanding physical health problem, live in an urban area, are economically inactive, and/or rent their home from the local authority or housing association (see Table 3.1).

The study in the Netherlands (NEMESIS) did not comment on physical disorder or social housing, but confirmed the other differences, i.e. the raised rate of depression and anxiety in lone parents, in lower income groups, in unemployed/disabled people, but also 'of people whose parents had mental problems, and of people who had traumatic experiences in their youth' (Bijl et al., 1998: 594). They also reported a raised rate of depression (but not anxiety) in urban areas.

There are some important clues here for prevention – something about close relationships is important, childhood family life, physical ill-health, something linked to housing for low-income families or being economically inactive, and living in the inner city. Each of these is pursued in subsequent chapters, to unpick the story behind these broad indicators.

Complexity of disorder: Comorbidity

Over half the US sample with one diagnosis also had another (such as depression with anxiety, panic disorder, drug or alcohol abuse) and a significant minority had three or more disorders. These people with high 'comorbidity' also form a high proportion of the subgroup whose difficulties are rated as 'severe', suggesting, in Kessler's words, that although 'psychiatric disorder overall is quite widespread in the general population, the major burden of psychiatric disorder is concentrated among people with high co-morbidity' (Kessler, 1994: 368). In fact they report that having had one disorder at any time is a major risk factor for subsequent

Table 3.1 Some distinguishing characteristics of people with 'neurotic disorders' or 'probable psychosis' (%), drawn from the UK National Morbidity Survey of 2000 (Singleton et al., 2001)

Percentage who are:	No psychosis N = 8520	Probable psychosis N = 60	No neurosis N = 7021	Neurotic disorder N = 1495
Separated or divorced	7	30	7	14
Living in one-person family unit	16	43	16	20
Economically inactive*	30	70	28	39
A single parent	5	7	4	9
Living in accommodation rented from LA or HA[†]	17	49	15	26
Living in an urban area	66	88	65	71
With longstanding physical health problem	42	62	38	58

* Neither working nor registered as seeking work (i.e. in full-time education, long-term sick, retired or looking after the family). [†] LA = local authority; HA = housing association.

disorder, particularly major depression (often preceded by a year or more by an anxiety disorder), and comorbidity is consistently associated with length of disorder (though both length and comorbidity could equally well be a result of the severity of the primary mental disorder). There is also a possibility that the high comorbidity found is an artifact of the diagnostic system. With the DSM having so many separate disorders, it is possible that different labels are given for complex disorders where differing symptoms predominate at different times. This criticism is noted by Kessler, who argues that this data is nevertheless useful. He notes that as anxiety, particularly phobias, precedes very many problems with alcohol and drugs, enabling people to develop coping strategies or overcome these anxieties would be a fruitful avenue for preventive intervention. The often lengthy period between development of phobias and other anxieties and the alcohol or drug use becoming problematic (often starting as a form of self-medication for continued fears) makes a preventive strategy all the more viable (Kessler, 1994).

What proportion seek treatment?

People with mental ill-health do not all seek or receive treatment of course, and personal circumstances, the nature of the symptoms, and their expectations of the benefits of doing so affect their decision to seek help. This means that those seen by treatment services are not a representative sample of all those with mental ill-health.

The UK National Morbidity Survey (Singleton et al., 2001) asked the 8578 people in its sample if they had consulted a GP in the past 12 months about being anxious or depressed, or for any mental, nervous or emotional problem. About 6% of those not rated as currently having a disorder on the CIS-r had done so, compared to 39% of those rated as having one or more disorders, and 71% of those with a 'probable psychosis'. Of those rated as having any disorder on the CIS-r, 3% had been treated in an outpatient clinic, 1% as an inpatient in the past quarter, compared to 28% and 6% respectively of those with a 'probable psychosis'. Only 24% of those with a neurotic disorder were receiving any treatment, rising to 47% if they had two or more such disorders, compared to 85% of those with a probable psychosis.

GP consultations were only slightly raised for those with an alcohol dependency, and only 10% were receiving any treatment for this. A quarter of those with a drug dependence (27%) had consulted a GP for a mental health related problem in the past 12 months; 15% were receiving some form of treatment.

Social factors and treatment

In 1980, Goldberg and Huxley suggested that there are four decision points or 'filters' in the pathway to inpatient care which operate in countries where there are general medical officers who are gatekeepers to specialist services. The first filter is whether the individuals themselves identify their problems as something that can be helped by medical or other services and seek that help; that is, their 'illness behaviour' (Mechanic, 1966). (Other options include confiding in a close family member, talking to a priest, self-medicating with alcohol or over–the-counter medicines, or retreating to bed.) The second filter is the recognition by the general medical practitioner (GP) consulted that the individual has a mental health problem that might benefit from some sort of treatment or support – their detection of symptoms and diagnostic practice. If they are the gatekeeper for further sources of help, the third filter is their decision to refer the individual for therapy and/or other specialist help. The fourth filter is the decision of the specialist (normally a psychiatrist) to admit the person for inpatient treatment.

The data cited above suggested that only 39% of those with symptoms of common mental disorders consulted about them during the year, but other data on GP consultations in the UK shows that more than 78% of patients consult their GP each year about something (McCormick et al., 1995), and on average those that do attend three to four times during the year. Clearly many of them do not mention their mental health concerns but consult for other reasons, a point noted by several other studies since Goldberg and Huxley (1980) drew this to our attention.

Data on patients attending general practice in the UK for any reason is regularly collected by the government's national statistics office (ONS) in order to inform service planning as well as profile the health of the nation. The 1992 survey (McCormick et al., 1995) involved data supplied by GPs on over half a million patients from 60 practices, 1% of the population of England and Wales. People employed in jobs categorized as class I and II (professional and managerial) and who own their own home consult least often. But after multivariate analysis controlling for other socio-economic factors, the excess among social classes IV and V was only 10%, with the main factors continuing to show a trend towards higher consultation being tenancy of accommodation rented from the local authority, or unemployment or permanent sickness (McCormick et al., 1995):

Other findings of relevance were as follows (McCormick et al., 1995):

- Unemployed adults have raised rates of consultation for all types of problem, but particularly mental health consultations, which were doubled in men aged 16–44.
- Children with unemployed parents or parents who were long-term sick had raised rates of consulting for mental health reasons.
- Boys, but not girls, living with a single parent showed raised consultation rates for mental health.
- Widowed, separated or divorced adults had raised rates of consultation, whether or not they had children living with them, particularly for mental health reasons.
- People in rural areas were less likely to consult for any reason.

Presentation factors and treatment

Some of the differences between GPs in diagnosis and referral relate to patient characteristics (how people express their distress) and to GP factors (how skilled an interviewer the GP might be, how well they identify with the patient, and their bias towards or away from seeing symptoms as diagnosed illness) (Goldberg and Huxley, 1980). Much mental ill-health goes undetected, and Goldberg (1992) described as *collusion* between doctor and patient the decision sometimes to keep the consultation away from psychological labels. He explains how patients can be quite satisfied with this in that doctors are usually kind and courteous, take all physical symptoms seriously so the patient is reassured that nothing important has been missed, frequently offering analgesics or other medication which provide relief, and avoid either of them facing up to the patient's personal difficulties (with which some doctors feel unable to help anyway). Non-detection is increased by the patient describing their problems only in physical terms (problems in sleeping or lack of appetite). On the other hand, a small proportion of patients are diagnosed when their questionnaire responses indicate a low level of symptoms, termed 'false positives', because the GP has treated them in the past for a mental health problem, and is expecting to see it again (Goldberg and Huxley, 1980).

Both detection and referral to specialist help are increased if the person draws attention to their difficulties, particularly if they do so in a way that others find challenging. This is frequently commented upon by researchers. For instance, Sorgaard et al. (1999) interviewed 2015 people consulting GPs for worries related to mental health in Norway, and found that referrals from GPs to psychiatry were more likely if, as well as having more marked symptoms, the patients described themselves as easily worried, inclined to speak out, and less willing to accept a 'below-par situation'.

Researchers in Bali, interviewing 8546 people in private households, identified 39 people with schizophrenia (giving a point prevalence of 0.4%), and only the 19 who had shown any kind of aggressive behaviour had ever received treatment (Toshiyuki et al., 2005). Similarly, Mechanic (1975: 393) commented, in relation to hospital readmissions, that: 'studies were consistent in finding that re-hospitalization was related less to instrumental functioning than to the manifestations of bizarre and difficult behaviour that significant others found hard to manage'.

Combining some of the evidence described above (Goldberg and Huxley, 1980; Sorgaard et al., 1999; Singleton et al., 2001; Kessler et al., 2005) suggests that having consulted the GP, those most likely to be diagnosed with mental ill-health are:

- those with severe disorders (psychosis); two or more comorbid conditions; phobias; and have been seen frequently before
- people who are separated, widowed, divorced; and female.

Of those diagnosed by the GP, those referred to a specialist are more likely to be:

- those with severe disorders (psychosis)
- those who are separated, widowed, or divorced; male; and inclined to speak out, less willing to accept a below-par situation.

Hence psychiatrists see a very small proportion of the total population with symptoms of mental ill-health, those they see are not very similar to those treated by GPs, and the decision on which people have a diagnosed mental illness has been made before the patient reaches the psychiatrist. GPs treat the full range of disorder, of which psychosis is a very small part, while psychiatrists primarily treat complex (comorbid) disorder and psychosis.

Since the study by McCormick and colleagues in 1995, the average number of consultations in general practice per person per year has risen steadily in England from 3.9 in 1995 to 5.4 in 2007 (QResearch, 2008). It is a similar story in the US: Kessler and colleagues had reported that of those with a disorder in the previous 12 months, only 1 in 5 had received treatment (from the National Comorbidity Survey). Those treated tended to have the most severe disorders. However, by 2001–3 their NCS replication was finding that 1 in 3 people identified as having some kind of disorder were receiving treatment (Kessler et al., 2005).

Following up the clues: More complex studies needed

Epidemiological evidence has provided many useful leads, but the story very often gains complexity on further examination, illustrated here first in relation to ethnicity, second with geographic location.

Given the higher rates of socio-economic disadvantage experienced by many ethnic minority populations, it might be expected that these would be reflected in higher rates of mental ill-health. But in the US National Comorbidity Survey Replication, when the sample was divided into 'Hispanics', 'non-Hispanic blacks' and 'non-Hispanic whites', both minority groups had lower rates of disorder than the non-Hispanic whites, particularly in 'internalizing disorders' (depression, anxiety, phobias) but also in some externalizing disorders such as substance use, and the lowest levels of ill-health were found among the least well educated (Breslau et al., 2006). In the UK, a survey of rates of both common mental disorder and psychotic symptoms among people from five different ethnic groups (African Caribbean, Indian, Pakistani, Bangladeshi, Irish compared to white British) has found the lowest rates in Bangladeshi women, despite their being the most socially disadvantaged group, having most 'chronic strains' and, along with Pakistani respondents, the most health difficulties (Sproston and Nazroo, 2002).

Bangladeshi women had significantly lower rates of common mental disorder (12%) than white British women (19%), while Pakistani women had much higher rates (26%), despite sharing many characteristics of the Bangladeshi women (often in manual work, high rates of unemployment, with low educational qualifications, young and married). Hence, as the US study found, this is counterintuitive. Among the men, rates of common mental disorder were similar for all ethnic groupings – around 12%, except for Irish men, who had raised rates of common mental disorder (18%), though their high rate was accounted for by high anxiety symptoms, not depression.

In relation to psychotic symptoms, once again Bangladeshi respondents had the lowest rates, and again these were very different to Pakistani women with whom they are so often grouped in surveys, which typically categorize Indian, Pakistani and Bangladeshi people together as 'South Asians'. Other differences were closer to previous findings, such as the over-representation of African Caribbean people in hospital admissions for psychoses, which has generated so much controversy over the years (Singh and Burns, 2006). In this community sample, raised rates of psychotic symptoms were reported for African Caribbean respondents, but not as high as usually claimed, and statistically significant only for women.

Despite this being one of the most extensive studies of the mental health of ethnic minorities in the UK to date, and the detailed exploration of a range of associated factors, no clear explanations for differing rates emerged. However, it produced a fascinating account of differences in idioms of distress, coping mechanisms, caring responsibilities and support networks, service use, physical health, and chronic strains (O'Connor and Nazroo, 2002). Bangladeshi women were the least likely group to be without a close confiding relationship or source of practical support, though often these were also problematic relationships. It suggests a further exploration of family and community support structures, but also a repeat survey to see if the differences might be explainable in terms of the methods of data collection, lack of equivalent concepts for translated CIS-r questions, or the stigma associated with acknowledging problems and the associated threat to the reputation of the family. There is clearly a great deal yet to understand.

Another variation in rates of mental ill-health that invites speculation is that between rural areas and inner cities. Each of the three major national epidemiological studies discussed above in the US, UK and the Netherlands found higher rates of mental ill-health in cities. Peen and colleagues (2007), analysing the NEMESIS data, showed that it is not just a numerical difference, but a difference in severity – more of those with complex problems lived in cities, particularly those with a comorbidity of four or more disorders. Categorizing their sample of over 7000 adults into five groups according to level of urbanization (based on population density), the gradient from most urban to most rural was clear: rates of major depression going from 7.9%, 6.8%, 5.4%, 4.9% to 3.6%. Paykel and colleagues did the same analysis of the UK data on nearly 10,000 participants in the 1993 UK National Morbidity Survey, and found the same result – higher rates of mental ill-health, alcohol and drug dependence in urban populations, least in rural settings, intermediate in semi-rural areas (Paykel et al., 2003).

Further exploration of this picture suggests that the city excess is largely explained by social disadvantage, but much remains unclear. Paykel and colleagues found that controlling for other socio-economic disadvantages reduced most differences, and those relating to alcohol and drug misuse were no longer significant. Similarly the US survey also showed that higher urban prevalence was only in complex disorder once other factors likely to explain the differences were removed from the analysis. This remaining difference may of course be linked more to those with severe and complex disorders 'drifting' over time towards the inner city (see Chapter 11).

An important study on emotional and behavioural problems in children suggests that 'social drift' is unlikely to account for all the urban–rural difference, given that children tend not to move home. In 1964 all children on the Isle of Wight (an island off the south coast of England with a population of 100,000 broadly representative of the population of England and living in small towns and rural areas) born between 1953 and 1955 were screened and a high-risk sample (those with a score above a given cut-point on a screening questionnaire) and a random sample were selected for study by Michael Rutter and his team. Two comparable samples (one high-risk, one random) in an inner London Borough were selected in the same way (Rutter et al., 1975a, 1975b). The random sample comparisons showed a twofold difference in the rate of disorder between the 10-year-olds in London and those in the Isle of Wight (25.4% compared to 12%) along with more children with a low reading ability.

The high-risk samples in both locations showed that four types of variable were associated with disorder – family discord and disruption, parental illness and criminality, social disadvantage, and certain school characteristics. The random sample showed that London had higher rates of fathers who had been in prison, mothers with poor mental health, large family size, children in care, marital discord, and overcrowding, and had lower rates of home ownership. Similar differences (with Isle of Wight a better environment) were reported in school characteristics (pupil turnover, teacher turnover, absenteeism, etc.). In other words, this type of two-stage epidemiological study has demonstrated that several family and school characteristics are correlated with emotional and behavioural difficulties, as well as the attainment of 10-year-olds, and that these 'risk' factors are also more prevalent in London than the Isle of Wight and largely account for the area differences (in a statistical sense at least). However, the reason London families have so many more social difficulties remains unclear. Some research suggests it may be the effect of living in run-down, impoverished neighbourhoods, or the lack of residential stability of many inner city areas (Silver et al., 2002, and see Chapter 11).

Clues or red herrings?

Some clues lead us to the wrong conclusions. Data on the prevalence of mental ill-health associated with the diet of a population eventually led to the discovery of pellagra about 100 years ago, but the many wrong turnings taken before the correct conclusions were drawn make it an instructive illustration. Pellagra is an illness that we now know to be caused by a deficiency of vitamin B3, for which symptoms include weakness, diarrhoea, weight loss, skin inflammation, and forms of mental ill-health (confusion, memory loss and depression), eventually leading to death. It was sometimes developed among people who were resident long-term in some of the asylums of the early 1900s and before, as well as a cause of new admissions. It was thought at first to be from some kind of poison, probably associated with Indian corn (unripe or mouldy), and was particularly widespread in Italy in the nineteenth century with thousands of people, mostly peasants, affected (Babcock, in Babcock and Cutting, 1911).

The prevalence in Italy of pellagra (40,000–50,000 cases per year according to Babcock, more than this according to Cutting, affecting 1 in 60 people in rural areas, and up to 1 in 19 in Venetia) preceded its appearance in the United States (initially in Louisiana and South Carolina) by about 100 years, but as it became more common in the US the American vice-consul in Milan, W. Bayard Cutting, forwarded his conclusions about the spread of the disease in Italy so that the US could learn from the Italian experience. The strong association between a diet of Indian corn and the spread of pellagra led to three rival theories to explain the link, all relating to the corn itself. From these theories, Cutting concluded that pellagra was a type of poison, resulting from eating a diet almost exclusively of corn, and consuming some that is spoiled or mouldy. Therefore the prevention of pellagra must include laws prohibiting the importation, sale or grinding of spoiled corn destined for human consumption, inspection of corn storage facilities, improved agricultural methods, and the education of the population about the dangers of bad corn, and best drying, storage and milling practices. In addition there were recommendations to prevent pellagra in childhood: 'to prevent pellagrous mothers from nursing their babies, or, if this can not be prevented, to see that the mothers are well fed; to treat a child the moment he or she shows the slightest symptoms of pellagra, and to send him or her away from the surroundings where the pellagra has been acquired' (Cutting, in Babcock and Cutting, 1911).

In fact, all the family needed was to eat other things as well as the corn – a slightly more varied diet, including high sources of niacin such as chicken breast and vegetables. Shepherd (1978) describes how Joseph Goldenberger, an American epidemiologist, became interested in the disorder, first noticing the absence of pellagra in staff eating with residents in the mental asylums where patients had the disease, also noting the higher rates in rural than in urban poor, and recognized the more varied diet of those escaping the disease. Hence finally the correct conclusions were drawn, and through introducing more fresh foods – milk, eggs, beans, peas and meat – into institutions such as orphanages where previously pellagra had been a common ailment, Goldenberger was able to prevent it.

In line with the approach recommended by Robins and cited earlier, that the best proof is that changing the risk factor changes the rate of disorder, Goldenberger completed his evidence with a study that would greatly distress the ethics committees of today – providing proof of his theory by inducing pellagra among prisoners by limiting their diet (Shepherd, 1978).

Conclusion

Epidemiological studies now use sophisticated standardized tools with interview guides, responses that can be analysed by computer, and methods to draw representative samples, to give a detailed picture of the distribution of the defined disorders in a given geographical location. However, the allocation of people above or below the chosen threshold into cases and non-cases has proved less reliable than hoped for the many borderline conditions. One implication here is that surveys should include a category of 'borderline' disorder or use a continuous measure. Nevertheless, Kessler and Merikangas (2004) argue that the recent national surveys of mental ill-health provide a firm descriptive foundation for further analytic and experimental epidemiological research.

The belief that the problems described here and which appear to be so wide-spread are ones for which medicine can offer some help appears to be growing in the West, along with the pressure on primary care services. Kessler and Merikangas (2004) attribute this largely to the direct-to-consumer advertising by the pharmaceutical industry, public education programmes on mental health, and the rapid expansion of information available on the internet. Those seeking treatment appear to be broadly representative of those found in community surveys to be more likely to need help, except for a subgroup who express their distress in a way that challenges, disturbs or frightens others, who move swiftly to higher levels of service support compared to others with comparable ill-health that is less of a problem to others.

Clues for preventive intervention from these broad-sweep studies are numerous, but are just that – clues only. What they mean, and what might be done to change rates of disorder, needs other kinds of research, and to explore why some people recover well while others remain unwell for long periods. Rates of mental ill-health are raised in people who live with a longstanding physical health problem, who are economically inactive, and/or rent their home from the local authority or housing association, have had a troubled childhood family life, and among those who are separated or divorced, live alone, or who are single parents. Most of these problems are more common among those living in urban than rural areas and there appears to be a raised rate of mental ill-health in cities in both adults and children associated with these social problems.

Those people defined as having more than one disorder may be a particularly important focus for preventive programmes. One such group is those aged 16–24 who have some symptoms of anxiety or depression, and are also dependent on alcohol or illicit drugs, whose numbers appear to be increasing.

Finally, the pellagra example was used to caution that when all clues seem to be pointing clearly in the same direction, the mechanisms through which the risk factor leads to disorder need to be understood to avoid arriving at the wrong suggestions for intervention. The corn may not be poisonous at all.

4 Preventing ill-health or promoting wellbeing?

> If normality and deviance are indeed independent then the "normal" majority are free to disapprove of the deviants. Heavy drinkers of alcohol are condemned, but moderation is beyond criticism. Obesity is bad, but average weight is socially acceptable (even in overweight populations). Football hooligans are deviant reprobates, but, in a market economy especially, less conspicuous aggression is usual and actually encouraged. In each case the population as a whole disowns the tail of its own distribution: hypertension, obesity, alcoholism, and other behavioural problems can then be considered in isolation.
>
> (Rose and Day, 1990: 1031)

> What is needed is an acceptance of collective responsibility for the population's health and social well being.
>
> (Rose and Day, 1990: 1034)

An important contribution to thinking about the differing approaches to reducing ill-health in the population in recent decades has come from the papers by Geoffrey Rose (1981, 1985, 1992; Rose and Day, 1990), who as a public health doctor has been able to step outside the traditional health preoccupation with the welfare of individual patients, and ask whether the best efforts of preventive advice and support to individuals can ever have the desired effect on the health of the population.

He makes several simple observations, which have important implications. The first and most important distinction is between prevention that focuses on tackling *causes of cases* and that which addresses *causes of incidence* (Rose, 1985). The discovery of causes of cases requires a comparison of those with a given condition in the population with those without the condition, or with lower levels of signs and symptoms, in search of factors which distinguish between those that might be related to onset or course and amenable to change, as discussed in the previous chapter. The risk factors identified, or protective factors, should confirmation of their importance be forthcoming, become the target of intervention for those at high risk. Rose draws on coronary heart disease as his primary illustration, and high blood pressure as a risk factor revealed by this method. People with hypertension might be defined as those with a systolic blood pressure above 150 mmHg, and the factors that appear to be associated with their hypertension include family history (genetic tendency) and lifestyle factors such as dietary cholesterol, stressful lifestyle or lack of exercise. Intervention will target those with the less healthy lifestyle, assuming nothing can be done about genetic susceptibility: more exercise, a healthier diet, less stress. This discussion can take place at the doctor's surgery when the patient is attending for any reason, or the point can be made through health education to the whole population, that those not exercising and not eating a healthy diet are putting themselves at increased risk.

Addressing causes of incidence – a slightly confusing term as Rose means by this the population rate of disorder, really prevalence rates – requires a comparison between the rate of disorder in one population (perhaps a country, perhaps a community) and that in another, and asks why is the disorder so much more common in this population than that one? It is the 'how many' question rather than the 'who' question, as discussed in the previous chapter in comparing rates of mental ill-health in cities in comparison with rural areas. The reasons for high numbers might be the same as the answer to the who question – more in one area or country exposed to the risk factor – or it might reveal something unsuspected. It might be, continuing the coronary heart disease example provided by Rose (1985), that it is common to drink a glass of full milk with each meal, as it used to be in Finland, so almost everyone in this population had higher blood levels of cholesterol than almost anyone in Japan. Coronary heart disease is common in Finland, much less so in Japan (Rose, 1985). A prevention programme in Finland might achieve better outcomes if the dietary custom were changed for everyone to be more like that of the healthier Japanese, rather than target those consuming the most dietary cholesterol to make their diet like the most healthy Finnish people. But this insight might not have been gained through examining within-population differences in risk if these were small or, if noted, might have been judged of minimal significance as so many healthy people drank milk regularly too. Coronary heart disease risk for one Finnish person more than another (the causes of cases) would have been related to a different risk factor, perhaps smoking, assuming there are smokers and non-smokers in the population.

Hence the causes of cases and the causes of population rates may have similar or differing explanations. However, the second issue that Rose raises relating to this is that whatever the factor of interest, it can often be more effective to aim the intervention relating to behaviour change at a whole population rather than at the high-risk group. This is so for several reasons. Asking those with unhealthy lifestyles to change when their peers do not need to change makes it far more difficult. Second, a population change is a more radical shift in habits that should sustain healthier populations in the future rather than help some high-risk people now, and the changes achieved now can also be greater. However, there are also significant difficulties with a population strategy in that for many individuals (those not at high risk), the benefits of changing are unimportant, they will have little motivation to change, and their doctors will have little motivation to encourage them to do so.

These two public health approaches will be discussed below in relation to preventing mental ill-health; that is, exploring targeting through the risk reduction and resilience promotion model; and exploring universal strategies through a population approach. However, unlike the position in physical health, there is now also a wellbeing perspective, a school of thinking that suggests it is possible to promote positive mental health and happiness, which does not take the prevention of ill-health as a necessary part of the benefit, nor the evidence on causes of ill-health as the evidence base for recommending action. Wellbeing proponents often recommend individual-level intervention, but offered to everyone, as there is no rationale for targeting.

Risk reduction and resilience promotion

The medical model aims to discover why *this* person gets *this* disease at *this* time, and to build up an understanding of how risk exposure and vulnerability combine to increase the relative risk of one person over another (Rose, 1985). Knowledge about the mediating processes, and about the critical periods when intervention might be most effective, and understanding how it is that some people cope better than others, informs proposals for intervention. Evidence that any of these components can be changed, and how exactly a programme should work in order to achieve the desired outcome, is also needed. Decisions to fund such a programme will also be influenced by a calculation of cost-effectiveness.

In the US, NIMH (the National Institute of Mental Health) chose this risk and resilience model as its preferred strategy in 1994. Three national consensus meetings were held between 1990 and 1994, and the results of these, together with the collation of work by five panels, were distilled into a 'National Research Agenda for the Prevention of Mental Disorders' (NIMH, 1994), arriving at what Reiss and Price (1996: 1109) describe as a 'cohering field of prevention science'. They group research and development into three fields – aetiological research (risk and protective factors and the mechanisms through which they increase risk or protect); strategies and opportune timing for effective intervention to reduce risk; and exploring implementation within communities.

Almost all ill-health is multifactorial;[1] that is, there are several contributing factors which act together to bring about the disorder. Some of these factors are not directly causal, but only become significant if some other risk factor is present. This type of factor is typically referred to as a *vulnerability* factor; that is, one that shows little or no effect on its own, but increases risk in the presence of another factor (see for instance, the Brown and Harris model of depression on page 61 showing that a severe life event can cause depression, but lack of a confiding relationship (a vulnerability factor) makes it more likely that it will).

Even in physical medicine, there are very few examples of disorders that have a straightforward linear relationship:

single cause $\rightarrow$ single outcome

Infections such as those producing a sore throat might be presumed to be caused simply by the action of streptococci in the throat. Yet a study of 15 American families over a 12 month period, providing throat cultures every two to three weeks and keeping a diary of events that disturbed family life, demonstrated that stress is also a factor, increasing vulnerability. Distressing events were four times more common just before illness associated with the presence of streptococci than in the two weeks afterwards (Meyer and Haggerty, 1962). A study by Cohen and colleagues (1998) replicates this finding (see Chapter 8).

For the vast majority of medical conditions, the model is more like the one in Figure 4.1. Disorders D1 and D2 appear to have causal factors B1 and B2 associated with physiological changes C1 and C2 which are antecedent to the appearance of disorder. These are probably poorly understood. But we may know that factors A1 and A6 are independently linked to a raised probability of the occurrence of B1 and B2, and are argued to play a causal role. However, A1 may very rarely lead to B1 without the presence of A3, but A3 never lead to B1 independently. It may be that A3 is even more potent if associated with A4. Both A3 and A4 are implicated in disorder D2 and probably many others besides. In fact, very many factors may contribute to very many different types of ill-health.

One advantage of this 'disease modelling' is that it can be used to narrow the target group to maximize the pay-off of action. For instance, screening through pap smears for early signs of cancerous changes in the cervix (e.g. at C1) could be offered more frequently to women who smoke (if this is A3) and not offered at all to women who have had no sexual relationships (A1). Mothers known to have had a previous post-natal depression (A6) whose new baby has a worrying health condition (A4) can be actively encouraged to attend the clinic's mother and baby support group to help reduce their anxieties (C2) and risk of depression (D2), while non-attendance by women thought to have few problems and a good deal of support at home (A3) would not be pursued.

Identification of risk through screening does not always lead to preventive action of course, as there will often be emotional or ethical issues to weigh, as in the raised risk of carrying a child with a genetic disorder (Emery et al., 1973). Similarly, some people at known risk of inherited disorder will decline to be tested (Lloyd, 1985).

The definitions of 'primary', 'secondary' and 'tertiary' prevention link directly to this model, as first used by the working groups meeting under the auspices of the Commission for Chronic Illness in the US in the early 1950s. Primary prevention was defined as practices prior to the biologic origin of disease, presumably then addressing the A and B factors; secondary prevention was defined as practices after the disease could be recognized but before it had caused suffering and

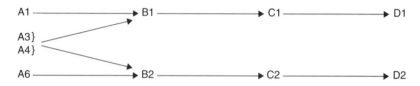

Figure 4.1 Traditional medical model of multi-factorial disorder (from Newton, 1988).

disability, presumably through screening for C factors, or shortly after the emergence of D. Tertiary prevention was added later, as action after the emergence of disorder to prevent further deterioration, recurrence or associated disadvantage (Commission on Chronic Illness, 1957). This three-stage classification became widely used in public health.

However, NIMH (1994) was persuaded by the recommendations of Robert Gordon (1983), special assistant to the director, that tertiary prevention should be excluded from the definition, and the terms primary and secondary prevention revised. He argued that these terms were unwieldy, with primary and secondary prevention often difficult to distinguish, poor consistency across disorders in the way the terms were used, and the origin of many disorders hard to pinpoint. He proposed restricting the word 'prevention' to:

> measures, actions, or interventions that are practiced by or on persons who are not, at the time, suffering from any discomfort or disability due to the disease or condition being prevented. This distinction would serve to eliminate most of what is now encompassed in the old category "tertiary."
>
> (Gordon, 1983: 108)

He also defined levels of prevention in a way that is not reliant on knowledge of the stage of development of the disorder, but is informed by cost-effectiveness, as follows:

- Universal prevention – for those strategies that would benefit everyone, i.e. wearing seat belts, eating a healthy diet, giving up smoking, 'for which benefits outweigh costs and risks for everyone' (p. 108).
- Selective measures are for use when the benefits for everyone do not outweigh the costs and risks, and where measures can only be justified for a high-risk group that is readily identifiable on the basis of age or occupation, or other clear criteria. For instance it might include rabies immunization for vets, flu immunization for older people or, say, subsidized work placements for all school leavers without a place in higher education or employment.
- Indicated strategies are those where personal characteristics of an individual lead to their risk; for instance, their elevated blood pressure, as indicated by a screening programme. Because these are at higher risk a more costly intervention can be justified, and may often be advised. These are the kind of interventions that might have been described as secondary prevention in the former terminology. Often the intervention will be a clinical one, as risk may have been identified through a medical examination.

The research report from NIMH (1994) was soon followed by a lengthy report by the Institute of Medicine (Mrazek and Haggerty, 1994), outlining the recommended way forward for the field. The 'prevention science' approach that emerged from these two reports suggested broad agreement that the way forward should be as follows:

1   Clarify the 'problem' (e.g. adult depression).
2   Review risk and protective factors that precede and affect its appearance, building a picture based on epidemiological evidence and aetiological theory, to explain how and why these factors link to this disorder.
3   The design of the intervention should then be informed as far as possible by this understanding, to modify these risk or protective factors and develop hypotheses related to the expected effect of doing so.
4   If possible, the intervention should be evaluated through use of a randomized controlled trial (RCT).
5   If evidence is positive, larger scale studies should aim to replicate the findings.
6   The findings should then be disseminated widely and the intervention built into the development of community services (Institute of Medicine, 1994).

There are both advantages and disadvantages with this approach.

Problems with the risk and resilience focus

Two problems were highlighted with the above list of six stages. First, Weissberg and Greenberg (1998) noted the difficulty of acquiring RCT evidence if testing an intervention that one has good reason to expect will have positive benefits for the intervention group. Subjects are unlikely to wish to be randomly allocated, those in the control group may develop something similar or find an alternative version of the intervention, staff responsible for control group subjects may also try to gain access to the intervention for a client they feel is particularly likely to benefit. A small-scale experimental programme led by enthusiastic pioneering researchers can often overcome such problems more easily than the larger scale study that follows.

Heller (1996) argued that neither of the two NIMH reports engaged adequately with the process of gaining community support and ownership for proposed strategies, suggesting that effective implementation needs a partnership with local organizations. For instance, a school-based programme that expects teachers to implement the programme as intended, despite the conflict it might create with their other teaching priorities and pressures on time, would encounter more difficulty than if adaptations to the programme were negotiated to fit better with school priorities. Identifying benefits to the school such as additional staff training or extra resources would also improve commitment (Weissberg and Greenberg, 1998).

But Rose (1985) has more fundamental concerns. He argues that the target of intervention is often a factor that moderates risk, rather than addressing the cause (e.g. improving coping skill rather than reducing stress), identifying those most likely to benefit is often costly, and exhorting them to do something the comparison group do not have to do is challenging. If most people in the individual's peer group are smokers, or regularly drink after work, it will be hard to quit or resist peer pressure to join them in the bar. Furthermore, while logical, Rose argues that targeting high risk will capture a small proportion of those who would have become ill as the majority of cases will arise from those with lower risk. One illustration of this is amniocentesis to screen for Down's syndrome. It was originally offered in the UK just to pregnant women over the age of 36, the highest risk group, even though the majority of mothers of children with Down's syndrome are under 30. Because most babies are born to mothers under 30, a low percentage of a large group is still a larger number than a high percentage of a small group. (Targeting has since improved through a blood test that can identify raised risk.)

However, the key issue in many types of ill-health is that those with a 'clinical' level of disorder simply represent the extreme end of the distribution. Heavy drinkers, obese people and those with high scores on scales measuring mental ill-health lie at the high end of the distribution tail. The numbers scoring above a given threshold can be predicted well from the average of the population to which they belong. There are fewer of them in populations where drinking is prohibited, average diet is low in fat, or other risk factors are low (Rose and Day, 1990). Exploration of potential preventive action should therefore aim to understand the behaviour of the whole population, with a view to changing the norm. Rose illustrates his point with graphs like the one in Figure 4.2.

Population B might be the distribution of scores of general mental health (the horizontal (*x*) axis) among the population of unemployed people (the average of whom at the top of the curve have a few symptoms of depression or anxiety

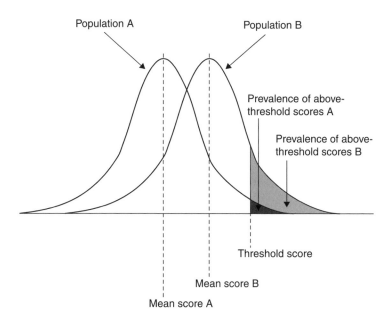

Figure 4.2 Score distribution in two populations where the variation or susceptibility is constant within each population, but varies between populations. From Anderson et al. (1993) (used with permission).

occasionally), while population A are in work. The vertical (*y*) axis is number of people. The average person in population A has less frequent and less marked feelings of mental ill-health. Or population A has an unemployment rate of 2%, population B of 20%. Those clinically depressed will be more numerous in B, and reducing the rate of unemployment may be far more effective in reducing the numbers with a clinical level of mental ill-health (above the threshold) than strategies targeting those at raised risk of ill-health among the unemployed.

However, the cost-effectiveness of a strategy to change the average diet, alcohol consumption or rate of employment depends also on the shape of the curve, the cost of the intervention, how easy it is to achieve change, and its acceptability to the whole population. Ahern and colleagues (2008) used mathematical simulations to try to calculate the relative costs and benefits of a targeted risk reduction strategy as compared to a population approach in relation to blood pressure and heart disease, and found it was not as clear as many might assume. Small differences in cost and the treatment effect could switch the best option from one to the other (targeted or universal). A cut point to focus on the very end of the tail was most cost-effective (cost per person providing savings on treatment) but produced the least population health benefit, but a general population approach needed to be very low cost or shift the mean substantially in order to bring more benefits (treatment cost saved) than costs, and Ahern et al. conclude that both approaches should always be considered.

In mental health, it may also be relatively low cost to identify those at high risk, as compared to the cost of pap smears, amniocentesis, or measuring serum cholesterol. It might mean asking teachers or midwives to refer people they are worried about, or working through an organization that works with street homeless teenagers, or pregnant care leavers. And the relative risks of those without risk factors and those with several may well be a larger difference than it might be in coronary heart disease. A young person who has had an abusive or rejecting early home-life, and as a teenager is failing at school and truanting, is a very high-risk candidate for adult mental ill-health. Furthermore, the change proposed for the high-risk group is also not as it seems to be in heart disease, to deny them something they enjoy (eating cake, smoking and drinking), but something it is assumed that they will wish to have – a supportive relationship, extra help of some kind. However, the difficulties of engaging and motivating participation of high-risk people of any age are not to be underestimated (see Chapter 10). And in the end, it is hard not to agree that the ideal is for the whole population to provide better parental care, so long as this does indeed reduce the population rate of neglect and abuse.

One issue that must be considered in mental health is that those people who are particularly vulnerable will very often have some symptoms already, though not over the cut point to be described as a 'case' of clinical severity, meaning that Gordon's definition will not work. An unemployed teenage lone parent whose family have rejected her and is not in contact with the child's father will be a good candidate for preventive support, but it would be surprising if she did not already have some symptoms of mental ill-health. Hence neither of the existing tripartite definitions is quite adequate. It would be helpful to retain a traditional public health distinction between intervention designed to prevent ill-health in those with and without symptoms of the disorder, as secondary and primary prevention, but also to distinguish targeted and population strategies, so that

- primary prevention is action intended to reduce the onset of mental ill-health in people who are not already experiencing discomfort or disability arising from the condition being prevented, and can be
  - universal – strategies that would benefit everyone, e.g. law to prohibit parents from hitting their children, rights to flexible working hours to care for a sick relative
  - targeted – strategies that aim to benefit those known to be at raised risk of mental ill-health, due to social, psychological or biological factors, e.g. practical and emotional support for young people leaving care, family support where children are born to parent(s) with mental ill-health
- secondary prevention is action intended to reduce the onset of disorder in those identified on the basis of existing risk factors and who already have some associated symptoms, e.g. emotional and practical support for a carer of a close relative with serious health difficulty who is reaching crisis point, or for a teenager regularly using cannabis or other drugs and with some symptoms of paranoia, or to prevent a relapse or recurrence of ill-health of the same type, e.g. supporting back to work someone recovering from psychosis.

The large literature on resilience, covered in later chapters, derives from this risk modelling approach, in that it explores how some people cope better than others when faced with life stresses that we know to be associated with a high rate of mental ill-health. It searches for vulnerability factors, or protective factors, and to understand the mediating process that led to one person coping well when another, facing similar adversities in their current living situation, did not.

Universal prevention: A whole-population strategy

As suggested above, universal prevention changes expectations for everyone – smoking is a less widely accepted activity, average consumption of alcohol is reduced, there is less tolerance of any physical chastisement of partner or child. A large number of people change a little (Rose, 1985).

Problems with a universal strategy – health education

Many universal strategies in the past in physical medicine have centred on a health *education* strategy, which although delivered to the whole population through mass media routes has effectively targeted those at the unhealthy end of the behaviour spectrum and can be experienced as judgemental. The critique by Becker (1993) reflects what has now become a widely held view, discrediting much of what was offered as part of this strategy as 'victim blaming'. Becker argued in his address to the US Medical Sociological Association in 1992 that health education encourages reasonably contented people to feel they ought to change, to expect that there may be harm or risk in many activities no-one worried about before, and that they themselves are responsible for their own poor health. In fact, he argued, the risk data is often controversial, and even when well supported, the benefit of change to each individual is very small. Promoting a long list of activities that are bad for our health may be counterproductive and work against the campaigns to change factors that are much more significant. Further, he argues, health education leads to the attachment of moral values to health behaviour, so that the person can be seen in a positive or negative light accordingly – smoking and relaxing in front of the TV being linked with ignorance, lack of willpower and laziness, for instance. He argues that health is linked to lifestyle, but this is largely determined by 'economic, political, cultural and structural components of society that act to encourage, produce and support poor health' (Becker, 1993: 4).

The first doubts about health education in UK policy came with the Black Report of 1980 showing a strong link between poverty and health. It suggested a shift in attention towards the reasons *why* some people drank more and smoked more, and ate high-fat foods, other than their own lack of will-power and ignorance. The association of one risk factor with many others brought a realization that as well as low income, many other socio-economic factors might also be relevant.

In effect, health education messages have largely followed the targeting risk model rather than changing whole population habits as envisaged by Rose (1985). They were focusing effort on the causes of cases, not the causes of incidence, to use Rose's labels. Rose was arguing for a change in individual *exposure to risk*, not universal approaches to changing individual response to risk. Relying on individuals to maintain their healthier lifestyle is challenging, as all those of us who have regularly broken our New Year resolutions know too well. Witness too the current rise in obesity in many Western countries, and associated rises in diabetes, suggesting it has been singularly ineffective.

The logic is clear, as Marmot (2001) has also argued. Not only is a clean water supply a more effective means of preventing a host of water-borne infectious diseases, compared to educating people to boil the water, but the water boiling is more likely to be done by those with better education and facilities to boil water. Hence a population strategy – an engineering project to supply clean water – is needed to reduce inequalities in health. A mental health example might be where illicit drugs are readily available, cheap and easily obtained in one neighbourhood, but in a nearby village it is less easy to obtain them, and they are more expensive. School-based education programmes may discourage some from using drugs, particularly those with supportive home lives where the message is reinforced and relationships are strong. Addressing the supply of cheap and plentiful drugs should reduce drug misuse more effectively, but also among those from all types of home background. It is often noted that those who benefit first and most from health education are those least at risk, and such methods can in fact increase rather than reduce health inequality (Doyle et al., 2006).

Universal changes can bring marked benefit – through policy and law

Governments can, of course, in theory, change population behaviour very rapidly, with a change in the law. Many countries across the world now prohibit smoking in public places, and this has been a notable success in achieving population health benefits. It has also changed cultural expectations about what is desirable, as well as what is acceptable. In most Western countries, few would now find it acceptable to sit for three hours in a smoke-filled train carriage. These changes are reducing rates at which people take up the habit. Siegel and colleagues (2008) showed, in a prospective study of teenage smoking in Massachusetts comparing those in cities with strong smoking bans in restaurants and those which had none, or weak regulation, that teenagers in the former, though being equally likely to try cigarettes, were significantly less likely to become habitual smokers. Juster and colleagues (2007) tracked the effects of a comprehensive smoking ban in New York State in 2003 on hospital admissions for acute myocardial infarction, and concluded that the ban led to an 8% reduction and a saving of $56 million of direct health care costs in 2004.

Benefits of this sort have accrued in reductions to self-poisoning, through changes to the supply of paracetamol (Hawton et al., 2004), now usually individually packaged in a box with a maximum number of 16. This makes it less likely that someone feeling suicidal will have a large quantity to hand at the key moment. Other policies with obvious benefit to mental health or suicidal behaviour include: those requiring barriers around frequently used jumping points, drink-driving restrictions, and legal restrictions on the availability of firearms and on the supply of alcohol and drugs. Stronger criminal prosecution of domestic violence, employment policy and school anti-bullying strategies should also bring benefits across the range, and lead to changes in attitude and expectations.

However, as the section below argues, in a democracy, such large changes in thinking that allow policy and law to change in the more contentious areas can take 30 years or more to achieve.

Problems in changing policy and law: Politics of prevention

Mills (1993) reminds us that what a society chooses to prevent, and how it does so, are political choices. Key players with some influence are the medical profession, producers such as the pharmaceutical and health food industries, but also the general public and lobby groups for particular interests. All have their interests to protect. The government itself also has a vested interest largely determined by a need to control spending and keep the population healthy and paying taxes, shaped in line with their particular ideological view, and remaining sensitive to popular opinion on what should be prevented, and what the role of the state in this should be. Mills (1993: 4) defines preventive health policy as 'strategies designed to eliminate, detect, predict or manage societal risks which would otherwise have deleterious health consequences'.

In relation to producers in the food, drink and tobacco industries, the government approach was 'non-interventionist', as Calnan (1991) described it. Industry was encouraged to respond to evidence on health risk through self-regulation to produce 'low-tar' cigarettes, health warnings on the packet, and alcohol-free beer. But according to figures sourced by Allsop and Freeman (1993), the drinks industry in the UK contributed 2% of all jobs and 5% of GDP in the 1980s, and the taxes on alcohol and tobacco were (as they remain) an important income source for government, hence industry lobby groups have been able to exercise some influence over decisions by politicians. Health education has on the whole been favoured (by producers) over legislative restrictions on risk behaviour. The government also prioritized health education strategies in a revised GP contract in 1991 to reward GPs for advising their patients, individually or in small groups, about risk factors.

When public concern is strong, politicians have been pressed to go beyond the evidence to do more than advise people how to minimize their risks. Hann (1993) notes that as breast cancer is the most common type of cancer suffered by women, causing early death, sometimes preceded by mastectomy, and is such an emotionally charged subject, women's lobby groups have been highly effective in campaigning for preventive programmes. Despite controversy over the superiority of mammograms over regular self-examination, or of the gains from earlier surgery, the pressure to show they were responding to the concerns led to policy that might otherwise have awaited a firmer evidence base. A parallel might be drawn here with the proposal to offer brief therapies for mental ill-health in primary care on a large scale.

On the other hand, powerful evidence on what government policy should contain has sometimes been very difficult to pass into law. Read (1993) illustrates this in relation to the politics around freedom of the individual and the introduction of seat-belt law. Despite the clear evidence of savings of life and disability through seat-belt use in cars, it was not until 1961 that law was passed in the UK to ensure seat belts were fitted to front seats of new cars, and it took a further 30 years before law was passed to compel all those travelling in cars' front or back seats to wear one. Concern for individual liberty was at stake. The evidence of preventable death and disability led to lobbying by the police, the Automobile Association, and the Spinal Injuries Association and to five attempts to pass new law in the 1970s, all of which failed (Read, 1993). One in four passengers in 1975 continued to choose not to use them. Much of the general population and many politicians felt that the public had a right to choose to take risks if they wished. This situation might be compared with gun use in the United States, and the large numbers of prevented suicides and homicides that might result from greater curtailment of the individual's freedom to own a gun.

Hence Mills and Saward argue that ideology should be seen as a key explanatory variable in prevention policy – for instance, ideology that maintains that individuals have a right to choose, and producers have a right to produce and make profits. The patriarchal public health role of the state, a concern for the 'common good' and the vulnerable, must somehow be reconciled with this. Individual choice and autonomy is a key feature of much of UK health and social policy, though some are beginning to question this (e.g. Doyle et al., 2006). For instance, the fact that in recent years a number of people have chosen not to immunize their children against measles, mumps and rubella in the UK was due to some controversy reported in the media over the safety of the triple vaccine, of which the negative evidence has now been discredited, but in the meantime this lowered immunization rates at one point to below 60%, seriously reducing the effectiveness of the immunization strategy which relies on high uptake. Individual choice allowed self-interest to take precedence over population benefit. Yet many countries have long ago passed law to allow compulsion. Colgrove and Bayer (2005) celebrated the 100th anniversary of a US Supreme Court judgement that upheld the right of a state to enact compulsory vaccination law, so that schools can today make up-to-date vaccinations an entry requirement.

Societal expectations that support the right of the individual to choose have particular relevance to mental health, and are more controversial than any of the examples discussed above. When the choices relate to marriage; having children; paying taxes; supporting people who are ill, disabled, unemployed or poor – the risk for government in countering aspirations for individual autonomy, to act in other than selfish best interest, can be a risk too far when reliant on democratic election. But we leave child protection social workers and others to grapple daily on our behalf with some of the dilemmas.

Promoting positive mental health

One might assume that if those studying people at high risk of mental ill-health seek factors that are associated with one tail of the distribution of mental heath in the population, then those seeking to promote positive mental health are arguably doing the same, at the other tail. However, Jahoda (1958), and others since (e.g. Huppert and Whittington, 2003; WHO, 2004), have suggested that health and illness are not in fact opposite ends of a continuum, but represent discrete concepts. Other terms describing related concepts are 'mental capital', 'mental wellbeing' and 'positive mental health', and there does not seem to be a strong consensus about what these mean.

It may be partly that – as Marie Jahoda (1958: 8) suggested – people can be happy or they can have a happy disposition, and these are not the same thing: 'Much of the confusion in the area of mental health stems from the failure to establish whether one is talking about mental health as an enduring attribute of a person or a momentary attribute of functioning.'

'Mental capital' has been used to refer to the former:

> a person's cognitive and emotional resources. It includes their cognitive ability, how flexible and efficient they are at learning, and their "emotional

intelligence", such as their social skills and resilience in the face of stress. It therefore conditions how well an individual is able to contribute effectively to society, and also to experience a high personal quality of life.

(Foresight, 2008: 10)

Mental wellbeing and mental health, on the other hand, represent respectively:

a dynamic state, in which the individual is able to develop their potential, work productively and creatively, build strong and positive relationships with others, and contribute to their community.

(Foresight, 2008: 10)

a state of wellbeing in which the individual realizes his or her own abilities, can cope with the normal stresses of life, can work productively and fruitfully, and is able to make a contribution to his or her community.

(WHO, 2001: 1)

Keyes (2002) further divides the concept of mental health into three independent domains – emotional, psychological, and social wellbeing, which are respectively: satisfaction with quality of life, and positive affect; self-acceptance and a sense of purpose in life; having a thriving social life, in local and broader communities (Robitschek and Keyes, 2009: 321). His measure of these dimensions allows a score with cut points for flourishing, moderately mentally healthy, or languishing. He cites evidence of correlation of this measure with: missed days of work; prevalence of cardiovascular disease; number of chronic physical health problems; and poor psycho-social functioning. The rating does not appear to be greatly different from the way mental ill-health is assessed, using psychiatric assessments (i.e. based on symptoms and social functioning), and in fact the authors themselves liken their scale to the upper levels of the Global Assessment of Functioning, a tool commonly used in research allied to the DSM IV.

Huppert and Whittington (2003) also base their measure of 'positive mental health' on a measure of mental ill-health – the GHQ-30. This consists of 15 questions with positive wording (e.g. Have you recently felt that on the whole, you were doing things well?) for which the usual scoring of the GHQ uses the negative responses, as well as agreement with the 15 items with negative wording (e.g. Have you recently felt that life is entirely hopeless?). The POS-GHQ instead uses the positive answers to the 15 positive items.

Drawing on the GHQ-30 data from over 6000 of the participants in the Health and Lifestyle survey, Huppert and Whittington (2003) compared its usual scoring with their POS-GHQ rating. As expected, the GHQ-30 was correlated with physical health problems and lack of social support, and indicative of depressive symptoms, anxiety and low self-esteem. But the POS-GHQ correlated more strongly than the GHQ-30 with unemployment, suggesting that unemployment is more strongly associated with an absence of positive feelings rather than a presence of depressive symptoms.

Yet they maintain that health and ill-health are separate dimensions. They support this claim with their finding that a proportion (17%) of their sample gained high scores on both positive and negative items, that is they were rated as both high on mental health and having a high rating on a number of symptoms of mental ill-health. These findings 'contrast sharply with the view that positive and negative wellbeing are at opposite ends of a continuum' (Huppert and Whittington, 2003: 114). They suggest that the fact that a number of people with disabilities linked to mental ill-health can also express feelings of competence or efficacy and coping or contentment needs to be addressed by assessments of quality of life, rather than assessing only the presence of symptoms. The two measures separately should be used in research and practice, they suggest, having shown elsewhere (Huppert and Whittington, 1995) that mortality is associated more strongly with the lack of satisfaction and enjoyment in life than the presence of psychiatric symptoms. While some might question the suggestion that the focus on improving symptoms through strategies such as cognitive behavioural therapy (CBT) should be complemented by 'wellbeing therapy' (Fava et al., 1998), the argument that practitioners should look for activities that foster feelings of well-being in their service users as well as addressing symptoms might be welcomed.

Aaron Antonovsky's interest in how people stay well is arguably closer to mental ill-health prevention in that the focus is on stress and coping (Antonovsky, 1979, 1987). He suggested that people have their own personal orientation about the extent to which environments are predictable, adequate coping resources are available, and the likelihood that events will turn out well. This orientation is pervasive but dynamic, and Antonovsky calls it 'a sense of coherence' (SOC). His SOC measure has been used in numerous cross-sectional studies since, demonstrating correlations with self-perception of depression, resilience under stress, and fewer circulatory problems (reviewed by Eriksson and Lindström, 2006). They note that the concept overlaps with optimism, mastery, learned resourcefulness and locus of control, and is negatively associated with measures of, for instance, anxiety, anger, hopelessness and depression. Longitudinal data suggests that it may also be protective against chronic illness and mortality (Surtees et al., 2003), mental ill-health and suicide (Kouvonen et al., 2010). But as yet, little evidence exists that intervention can strengthen SOC and thereby reduce mental ill-health.

By contrast, there is some limited data to suggest that positive psychology, as conceptualized by Martin Seligman, can be taught, and can help to improve mental health, though the outcomes reported are often reductions in depressive symptoms. Seligman breaks down the concept of happiness into three components: positive emotion, engagement and meaning. While his early work on learned helplessness was valuable in the development of CBT, his work on learned optimism has been developed into 'positive psychotherapy' (Seligman et al., 2006), a taught structured programme to rehearse strategies to enhance mental health, which he has shown to be an effective treatment of depression (see Chapter 8).

The number of contributors to this field is substantial and only a few are mentioned here. They do not yet share a unifying theory to guide intervention, as differing concepts are emphasized by different contributors. Hence, the implications for action are extremely wide-ranging, and the potential measures of effectiveness equally so. Some of the ideas and research remain controversial and attract hostile discussion between critics; see for example Lazarus (2003). The areas that link with the concepts of optimism, coping and adapting to stress are discussed further in relation to coping and resilience in Chapter 7. Positive psychology is revisited in Chapter 8.

Cost-effectiveness

The concern to prevent mental ill-health has grown as the recognition by the public and by governments of its prevalence and associated cost to individuals, families and society has increased, as discussed in Chapter 1. Mechanic (2003: 13) argued that this could lead to more resources, or it may give the impression that supporting those with mental ill-health (let alone those seeking happiness and mental wellbeing) is a bottomless pit. As he argues, 'if we reported medical disorders the way we report mental disorders, the headlines would have to declare that almost everyone is sick much of the time. Such headlines would not be incorrect but trivial. Dandruff is a disease, but it need not necessarily be treated in most instances.' Much of what we now describe as one of the 'common mental health problems' would not have received any treatment before the mid-twentieth century other than the care of friends and relatives and perhaps conversations with a family GP.

Hence it may serve the field better if ill-health prevention remains focused on serious consequences that should, if not prevented, be the concern of health and welfare services, and that positive wellbeing promotion is more firmly separated, and placed fully outside the domain of such provision. Promoting wellbeing may fit better with policy and practice allied to human rights, community development, morality or spirituality, rather than being seen as part of health policy.

Spending on health and welfare by any government must always be informed not only by population need, but also by the benefit that intervention might bring, and its affordability. There is never enough money, and there must be a means for rationing. Inevitably this involves moral judgements: Who should gain access to the limited service resources, and for which type of help? Making those judgements requires an evidence base – of need, benefit and cost, none of which are straightforward concepts. They are value-laden and contested. Which cost is more important? The individual cost to quality of life, the cost to families, employers, or the state? What do we mean then by cost-effectiveness, and what are the implications for our approach to prevention?

For ill-health not prevented, which then requires treatment by the health service, the simplest comparison is between medical costs incurred and medical savings only, though of course in mental health it is unlikely that either cost incurred or savings achieved by the state will be by the health service alone. But to simplify by way of illustration, take the example given by Russell (2009), who demonstrates that 'hundreds of studies have shown that prevention usually adds to medical costs instead of reducing them'. Diabetes can be prevented in middle-aged overweight people judged high-risk on the basis of oral glucose tests, through guided diet and exercise plans. She cites a cost-effectiveness analysis (CEA) which showed that after four years 11% of the intervention group had diabetes compared to 23% of the control group. The additional cost was considered worth the money, so it was judged cost-effective but added medical costs of $143,000 dollars per healthy year at 2000 cost levels.

Treatment savings are higher for those at higher risk, and of course for lower cost preventive interventions. Newton (1992) argued for support to maximize the use of naturally occurring and community networks of support where these can bring benefits within targeted strategies. Cervical screening has been judged cost-effective when done every three to five years, but cost-effectiveness declines significantly with more frequent screening, with annual screening a very significant cost (Russell, 2009). Russell's analysis of 599 CEAs published between 2000 and 2005 showed that less than 20% of prevention programmes save more than they cost, and that careful choices are needed 'about frequency, groups to target, and component costs' to ensure cost-effectiveness (Russell, 2009: 42).

However, once other types of cost are considered this can change the balance for the state, though not for the health budget. Richard Layard (2006b) advised that as national psychiatric surveys show such high rates of chronic anxiety and depression, costing society dearly in terms of lost productivity and welfare benefits, the government can justify spending on counselling. He argues that the evidence is strong enough to expect that a short course of CBT would lift half of those people out of their depression or anxiety, so with sufficient therapists, this could be achieved in the UK for just £750 per person (2006 prices). He claims that this treatment would pay for itself in one month of saved cost of incapacity benefit (IB), which many may be claiming, given that over one third of IB claims are due to mental ill-health, and this bill now outstrips the cost of unemployment benefits. All we need, he argues, is to train another 10,000 therapists.

The calculations become ever more complex, and the benefits more important, when the intervention is with families with babies or young children and intervention might not only benefit the adults, but make a significant difference to their children's lives. Similarly when considering work with adolescents who are likely to become parents quite soon, the benefit must be considered both for the adolescent and their future offspring. For this reason, it is tempting to brush aside financial calculations, as such potential gains are inestimable. But what cannot be brushed aside is the evidence of benefit. This needs to be established not simply from small-scale experimental interventions led by pioneering researchers, but from evidence that they are effective in practice – a much greater challenge, as discussed in Chapter 12.

Hence the choice between population measure or risk and resilience strategy will take account of cost-effectiveness, but might primarily be driven by evidence of benefit. Some of the most important factors relating to prevention are societal ones – social norms and expectations, and legislation – but some of the best evidence comes from targeted intervention. The risk and resilience focus in relation to the 'cases' at the end of the distribution is undoubtedly the approach required to gain greater insights into the processes through which some people come to be at greater risk than others, and why some cope better than others, and this is needed not only to target effectively, but also to understand between-population differences and to ensure that universal measures work.

The political cost of then moving from attention to 'sick individuals' to 'sick populations', as Rose described it, may mean a more serious investment by all of us than we might realize. It means, as he suggests, that we can no longer require the heavy drinkers to moderate while condoning moderate drinking for the majority, nor expect to reduce domestic violence or child abuse by simply continuing to focus on a small minority of troublesome people. We will need to look at factors that affect aggressive behaviour and parenting skills throughout society.

Polarization in the stance of contributors to the field in relation to illness prevention versus health promotion in the past has been an unhelpful distraction from making progress in what is an agreed goal of ensuring a minimal level of mental ill-health in the population, and a thriving, well-functioning society. This has sometimes characterized debate about priorities. Instead the divide should be between what individuals can do for themselves and their close networks (peers, work colleagues, clients, communities, about which we will learn most from studying risk and resilience) and what politicians can do, through policy and law; also between what is legitimately part of the role of the health service and what is not.

The chapters to follow will have this split in focus – not between prevention and promotion but, taking the lead from Geoffrey Rose, examining *between-*population differences and *within*-population differences and the insights they provide about mental ill-health, and associated risk and protective factors.

Note

1 This discussion closely follows that in Newton (1988).

5   Depression

Those who have experienced a marked depression describe first and foremost their lack of energy, or desire to be bothered to do anything. Even talking may seem to take effort. Instead there might be a desire to retreat to bed, to sleep and perhaps to cry. On the other hand, sleep may be difficult: the person may wake in the early mornings and lie for long hours unable to get back to sleep, feeling particularly low at this time. Appetite and enjoyment of food can also sometimes be affected.

Few people with depression feel good about themselves or see anything to which to look forward. No point in studying, as would not get to college anyway. No point in trying to complete those extra tasks at the office, as stand no chance of being considered for that more senior position at work. But the depressed person may also have much suppressed anger, resentment, fear or anxiety, which can be reflected in some agitation and in irritable behaviour, perhaps snapping at those close to them (see Gilbert, 2007). In fact, a mixture of anxiety and depression is even more common than depression alone (see Chapter 3). The experience of most or all of the symptoms described above for at least two weeks would lead to a diagnosis of major depression on both the ICD and the DSM. On the ICD, the diagnosis would describe it as moderate or severe, based on the number of symptoms.

At the other end of the range, a mild depression has a fairly ordinary quality about it that most of us understand, as we have all experienced at least the short, transient feelings of misery, apathy and hopelessness which are a prominent part of the picture. But if these feelings endure – and some people have low–level symptoms on and off for years – then the DSM and ICD might label this 'dysthymia' (if two years or more). It is possible – indeed quite common – to experience a major depression on top of dysthymia (Hammen, 1997).

As well as weariness, people often describe a sense of feeling trapped or imprisoned (Rowe, 2003), and alone, but past caring too, as Beck (1973) has famously described it; feeling oneself to be worthless, in a meaningless world, the future hopeless. As Chapter 3 showed, it is very common, particularly the milder forms (the most prevalent of all diagnoses of mental ill-health) the 'common cold' of psychiatry, though this comparison underplays its effects on the individual and those close to them. It affects people of all ages, women more than men, from childhood to extreme old age, though it is most common from age 16 to 55. The most severe 'melancholic'[1] form that is more likely to be encountered in a hospital setting is much less common. Most people who are depressed carry on their lives at work, at home, with their families, but much less competently than normal, with or without treatment from their GP, dwelling on the negatives in their life.

All forms of depression can recur, and frequently do. Hammen's review cites longitudinal studies demonstrating that between 50% and 85% of people who have had one episode will have another at some point, and the first few months following recovery from the first is the time when it is most likely, particularly if the person also has other physical or mental health problems. A substantial minority of people (about one in four; Brown and Moran, 1994; Hammen, 1997; Spijker et al., 2006) remain depressed for a year or more, in which case they are considered to be 'chronically depressed'. Depression frequently occurs alongside physical ill-health (Singleton et al., 2001). This seems to be a two-way process – physical disorder and disability can lead to depression, but also depression and life stress affects immunity to infection and disease (Martin, 1998, and see Chapter 8). Roughly one in nine people with major depression eventually kill themselves, and about half of all suicides have a diagnosed depressive disorder (Hammen, 1997). On the other hand, most depression (over half) clears up even without treatment within four to six months, and three-quarters by 12 months (Hammen, 1997).

There are many types of theory about why anyone gets depressed, drawing on psychology, psychoanalysis, biology, evolutionary theory, sociology and personal experience. As much as we can say we 'know' what causes the more common types of mental ill-health, the concept of 'stress' features in almost all explanations, but so too does the recognition that some people cope better with these 'stresses' than others – that some people are seemingly resilient. As Chapter 1 illustrated, there is a longstanding assumption that the origins of resilience or vulnerability lie in childhood, or even parental life pre-dating conception. The various explanations are not necessarily alternatives, and most researchers now believe that all are useful, and what is needed therefore is a bio-psycho-social model.

The chapter will explore what more we know about this – who is likely to become depressed in the context of life events and difficulties, and why? Why do some people recover quickly, while others have recurrent episodes or remain continuously depressed for years? What might lie behind the large variation in rates of depression between populations? And what are the implications for prevention?

Variations in rates: Between-population comparisons

There are substantial cross-national differences in the prevalence of depression. Two major studies found high rates in South American cities, low rates in south Asian cities, with Europe and the US between these two extremes. For instance, Weissman and colleagues (1996) found rates below 3% in Taiwan and Korea.

Although not strictly comparable (as the samples were drawn from primary care centres, hence rates influenced by reporting or treatment-seeking decisions), Simon and colleagues (2002) found similarly low rates in Shanghai and Nagasaki. The former study reported 16% in Paris and 19% in Beirut; the latter 13.5% in Paris, but highest rates in Manchester (17%), Rio de Janeiro (18%) and Santiago (26%). Weissman and colleagues speculate on differences in rates of stressors to account for the variation: perhaps linked to political differences affecting freedom of the individual, threat of violence, deprivation, rapid cultural shifts, and perhaps ethnic difference in vulnerability.

Brown (1998) cites comparative rates of depression in women only, assessed using the same measurement method as that used by his own research group – a shortened version of the Present State Examinaton (PSE) and the Bedford College criteria to determine 'caseness' (closely similar to the definition of DSM, Third Revision – DSM3R) – to give 12 month prevalence rates in six differing populations of women aged 18–65. The findings (Table 5.1) reflect the major differences found elsewhere between urban and rural populations, but marked differences between urban centres. The highest rate (of 30%) was found in the study of Shona-speaking women in a township in Harare (Zimbabwe), twice as high as inner city London, but more than 10 times as high as the highly integrated community of Basque-speaking women in the Basque region of Spain. Abas and Broadhead (1997) note that two thirds of the Zimbabwean women they interviewed showed anxiety as well as depression; the same proportion recovered partially or fully within 12 months, most explaining their symptoms in terms of specific social stressors. More of the London sample had a long-term depressive disorder. Reflecting on the results of these and findings in related research in other countries, Brown (2002) notes first of all the strong confirmation in all studies of the role of adverse life events and difficulties. He also notes the regular finding that difficulties in core relationships, usually marriage or cohabiting, have a significant relationship with depression, and that indicators of social integration in rural areas, and social class in urban areas, also appear to be associated with markedly differing rates of depression, though not always with anxiety. One further population difference revealed by his comparisons was that having children in inner city London in the 1970s was associated with raised rates of depression, particularly among mothers of three or more children, whereas there was no such association

Table 5.1 Differing population rates of depression from four studies using the same methods (from Brown, 2002)

Harare, Zimbabwe[1]	Camberwell, London[2]	Bilbao, Spain[3]	Outer Hebrides[4]	Basque, Spanish-speaking[3]	Basque, Basque-speaking[3]
Urban	Urban	Urban	Rural	Rural	Rural
30%	15.1%	10.3%	10.6%	11%	2.4%

[1]Abas and Broadhead, 1997; [2]Brown and Harris, 1978; [3]Gaminde et al., 1993; [4]Prudo et al., 1984.

in Spain or Italy, suggesting that there may be some benefits to mothers of living in a more family-oriented culture (Brown, 2002).

In all countries compared, the higher rate in women than in men (usually double) persists.

Stressful events and long-term social difficulties cause onset

As Chapter 3 and common sense tell us, a long list of adverse life experiences can make us depressed – becoming unemployed, living with physical ill-health, struggling to manage a low income, going through separation or divorce – and it would seem likely that these account for a good deal of the population variations mentioned above. Some 40 years of studying the role of events and difficulties by Brown and Harris and their colleagues through interviews with samples of inner city working class mothers shed further light on the quality of such events. They combined an almost anthropological examination of women's lives with measures that permit statistical testing of the ideas arising, producing data that not only is invaluable to those wishing to plan preventive intervention, but also stands the test of methodological rigour, widely recognized as such by other prominent researchers in the field (see Harris, 2000).

In their first investigation in Camberwell, a working class area of south London, they interviewed a random sample of 458 women, plus 148 women receiving inpatient or outpatient care at one of the three local hospitals or from a local GP. They found that 15% of the random sample were clinically depressed in the three months prior to interview, half of whom had been depressed for more than a year (hence termed 'chronic cases'). A further 18% had borderline levels of symptoms (Brown and Harris, 1978). Severe life events were three times more common among both the depressed patients and the depressed women in the community as compared to the community sample without depression (61%, 68% and 20% respectively).

'Severe' events constituted a marked or moderate loss or disappointment with long-term implications, and focused on the woman herself or jointly with someone else. Onset of depression usually followed a severe event quite rapidly – within weeks or sometimes days. Long-term difficulties could play a similar role (living in overcrowded home conditions, a partner's drug addiction) if they had been ongoing for at least two years, and were rated as major (1–3 on a six-point scale). Two thirds of both patients and community cases experienced major difficulties, compared to only 20% of non-depressed women (Brown and Harris, 1978).

The meaning of an event to the individual is core to its effects; for instance, an event which matches an area of life to which the person is particularly committed, or reflecting a long-term difficulty (Brown et al., 1987). Among the 404 Islington women in this longitudinal study, the discovery of, say, a child truanting from school and stealing from her would have greater effects on a woman whose view of herself as a good mother was core to her identity. Had she been less committed to her parenting role, perhaps because her partner undertook most of the childcare, there would be less chance that the event would be so threatening. Examples of events matching difficulties might include a partner leaving home after several years of arguing and discord, a child arrested for burglary after a long period of difficulty at home and at school, or a substantial fine after a long period of financial difficulty.

This study later led to further insights suggesting that it is not therefore loss that was the central feature of life events, but the sense of defeat and/or the 'message' from an event that the way forward is blocked that conveys a sense of hopelessness about the future – that the person is trapped in a miserable situation, having no control. The authors describe the quality of events thereafter as most damaging if conveying a sense of 'entrapment and humiliation' (Brown et al., 1995; Brown, 1998). When recategorized in this way, 34% of events in their Islington sample led to depression. Death was the only uncomplicated loss that provoked a depression almost as frequently (in 29% of occurrences). Otherwise a loss such as in separation where the individual was the partner who left, and other lesser losses were much less likely to provoke a depression (11% and 7% respectively; see Brown, 1998).

Research into the role of life events in depression must address at least three problems. First is the time sequence – which came first, depression or event – and the time delay; second that depressed people reporting events are more likely to recall them negatively than they would had they not been depressed; third that depressed people may by their behaviour cause some of the negative events that arise. The Life Events and Difficulties Schedule (LEDS) was developed to overcome some of these methodological challenges, allowing the interviewer to explore the context of the event and apply their two-stage process to rating the likely meaning of the event to anyone facing a similar situation (Brown and Harris, 1978). Hence the first stage was to decide if a situation was eligible for inclusion according to a set of highly developed criteria provided to the researcher. The second stage involved an exploration of the context – details of the event, the person's prior experience and preparation, their immediate reactions, the consequences and implications. The event and its context were then rated by a research team with no knowledge of the woman or her responses, to arrive at a judgement on how much of a long-term threat it would pose to the average person under the same circumstances.

The lengthy interview method also enabled the start of both the social difficulties and the mental health difficulties (using an adapted version of the PSE) to be clarified, dating the time when an increase (or decrease) in the number and severity of a woman's symptoms led to a noticeable change in her mental health. Finally, they could check whether their findings held if they considered only those events that were unlikely to have been caused by the person who was depressed, such as a woman's husband being made redundant, and excluding events that may potentially have been caused by depressive symptoms, such as family arguments.

Most people do not get depressed after stressful life events and difficulties

Most people cope with markedly stressful experience without becoming clinically depressed. This is illustrated in all studies; for instance, in the first Brown and

Harris (1978) study, 80% of those experiencing a severe event or difficulty (together termed 'provoking agents') did not get depressed. Brown and colleagues (1987) reported on 10 other studies that had used the LEDS which together suggested that at least 76% of depressive illness in the general population is brought on either by severe events or by major difficulties. However, the story is rather like smoking and lung cancer – while almost all those who develop lung cancer are, or have been, smokers, most smokers do not in fact develop lung cancer. Life events should be considered as important to depression as smoking is to lung cancer.

But continuing the smoking and cancer argument, almost all depressive episodes followed a provoking agent. In their Islington sample, 303 of the 404 women were followed up after 12 months (i.e. those not already depressed and willing to be interviewed) and one in 10 became depressed during this interval. Of these 32 women, 29 did so following a severely threatening event, one other after a major difficulty only (Brown et al., 1987). Kendler and colleagues (2003: 789) have substantially confirmed this picture in an analysis of data from the Virginia twin study involving 7322 adult twins, and showing too that the categories are as applicable for men as for women. 'In addition to loss, humiliating events that directly devalue an individual in a core role were strongly linked to risk for depressive episodes.' Their evidence also confirms that the association between events and depression is a causal one.

Life events often also cause first onset of severe types of mental ill-health

The most severe melancholic depressive disorders seen by psychiatrists were at one time described as 'endogenous', as they were thought to be unrelated to life events. However, several studies have shown that the first episode in particular is usually provoked by a severe event, although subsequent episodes may be more likely to 'come out of the blue' (see Brown et al., 1994; Stroud et al., 2008). A good illustration of a humiliating event that provoked a bipolar disorder is given in an autobiographical account by Sutherland (1976). A university professor in England, with no mental health history throughout his adult life, he quite rapidly developed a severe depression in his mid-40s, after learning new details of his wife's affair. He and his wife had both had relationships outside marriage, which they did not disguise from each other, but when he discovered that his wife's lover was not, as she had told him, a stranger, but one of his own friends with whom he had an ambivalent, rather competitive relationship, and in whom he had confided details of his wife's affair, a major depressive illness followed from which he did not recover for years – an acute episode followed by a period of mild elation, and a longer, less severe depressive illness after this.

Differing types of disorder appear to be linked with differing qualities of event. Finlay-Jones and Brown (1981) showed a markedly higher rate of events characterized by danger (as opposed to loss or humiliation) in the lives of general practice patients consulting with symptoms of general anxiety. A large range of physical disorder is more common in the lives of those with stressful lives, from the common cold to coronary heart disease (Lovallo, 2005; and see Chapter 8), where chronic stress is sometimes more important than acute events. Brown and Harris (1989) show there are links between differing types of event and schizophrenia, inflammatory bowel disease, multiple sclerosis and menorrhagia, as well as anxiety and depression.

However, as the minority of those experiencing all types of stress develop a clinical disorder, and even in the case of depression it is only one in five, this means that something else is also required. Many alternative explanations exist for what this something might be, and how it shapes vulnerability.

Vulnerability and resilience

The contributions to the analysis of who gets depressed and why can be examined from the deliberations deriving from five schools of thought:

- *genetics* – we inherit a susceptibility to some disorder, or a personality that makes us more likely to respond adversely to stressful experience
- *psychoanalytic theory* – our childhood has created specific sensitivities to later loss experience
- *cognitive psychology* – early experience or personality characteristics can produce a propensity to negative evaluation of events
- *social psychology and sociology* – childhood adversity and current circumstances leave us short on resources to cope with difficulties
- *evolutionary perspectives* – it is an adaptive and a necessary response to defeat.

Of course these are not alternative explanations, and the evidence to date suggests that the insights derived from all of these play a part. There is also a strong interaction between them, as will become clear.

Genes

Most of us can recognize some aspects of our personalities in our parents or our children, and it seems likely that these same types of inherited attributes contribute to vulnerability to common mental health problems such as anxiety and depression, and to childhood behaviour. That is, our genes contribute to our shyness, fearfulness and impetuousness rather than there being specific genes for specific disorders. Kendler et al. (1987) concluded from their study of 4000 Australian twins that the genetic susceptibility to anxiety and depression is similar, whereas the environment has specific effects. They replicated this finding in a twin study in Virginia (Kendler, 2004), showing that general anxiety disorder (GAD) (but not phobias or panic disorder) and major depression (MD) share a similar genetic profile, but that 'pure' anxiety and 'pure' depression are linked to some different environmental factors. The studies of Kendler's team have in fact shown how anxiety is both a risk factor for depression (doubling the risk) and, in acting to sensitize people to the effects of stressful life events, can have an interactive effect that further increases risk (Hettema et al., 2006).

Recent developments in molecular genetics on mechanisms that regulate gene activity have revolutionized work in this area, as it has become clear that the environment can influence how genes are 'read', without a permanent change in the DNA sequence itself. This adds to the already complex possibilities for how genes and environment interact (G × E). The effects with which we are most familiar include the way the characteristics of the individual can shape the behaviour of close others, and the way we differ in our response to a negative event. More recent interest has been in the way in which prolonged exposure to certain environmental conditions actually *changes* the expression of the gene, described as epigenetic effects. Meaney (2010) explains that the development of the individual is best considered as the emergent property of a constant interplay between the genome and its environment (see Chapter 9).

The main environmental factors identified in shaping risk of depression are: support from close others, child maltreatment, and stressful life events. To date, the G × E studies have focused primarily on the latter two; that is, how our genes may increase the risk of depression and other common mental health problems for those of us maltreated as children, and/or who are struggling to cope with stressful life events.

The gene variant/polymorphism identified so far as likely to play some role in depression is known as 5-HTTLPR (a gene that transports serotonin, which is a neurotransmitter that appears to play a role in depression, and is positioned on chromosome 17). We inherit a gene from each parent, and if we inherit the short as opposed to the long allele of the 5-HTTLPR gene from both parents, this seems to raise our risk of depression (Caspi et al., 2003). About 17% of the population have the short/short version (as opposed to short/long or long/long) (Caspi et al., 2003), and among this group, the risk of depression at age 26 was raised only in those who had either experienced more than three events in the past five years, or had experienced child maltreatment between ages 3 and 11. Among those without either social risk factor, there was almost no difference in rates of depression associated with the short allele on the 5-HTTLPR gene, indicating that the gene affects response to stress, rather than directly affecting depression. This study was a careful, detailed analysis of a sample of 847 people from the Dunedin cohort in New Zealand, studied from ages 2 to 26.

The findings so far are fascinating, but the research is at early stages, producing as many questions as answers. It may be that the same genetic factors that increase risk are in some situations protective, or bring other advantages (see below), and it is not clear that there are implications for population rates of disorder. While the role of these genetic variations in the onset of common forms of depression appears to be small, and relevant primarily in their interaction with environmental factors, there is growing evidence that their role is greater in chronic (i.e. long term) depression (Brown and Harris, 2008).

Genes and severe or bipolar depression

Many of the people who write about their own depression argue that inheritance plays a major role. However, they are more usually referring to bipolar disorder than to the more common depressive state. Jamison (1993), a psychiatrist, researcher and writer who has lived with bipolar disorder all her adult life, reviews twin studies of bipolar disorder completed by the time of her writing, and concludes that evidence for a genetic link is much stronger for bipolar disorder than for unipolar depression, citing evidence for high rates among children where both parents have affective illness, at least one being of the bipolar kind. But she is most persuasive in her analysis of the link between creativity and bipolar disorder, and the overlapping personality traits of family members. Her thesis is that there is a large overlap in the artistic and manic-depressive temperaments, and both run in families. She traces the family trees of Tennyson, Schumann, William and Henry James, Coleridge, Hemingway, Woolf, Shelley and Van Gogh in detail, and lists nearly 200 other writers, artists and composers with probable cyclothymia, major depression or manic-depressive illness, starting at Hans Christian Andersen and ending with Emile Zola in the writers category, and going from Antonin Artaud to Walt Whitman in the poets list.

She is able to trace Lord Alfred Tennyson's (1809–92) relatives through the largest number of generations, showing that Tennyson had recurrent depressions requiring treatment and was one of 12 children: four others had similar problems, two others had an unspecified psychosis, and one further sibling was affected by manic depression and confined for 60 years in an asylum. They were children of Elizabeth (sweet-tempered and easy-going) and George, clearly manic-depressive, whose own father George had an unspecified psychosis (involving 'choleric rages' and recurrent melancholia) and was son to a couple seemingly free of mental ill-health, but who both had a father with violent rages or major depression. Some families in Jamison's analysis also had a strikingly high rate of suicide: Ernest Hemingway, for instance, shot himself in 1961, shortly after an inpatient stay and ECT for psychotic depression, 34 years after his father did the same, and two of his siblings also killed themselves. Both of Hemingway's two children by his second wife had severe mental health problems, one with bipolar disorder, the other a psychosis apparently triggered by a head injury sustained in a car accident.

The families Jamison describes share many devastating mental health problems, but also destructive patterns of drug and alcohol misuse and financial chaos. They also share uncommon ability and originality.

Jamison's argument is that manic-depressive illness confers an advantage, 'but often kills and destroys as it does so' (Jamison, 1993: 240), and she asks what would be lost by prevention. Many of the artists she quotes state openly that they avoided treatment, as they felt that their madness was central to their creative talents. She asserts that 'Missing the highs of hypomania is, in fact, an important reason why many patients stop taking lithium against medical advice' (p. 242), and that many artists 'fear that psychiatric treatment will transform them into normal, well-adjusted, dampened, and bloodless souls – unable, or unmotivated, to write, paint, or compose' (p. 241). She debates how medication can best be managed to facilitate creativity and concentration, as she knows too well, from personal experience as well as clinical practice, how destructive and devastatingly painful the acute phases of untreated bipolar disorder can be, and how frequently suicide can result (and did result for 42 of her 195 listed writers, musicians and artists). But she raises her greatest concern in relation to gene therapy, or genetic screening in order to consider primary prevention through selective abortion. The gene, or genes, involved in manic-depressive illness 'can confer advantages on both the individual and society' (p. 251), and Jamison notes that other 'disorders' also have hidden benefits – the sickle-cell carrier seeming to have relative immunity to certain types of malaria. It is a balance that must give pause for very careful thought to those considering the potential for prevention.

Despite these family histories, the evidence discussed earlier for a genetic contribution to the far more common and less severe depressions, and even to the severe melancholic disorders, shows it as playing a much smaller role, and the mode of genetic inheritance as far more complex. In fact researchers and psychiatrists have for decades debated whether the severe unipolar or bipolar disorders are part of the same condition as the major depression experienced by up to a quarter of us at some time in our lives. Despite the evidence that life events are implicated in the first episode of all types of depression, there appear to be fewer social vulnerability factors. For instance, in the beautifully written and scholarly self portraits of severe depression such as those by novelist Andrew Solomon (*The Noonday Demon*) or psychiatrist Kay Redfield Jamison (*An Unquiet Mind*), biologist Lewis Wolpert (*Malignant Sadness*) or lecturer Stuart Sutherland (*Breakdown*), it appears they all had good jobs, high status, loving relationships, happy childhoods, plenty of money.

Hence the likelihood is that the inherited genetic factor is particularly important in these severe disorders. Jamison notes her own father's black moods. But perhaps surprisingly to readers of the graphic accounts of the terrible depths of despair, the thoughts of and plans for suicide, she is not alone in seeing a positive side to her experience. 'I have discovered what I would have to call a soul, a part of myself I could never have imagined until one day, seven years ago, when hell came to pay me a surprise visit. It's a precious discovery' (Soloman, 2001: 443). And from Jamison:

> I have often asked myself whether, given the choice, I would choose to have manic depressive illness . . . Strangely enough I think I would . . . I honestly believe that as a result of it I have felt more things, more deeply; had more experiences, more intensely . . .
>
> (Jamison, 1997: 217–18)

They have also found effective ways to manage their symptoms, and recovered in the sense described in Chapter 2. Seeing value in the experience has been argued to be an important stage in the recovery process. Herman quotes Freud on psychoanalysis, who advises that the patient must find the courage to direct his attention to the phenomena of his illness. His illness must no longer seem to him contemptible, but must become an enemy worthy of his mettle, a piece of his personality, which has solid ground for its existence, and out of which things of value for his future life have to be derived.

(Herman, 1992: 175)

Psychoanalytic theories – childhood loss, poor parent–infant bonding

Loss and grief, and the idea that difficulties in coping with them in adult life have their origins in childhood, have been one of the central themes of psychoanalytic schools of thought since Freud's influential text *Mourning and Melancholia* in 1917.

One of the most well-known British scholars to have taken forward these ideas in more recent years is John Bowlby (1969, 1973, 1980). His reflections about loss, depression and early childhood departed somewhat from the Kleinian school of psychoanalytic thought, with which he was affiliated, in terms of the way early separation experiences were important. His explanations have now achieved wide acceptance.

Bowlby's focus was on the importance of the bond, the closeness and warmth, established between mother and child in the first years of life, and its link with later vulnerability if disrupted or poorly established. But he also saw grief reactions to separation and loss as the same process for adults and children. The importance of the childhood experience of loss in Bowlby's terms is a real, not an imagined loss, derived from the failure to make or sustain a stable relationship with the care-giver, usually the mother.

His ideas are close to evolutionary psychology, as he argues that we have an instinctive (inherited) need to maintain proximity to attachment figures, because this has had evolutionary survival value. We have therefore developed behaviours such as distress calling and clinging designed to maintain proximity to, and gain care and protection from, care-givers when those relationships come under threat. Most parents will have seen this on any separation from their very young child, but Bowlby's 'attachment theory' suggests that excessive separation anxiety can result from more marked adverse family experiences, such as threats of abandonment or threats of rejection, or perhaps by illness in family members for which the child feels responsible, and this in turn leads to a sensitivity to separation and loss events in adult life, and can impair the person's capacity to establish or maintain affectionate relationships.

A continued propensity to interpret information in a negative way can result for those who as young children did not develop a secure attachment; for instance, feelings of helplessness, an expectation of irretrievable loss. This insecure attachment may have resulted from the child finding himself unable ever to meet his parents' aspirations for him, or who had been repeatedly told he was unlovable and incompetent, or who experienced an actual loss of parent. By contrast, the securely attached child has better relationships with peers, is more sociable, and develops a more positive self-concept. These ideas, developments of those from the psychoanalytic school, have continued to feature in theories of depression. In particular the concepts of loss, attachment, self-esteem, anger against the self and helplessness have been important.

In a review of the evidence for these ideas, Rutter (1981) concluded that the circumstances surrounding the loss of mother (the disruption caused by the discordant relationships leading up to the loss) needed to be taken into account, and it is this family discord that often explains a good deal of the damaging effects. Bowlby (1980) gave greater weight to the disruption of the mother–child bond itself, which he suggested led to particular 'cognitive biases'. These biases, resulting from disordered mourning, might involve compulsive care-giving to others, ambivalence and anxiety in relationships, or a show of independence from close ties. Rutter's analysis also questioned the assumptions in Bowlby's work that the bond must be between one continuously present mother figure and her child, and that other parenting figures were unimportant. He confirmed that in fact the child benefits from multiple attachments, and mental health does not hinge on the security of the one. Nor is the separation so crucial if the bond or bonds are strong, and the separation is not due to, or interpreted as, rejection.

This position has not changed, and there is good support for the assertion that a markedly poor early relationship between the main parent and child, through which the child experiences a sense of rejection, plays an important role in mental health during childhood and later. Separation and loss are more likely to be inter-preted as rejection if occurring in the context of a poor relationship with the main parent.

Psychological theories – negative thinking

Various 'cognitive vulnerability' explanations for depression have gained wide recognition, particularly the development of a negative view of the self, and of 'learned helplessness'. As in Bowlby's theories, the origins of these maladaptive thinking styles are assumed to originate in childhood experience. The recent rise in popularity of cognitive therapies as both therapeutic and preventive in a wide range of circumstances is underpinned by these ideas.

Years of careful clinical observations and experimental studies with depressed hospital patients led Aaron Beck to describe the thinking of the person with depression as comprising a 'cognitive triad' – the tendency to see himself as worthless (attributing his unpleasant experiences to defects in himself), to see his world as presenting insuperable obstacles to achieving his life's goals (and misin-terpreting his interactions with his animate or inanimate environment as repre-senting defeat or deprivation even when more plausible alternative explanations are available), and his future as hopeless, as he expects unremitting hardship and frustration as all efforts will lead to a negative outcome (Beck et al., 1987: 11). A set of relatively stable beliefs, formed in childhood, is used to justify or explain his negative views and expectations, or mental 'schema', and can lie buried in the memory until stressful experiences occur when they return to the fore of his or her thinking. Information, events, situations will be distorted in line with these schemas. While the mildly depressed person has some insight into this distortion, someone who is severely depressed may become obsessed with negative thoughts and increasingly unable to see them as erroneous.

This schema was assumed to derive from an important loss event in childhood (something, someone, or an important unfulfilled aspiration) leading to a generalized negative appraisal of the self (Beck, 1973), so the person might come to view himself perhaps as 'a loser', lacking in skills and in opportunities to make the future rewarding. This thinking does not apply to all events – otherwise he might be permanently depressed – but only in relation to the pursuit of important goals, and particularly when the situation bears a similarity to the childhood loss. Rejection and taunting by childhood peers on account of a physical impairment may in adulthood lead to an over-reaction to rejection – a rebuff from someone he hoped to date, perhaps. Repeated humiliation in school athletic activities in childhood may lead him to make a negative judgement about himself each time he experiences difficulty in any competitive situation in the future. The judgement made is an extreme and absolute judgement of his worth, and each time the judgement is made, it reinforces the negative self-image. The key notion is that it is not the events themselves that produce depression, but their meaning to the individual person, and this meaning is arrived at through the person's own cognitive schema.

Martin Seligman linked his ideas more closely to problems in the parent–child relationship, and the child's experience of unpleasant events that he or she was powerless to change. This was argued to lead to a learned expectation of helplessness based on finding that his own 'good' behaviour could not protect him or bring a more rewarding response from parents. The ideas were developed from experiments with dogs, then rats, in which the animals were confined in a small space and given electric shocks. In some instances the animal learned that, following a particular response, it could prevent the delivery of the shock. In others, no response could affect the arrival of the shock. Similar types of experiment were tried with students, for instance confined in a room with a loud noise. The findings were, essentially, that those dogs, rats or students receiving the uncontrollable unpleasant experience began by making determined efforts to stop or escape it, but, after a lack of success, eventually became passive and helpless. What was of most interest, however, was that these subjects then performed less well in subsequent trials when the outcomes were made controllable than those animals or students who had previously been in controllable situations (Seligman, 1975). This passivity and intellectual slowness, the expectation that one's actions are doomed to failure and the depressed mood reflect the main negative attributes of a depressive illness. Again, it is not the uncontrollable event that is the crucial determinant of depression, but the *expectation* of a lack of control over stressful experience that is considered a sufficient condition for depression (Seligman, 1975).

Although initially arguing that the person saw events as impervious to his influence, a reformulation of these ideas changed the emphasis to self-blame for the failure, bringing this theory in line with the ideas from Beck. Drawing on attribution theory, the person prone to lasting helplessness and depression was seen as one who tends to attribute failure to global, stable and internal factors (Abramson et al., 1978). That is, when a person is unable to resolve a problem, he expects this as his poor performance applies to a wide range of tasks, and he attributes his helplessness to the difficulty of the task or his own poor skill rather than to bad luck, and the source of the problem is seen to lie with himself rather than elsewhere.

These two research groups have since joined forces to test their theories. They interviewed new students at two US universities and conducted follow-up assessments and interviews on a range of relevant variables over the following five years on two groups – students (83–90 in each group at each university) in the highest and lowest quartile on scores of negative cognitive style (Alloy et al., 1999). They found that their high-risk group – those in the highest quartile of scores for negative cognitive style – had markedly higher lifetime rates of major depression, and more severe depressions, and their raised rates were not mediated by current symptoms.

Preventive proposals arising focus primarily on the use of cognitive therapy aimed at reducing negative thinking. Second, those who also experienced abusive or neglectful childhoods could be helped to come to a more benign interpretation of their past in terms of deficiencies in their parents' psychological competence, rather than having been maltreated because of any defective or bad behaviour in themselves. Third, there may sometimes be possibilities to change the environment to be less 'hopelessness inducing'. Finally there are primary prevention possibilities – first in helping parents learn better parenting to reduce maltreatment, but also in helping parents to model and provide feedback about more benign attributions about experiences proving stressful for their children. Similar programmes can be offered in schools to help children directly to avoid or reduce negative interpretations (Alloy et al., 1999). An earlier paper by Garber and colleagues (1979) had also described strategies to help children rehearse coping with a stressful experience over which they have some control, so that when they later experience uncontrollable stress they may be less helpless.

These theories have generated a great deal of research, and have been incorporated into other models of depression (described below). Although initially criticized as only applicable to sad affect and minor depression, the results of the studies described by Alloy and colleagues (1999) indicate a broader relevance to more serious depressive illnesses too.

Psycho-social explanations

Psycho-social explanations have been developed, primarily through detailed epidemiological studies comparing those who do and do not become depressed following a severe life event. Brown and Harris (1978) initially identified social support as the most important difference, finding that only 10% of women who had a close confiding relationship with someone in their household (e.g. with their partner) became depressed. This compared with 26% of women without an intimate tie, but reporting a confiding relationship with another person (seen weekly), and with 41% of those who had a confidant seen infrequently or without any confiding relationship.

Good social support was found to be particularly important to women who had low self-esteem (a 'negative evaluation of self') or already existing low-level symptoms of depression or anxiety. Negative evaluation of self, measured through the negative comments the person makes about themselves during an interview, was associated with more than a twofold increase in depression (33% compared to 13% without negative evaluation of self) following life events in the prospective study by Brown and colleagues (1986a). With both low self-esteem *and* low social support, a woman's vulnerability to depression increases markedly. (For lone mothers, the absence of any close relationship was counted as negative support.) In fact, without one or the other (low self-esteem or low support), none of the women became depressed; with one of them, 20% of those experiencing a humiliation or entrapment event became depressed; with both of them, 45% did so (Brown, 2002).

While early findings suggesting separation from or loss of mother before the age of 17 produced a raised risk of depression, it is now understood that the key experience associated with this was neglect. Brown and colleagues (1986b) described it as a 'lack of care', if indifference (neglect; lack of interest and attention) was combined with lax parental control and lasted at least 12 months. This produced a threefold risk of depression as an adult in the face of later life events or difficulties. Since then, numerous studies, by both this team and other research groups, have included abuse and rejection, as much as neglect, as key factors (see Chapter 9).

Green and colleagues (2010) drew on data from the National Comorbidity Survey (replication) of adults in the US identifying three main clusters of childhood adversity linked to both childhood and adult disorder (not just depression): abuse (physical, sexual, neglect), family maladaptation (mental illness, substance abuse, criminality, violence) and loss of parent (by death, divorce, separation). The first of these appears likely to be the most important (Brown et al., 2007).

However, there are broadly three 'routes' through which childhood adversity affects adult mental health, one through cognitive effects (as discussed above – expectation of failure, of a lack of control), and a second through an 'experience' pathway, where further adverse experiences become more likely. A third links to the gene–environment interactions, including epigenetic effects on the person's response to stress, increasing vulnerability to chronic depression.

Some illustration of the complex interweaving of risk factors is provided by the study of 225 women selected from GP registers as likely to have experienced early lack of care. Brown and colleagues (1986b) found that if they had both a lack of care in early childhood and an unplanned pregnancy in their teenage years (or married early), their likelihood of adult depression was raised. A period of institutional care increased the risk of an unplanned pregnancy. It is likely that there are many other such associations given that living in care and having an early pregnancy may mean the young woman is at risk of finishing school without the qualifications she might otherwise have gained, of meeting and staying with a young man from an equally disadvantaged background (Quinton et al., 1993), of remaining in low-paid work, and experiencing a high rate of stressful events. The bad start in life too often creates the circumstances for further disadvantage, and helps to explain the social class differences in mental ill-health. Harris and colleagues (1990) have sometimes referred to these links as a 'conveyor belt' linking early disadvantage and adult mental ill-health, where each stage along the path makes the next type of risk factor more likely to occur, and they have since argued that a life-course perspective on depression is essential.

This interplay of cognitive and experience pathways is also illustrated by the way the young person copes with an unplanned pregnancy. She can avoid becoming trapped into an unsatisfactory lifestyle by arranging adoption or termination of pregnancy, arranging family support, or she might decide to make a home with the child's father for positive reasons. An internalized sense of helplessness resulting from childhood lack of care may contribute both to lack of action to prevent pregnancy and to ineffective coping responses after becoming pregnant. She is then likely both to face more adverse events and to have reinforced her negative view of herself (Brown et al., 1986b).

Hence this model suggests that severe life events and major difficulties invariably precede depression, most commonly conveying humiliation or entrapment, though bereavement or other major loss can also lead to depression. But it is unusual to become clinically depressed after such events unless the woman has a low evaluation of herself and/or she has poor social support (or, if a lone parent, has no 'close other' seen regularly). These vulnerability factors are in turn often the result of experience in childhood of parental neglect, rejection, or physical or sexual abuse. The early childhood adversity can also, through a chain of other problems that have been made more likely, contribute to a raised rate of humiliation and entrapment experiences in adult life.

Evolution – depression is needed to maintain group inclusion – it's adaptive

As Randolphe Nesse (2008) explains in *The Lancet*'s tribute issue to Darwin, ill-health needs two kinds of explanation: a contemporary one, exploring the bodily mechanisms of the individual and the factors in their lives, past and present, that may bear on this; and an evolutionary one, which instead of looking for differences asks why we are all the same in ways that leave us vulnerable to such ill-health. In relation to depression – which appears utterly useless – he asks

> How can it possibly be helpful to feel hopeless, worthless, and lacking all motivation? In general it is not. Much depression is a disease. However, depression is not a disease like diabetes or cancer, it is more like chronic pain,

a dysregulation of a response that can be useful in some situations. Studies are just beginning to identify what those situations are, but there is a general consensus that low mood offers advantages in inauspicious situations in which all efforts are wasted or risky, and some depression arises from dysregulation of this system.

(Nesse, 2008: S25)

Price (1968) has long argued this point; that is, that depression must have advantages in evolutionary terms, for instance in maintaining the stability of a community in a dominance hierarchy, in which elated behaviour is associated with a rise in status in the group, and a depressive response with a fall. The importance of the behaviour is that the person 'should stay down quietly and not try to make a comeback for some considerable time'. Its advantage was also suggested to derive from its role in de-escalating conflict, through appeasement behaviour, or the obvious signs of apathy and low mood that show that the individual is hardly likely to threaten the more dominant member of the group in the near future, and so will not attract further aggression.

Price has continued this exploration of the adaptive functions of depression in the ensuing 40 years, but despite the numerous contributions to theory, a number of problems remain, not least the fact that many low-ranking people are happy and many high-ranking people are depressed (Price et al., 2007). However, Gilbert (2007: 330) has used an evolutionary perspective to develop suggestions for therapeutic intervention (see below), arguing that 'Happiness lies in securing important evolutionary goals, especially social ones'. He reinforces the evidence on the importance of shame in depression, and urges those aiming to be supportive to avoid language that may contribute to shame, such as 'distorted thinking' or 'maladaptive beliefs', and rather to use less pejorative terms such as 'biases in thinking' and 'unintended consequences'.

Evolutionary analyses are closely aligned to the position of those who argue that social status is core to mental health and wellbeing, and therefore reducing inequality and social exclusion should be policy priorities. These ideas are discussed further in Chapter 11.

Why do some people remain depressed, while others recover quickly?

A substantial proportion of acute depressive illness clears up quite quickly, within a matter of a few weeks or a few months, very often without treatment (Goldberg and Goodyer, 2005). But the people who do not recover quickly accumulate in the population so that surveys tend to find that about half of those depressed at any one time have been depressed for more than a year. It appears that the same factors that contribute to onset of depression are implicated in its course.

A substantial reduction in difficulties, or a positive event that brings hope of a reduction in problems, can shorten time to remission (in women but not men), according to a follow-up over 3.5 years of 86 primary care patients diagnosed with depression by Oldehinkel et al. (2000). Brown and Harris found that about 60% of remissions followed a 'fresh start event' conveying hope, such as securing a job after a long period of unemployment, the chance to move into much better accommodation or a new romantic relationship (Brown et al., 1988; Harris et al., 1999b).

Conversely, when there seems to be little chance of improvement in social difficulties, the depression also tends to persist. Hence the association between low socio-economic status and depression is stronger with persistent depression than with first onset (Lorant and colleagues, 2003). Spijker and colleagues (2006) drew on the prospective NEMESIS study sample in the Netherlands in which 4796 people from the general population had been interviewed at three points in time – 1996, 1997 and 1999. They studied 250 people with onsets of depression between 1997 and 1999, including first and recurrent episodes, and found that 23% lasted over 12 months. People with these long-lasting conditions were more likely to also have a chronic physical health problem, low social support, a lengthy episode previously, and more severe and extensive symptoms.

The same is true for vulnerability factors that raise risk of an onset of depression: they also play a role in its course. For instance, child maltreatment almost doubled the risk of onset of depression following a humiliation or entrapment event, but quadrupled the risk that it would take a chronic course in the two-year follow-up of their Islington sample by Brown and Moran (1994). This finding was replicated in a study of sisters (Brown et al., 2008b), and showed that the link between child maltreatment and chronic depression endured after all other vulnerability factors were controlled, so having an independent role, as well as being linked via its effects on other social disadvantage. In addition, a current severe interpersonal difficulty that was present at the start of the depressive episode was also strongly linked with the depression taking a chronic course.

Preventing chronic depression

Gilbert (2007) offers a model of what might help, in terms of preventing depression becoming a chronic condition, and links clearly with the ideas discussed here. Although his advice is for therapists, they are the types of changes that might be achieved in other ways too, through supportive relationships or preventive interventions that aim to help people reduce social difficulties, find a fresh start or build more support.

Gilbert's strategies are informed by his evolutionary perspective on how depression has evolved, that is as a way of adapting to threats in order to protect oneself from further harm. He suggests that it causes the person to narrow down their attention onto the threat, and to lose their ability to create a feeling of safeness and to reassure themselves. He proposes ways to help the depressed person to 'tone down' their threat responses, to reduce the effect of the stressor, and to strengthen their coping, through:

- creating personal space – respite from caring roles, some emotional distance from critical relationships, and the reduction of negative signals. This can also include attending to rest, sleep, eating well.
- exploring any sources of 'put-down' – in critical, bullying or abusive relationships, and what might be done to improve or escape them, and improve the person's sense that they can do so.
- developing problem-solving strategies to replace angry responses or the feelings of needing an escape, and assertiveness to be able to tackle the causes of difficulty constructively rather than seeking to escape them.
- examining the person's tendencies to certain negative styles of thinking – automatically assuming the worst, seeing problems as failures, and failures as meaning they are stupid – thinking linked to feelings of shame.
- finding activities or coping methods to reduce the person's tendency to ruminate on the difficulties.
- learning to accept feelings of anger, shame and guilt, as well as traumatic memories, and work through them, accepting too that their problems, trauma, conflict are a part of life, and not uncommon.

On the positive side, Gilbert suggests that the person needs:

- to see hope in the future, so efforts to help them do so can be beneficial, as may support gained through engaging in pleasurable activities with others, or taking part in self-help groups
- to learn to be compassionate to oneself, speaking in one's head in a warm, caring voice rather than an angry, reproachful way, and learning to recognize and reward oneself for small achievements.

Of course changing the social circumstances is what usually needs to result from these deliberations, or at least a realistic hope that such change is now achievable, and could be a result of, or a trigger for, further psychological change, and there is every reason to believe that the changes listed above can be brought about through:

- helping people to find positive events that bring hope for a better future, a way out of misfortune, and to act on these.

Such 'fresh start' events have been described by Harris and colleagues (1999b) as one of the means through which a befriending project reduced rates of depression in an experimental inner London study.

A multifactorial model of depression

To bring together the above discussions, it can be seen that there has for some time been broad agreement that life events and major difficulties can bring about a depressive illness in vulnerable adults; that is, they play a causal role. Events that are humiliating and reinforce a sense of entrapment are particularly powerful (which concurs with Seligman's original thesis), but an event cannot be defined in this way in the absence of context, for it is the meaning of the event to the person in the context of their commitments and convictions, in relation to things that really matter to their sense of who they are, that makes it so. Neglect and abuse are, as Freud, Bowlby and Beck suggested, key in shaping the meaning of current events and difficulties, making it more likely that an event will be pernicious in its effects through finding a match with a schema linked to low self-worth.

A vulnerability factor, on the other hand, is one that has little or no effect on its own, but increases risk in the presence of another factor. In its opposite it is a protective factor. Childhood maltreatment, probably linked to other family problems, features in all explanations as a key vulnerability factor, raising risk through psychological and social pathways. There is an interactive effect with genetic susceptibility and gene expression. Particularly important is the role played by subsequent relationships, hence the potential for a harmonious, caring relationship to break the chain of adversity leading to later depression, while one with strongly negative features will not only raise risk of onset, but also perpetuate a depression. Also contributing to a person's vulnerability is low self-esteem, or pre-existing low-level symptoms.

Kendler and colleagues (2002) have integrated what is known about the onset of depression into a comprehensive bio-psycho-social model of depression, drawing on their longitudinal study of Caucasian twins in Virginia. Brown et al. (2008b) have done the same, including more detail about factors involved in the perpetuation of depression. There is broad agreement between them, with both increasingly recognizing that events that cause depression are often in fact dependent rather than independent, due to the raised rate of problems brought through early vulnerability factors. They demonstrate powerfully that the major risk factors accumulate from early in life: genetic risk, child maltreatment and family adversity, both separately and in their interaction, increase risk in early childhood of low self-esteem, behavioural problems and anxiety. These same factors also contribute separately and together in increasing the likelihood of educational problems, adolescent interpersonal problems and substance misuse. The contemporary factors in onset are primarily the interpersonal difficulties, social difficulties and severe life events. Together, Kendler et al. (2002) calculate that the model can account for 52% of the liability to episodes of major depression, but can plot 64 differing paths to depression through these various risk factors. Some of this is illustrated in Figure 5.1, which illustrates some of the complexity of the task facing those planning to provide preventive intervention.

Implications for prevention

The model below shows there are three areas to consider, although in all three areas the prevention of child maltreatment is the most important.

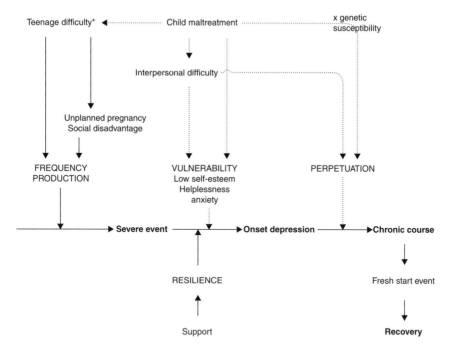

Figure 5.1 Overview of core components of a multi-factorial model of depression.

(i) Frequency production

The first consideration is the disadvantage that accrues to young people who start out in life with poor family support, particularly that involving abuse, neglect or rejection. This 'frequency production' pathway in Figure 5.1 shows how the consequences of childhood adversity can increase the likelihood of a host of other problems through childhood and adolescence that result in a high rate of adverse events and difficulties. The aim of any intervention would be to help them reach adulthood with a risk of adverse events no higher than the person without this poor start.

There are implications for schools to ensure that the young child known to have poor support at home gains a sense of achievement either from academic work or from other aspects of school life. Existing behavioural problems, whether or not these have their origins in a troubled home life, are an appropriate target for support to prevent their continuation or escalation, by addressing school achieve-ment and peer relationships, and to prevent substance misuse as they move into their teenage years. Troubled adolescents can generate a good number of stressful life events for themselves and others, and experience many social difficulties. High on the list of problems to avoid are unplanned pregnancy, truanting from school and leaving without qualifications. As they approach school leaving age, the development of realistic plans for a secure future is an obvious priority: accommodation, further education or employment, avoiding damaging interper-sonal relationships. For young people beginning to establish romantic relation-ships, primary prevention might aim to influence the acceptability of aggression, bullying or controlling behaviour between couples, and help young people develop 'planning' skills to think carefully before entering partnerships that may not provide the support they need.

(ii) Vulnerability

The second area of focus is vulnerability to the effects of life events and difficulty. A negative evaluation of the self, a pre-existing level of anxiety, combined with early childhood adversity will mean that a humiliating or entrapping event is much more likely to lead to depression. If combined with interpersonal difficulty the risk of depression after a severe event may be as high as 50%. Implications for intervention would relate to any of these vulnerability factors. For instance, after an event such as assault, bullying, or the break-up of a relationship, help would need to reduce their negative appraisals of events, to reduce self-blame, perhaps offer assertiveness skills, and increase support available from other sources.

A sense of helplessness not only is a result of adverse early experience, but can also be a product of living circumstances, or dependency due to age or physical impairment. It is possible to improve the sense of control people have, and the support available. Examples of these in later life include the design and management of residential care homes and sheltered accommodation, and ensuring people have control over the timing of visits made by support workers, or at least know in advance when they will be. Arrangements for care and support should not place people in positions in which they feel they have no control over their lives.

People living with long-term difficulties, such as caring for a disabled young child, or an older person with dementia, who do not have a supportive partner or close relative able to help them regularly are particularly likely to benefit from reliable support from other sources.

While these are a small selection of the types of situation where adverse events and major difficulties are apparent, and vulnerability to those events is recogniz-able, the general principles are the same. People with existing anxiety, low self-esteem, a sense of powerlessness and problems in their closest relationships are at raised risk of becoming depressed, and intervention that addresses any or all of these factors could be justified.

(iii) Perpetuation and recovery

In some ways, secondary prevention might be more straightforward, targeting those who have been depressed for about three months already, whose confidence is further undermined by a negative close relationship. Particularly if they also have experience of childhood maltreatment, they are at high risk of chronic depression, and if they are mothers of young children then there are potentially primary preventive benefits for their children too. It may be possible to identify them through general practitioners or health visitors. Intervention might involve strategies to build new supportive relationships, help to minimize any feelings of self-blame, to see that they need not be trapped by their adverse events or difficulties, that there are options and choices, and help to make them.

While targeted programmes are important to help those at high risk of depression within any population, a universal strategy will need to look more closely at what it is about life in south Asian cities, or in a Basque-speaking rural community, that ensures that rates of depression stay low. One might then speculate on the social and economic policy required. Do South American societies leave a large proportion of the population excluded, financially struggling, with high rates of humiliation and entrapment events in a way that south Asian societies do not? Are there social policies that might strengthen family life, reduce domestic violence, improve the support partners provide to one another, reduce the many social difficulties that link to high rates of child maltreatment?

Both targeted and population strategies that support family life will be considered in the chapters to follow, after first turning to what we know about psychosis.

Note

1 Those depressions where physical symptoms are particularly marked, i.e. agitation or slow movement, early morning waking, loss of appetite and weight, worse symptoms in the morning, as well as other symptoms of depressed mood and thinking, and loss of pleasure.

6 Psychosis

The types of symptom that have been grouped together, by psychiatric convention, under the term 'psychosis' are those which suggest that the person does not have the same sense of reality as most of those around them. They experience hallucinations and/or delusions. Two main groupings are usually identified – the affective and non-affective psychoses, the former where extremes of mood are prominent features, the latter where in fact the emotions may be 'flattened'. Manic depression and schizophrenia are the two labels with which most people will be familiar, diagnosing conditions that can sometimes be quite difficult to distinguish, particularly in a first episode, as there are overlapping symptoms. Both are 'functional psychoses' where no medical explanation (such as fever, brain damage or drug misuse) appears to account for the symptoms. This chapter will focus primarily on research on the latter – the non-affective psychoses, particularly those diagnosed with schizophrenia, for whom 'first rank' symptoms include hallucinations, delusions or paranoid thoughts, disorganization of thoughts, or a belief that their thoughts and actions are influenced by or controlled by an external agent. Such symptoms are described as 'positive symptoms', and occur alongside 'negative symptoms' such as apathy, social withdrawal, lack of motivation or poor concentration.

For some (about half; Warner, 2004), the first onset develops rapidly, over a period of six months or less, in which case it is described as an 'acute onset', while others may have a slow, 'insidious' development of symptoms over several years. The course is also variable, from complete recovery after a few acute episodes to a continuing difficulty lasting for many years. One account of some of the symptoms and life difficulties that can be experienced is provided by Canadian Ian Chovil on a website he maintains to inform and help others with similar problems (www.chovil.ca). He described how, 36 years after the beginnings of what was eventually diagnosed as schizophrenia, he was recovering well, but still finding it hard to 'unbelieve' completely the delusions he held for so long.

> I got a lot of messages and was in constant telepathic contact with someone most of the last five years. I discovered antigravity and understood human evolution and my imaginary wife and I were going to become aliens and have eternal life travelling to the end of time where all matter had turned into

energy and all that remained was music and space. I knew I was going to become an alien in 1991 because I saw a book written by Nostradamus entitled 3791. I turned 37 in 1991 so that was obviously his message to me from the 1500s. I was living in a cockroach infested illegal rooming house and changing light bulbs as they burned out in the Hudson's Bay department store, afraid of my enemies who wanted to take my place as the most important man in human history.

The experiences are quite frequently frightening. They can include problems with sight and speech: Cutting (1985: 182) quotes someone describing the bright colours that frightened him, and his inability to make the thoughts in his head come out in a language that he understood.

Although we recognize these accounts as bizarre, some of these experiences are not completely unknown to many of us. Bentall (2004) notes one large general population survey that found nearly 8% of men and 12% of women in the UK reporting at least one vivid hallucinatory experience (often with religious or supernatural content, or of a living person not present at the time), and describes a US study of university students of whom 39% reported having heard their thoughts being spoken aloud. Both these findings have been repeated in later similar studies (see Bentall, 2004). Similarly, according to a Gallup poll of 1236 US citizens cited by Bentall, about one in four US citizens believe in ghosts, a similar proportion reported telepathic experiences, and one in seven say they have seen a UFO. While not intending to minimize the devastating effect a psychotic disorder may have on someone's life, Bentall aims to 'humanize' the person experiencing psychotic symptoms, to help reduce the distinction between 'them' and 'us'.

But Bentall's suggestion that schizophrenia consists of groups of symptoms that are not unique either to this disorder or to psychotic patients more widely, but are shared by others without a diagnosis, is a markedly different view to that which has prevailed for the past century or more. By contrast, depression and anxiety have been acknowledged as problems experienced by everyone to some degree some of the time, those diagnosed as 'cases' being at an extreme end, so this argument is well accepted for these types of disorder.

People diagnosed with schizophrenia can have very different experiences one from another, depending on the prominence of each of the associated symptoms, the differing extent to which these interfere with their everyday life, and the variability in course and recovery. This has always been acknowledged within psychiatry, such that it has often been mooted that schizophrenia might really be a group of closely related conditions rather than a single disorder. In his analysis of the course of schizophrenia, Warner (2004) emphasizes the psycho-social aspects, and he shares the concerns expressed by Bentall about the damaging effects of the label. But his suggested responses are focused on social factors, Bentall's more on psychological support. Warner argues that to render the condition less damaging requires a greater focus on social inclusion and employment. These writers reflect a renewed challenge to narrow biological perspectives on psychosis, arguing that psycho-social factors are just as important in preventing recurrent episodes.

Warner's thesis has been built on the very different recovery rates found for psychosis around the world.

Within- and between-population differences in incidence and prevalence

McGrath (2005) produced a systematic review of the epidemiology of schizophrenia, finding 55 studies providing traditional data on incidence from 25 nations, showing that while the disorder is recognized everywhere, rates of new cases vary from about 8 to 43 per 100,000 (a fivefold variation between countries). They usually find significantly higher rates in men than in women; several find an excess among migrants and among those born in the winter–spring or in cities. McGrath and his colleagues did not find these variations to be explained by economic differences between countries (Saha et al., 2006).

By contrast, data on the *course* of the disorder, reflected in prevalence data, does appear to show a difference between the developed and developing worlds. The World Health Organization has co-ordinated an International Study of Schizophrenia across 16 sites in 11 collaborating countries over 25 years (Hopper et al., 2007). Three phases have been undertaken to date: an initial pilot study, a study of determinants and outcomes, and an exploration of reduction of associated disability. An unexpected finding of the first follow-up of the pilot study sample in each country during the 1970s was the significantly better outcomes for the samples in Nigeria and India, at two years and at five, as compared to the samples in developed countries.

Because of criticism surrounding sampling, and to better understand the differences revealed, the second study in the 1980s strengthened the epidemiological design, ensuring greater consistency in methods and use of standardized measures to identify first-episode incident cohorts, with high inter-centre and intra-centre reliability in assessing symptoms, disability and social functioning (Jablensky and Sartorius, 2008). The research teams actively sought all people with a first onset in all types of facilities, from primary care, traditional healers, religious shrines and prisons as well as mental health settings. Twelve sites in 10 countries were involved in this part (Colombia, Czechoslovakia, Denmark, India, Ireland, Japan, Nigeria, Russia, United Kingdom and United States). The 1379 individuals identified, and other key informants, were interviewed at baseline, and nearly 80% at one-year and two-year follow-ups. At eight of the centres, a large proportion were traced and re-interviewed 15 years later.

They found a diversity of outcomes, showing an overall more favourable prognosis in developing countries – though not uniformly so – and more of those in developing countries making a complete clinical recovery (37% as compared to 15.5% in developed countries), and slightly fewer of the developing country samples were continuously affected, though not significantly so (11.1% versus 17.4%), meaning that despite the much smaller proportion taking anti-psychotic medication (16% compared to 61%), those in developing countries experienced longer periods of unimpaired functioning in the community (Jablensky and Sartorius, 2008). Across all centres, outcomes were significantly worse for an insidious than for an acute onset, and outcomes at two years were the best predictor of outcome at 15 years. Despite discussion by Warner (1994) of the idea that part of the variation might be explained in terms of the debased status of someone with a diagnosis of schizophrenia in the West, their final report did not find their assessment of stigma reached statistical significance, but social exclusion, gender, marital status and drug misuse did.

Their conclusions have been challenged by Cohen and colleagues (2008), drawing on 23 longitudinal studies conducted in 11 low and middle income countries. They argue that the many sociocultural factors such as family support and styles of interaction, industrialization and urbanization thought to contribute to these differences in course and outcome are not well supported by their evidence, and that the 'black box' of culture needs more sensitive analysis. They find poor care associated with poor outcomes wherever they occur, and both within- and between-country differences that are more complex than the WHO studies suggest. For instance, families might accommodate their relative, but may also be harshly critical, and what is meant by employment and unemployment varies greatly. They found evidence to confirm that outcomes in India appear to be good, as WHO studies suggest, but in Brazil and China they are far less positive; social functioning was found to be good in India and Indonesia, but poor in Nigeria.

Jablensky and Sartorius (2008) address the criticisms of their methods, and defend convincingly their finding that outcomes in poor countries are indeed frequently better than in rich countries. However, both sets of researchers emphasize that there needs to be further detailed ethnographic research to explore the ways in which the factors identified shape outcomes within differing cultural contexts, and that generalizations about marriage, employment, gender, or families in the developing world being more supportive should be avoided.

Harrison and colleagues (2001) bring WHO data together with data on samples in three invited cohorts (Hong Kong, Madras and Beijing) and four samples that were part of the initial pilot, so 18 centres in total, to explore long-term outcomes over 15 and 25 years. They found that death rates of the samples, as compared with the average of their own country, were highest in eight samples from developed countries. These were highest in young men, more often from unnatural causes, mainly suicide. In terms of the course of the disorder, about half of the samples experienced two or more florid episodes, with full or partial recovery between these times, and many then stayed relatively free of troubling symptoms. Others followed a more continuous pattern of ill-health, and a larger proportion of these then had a less favourable outcome. Family involvement in treatment appeared not to improve recovery, and young people, drug users and those losing touch with friends seem to do less well (Harrison et al., 2001).

Numerous clues for preventive intervention meriting further exploration have been suggested. One that has led to service development for early intervention is the better outcome at 15 years for those people experiencing symptoms for the lowest proportion of the first two years. A second set of clues derive from the possible cultural differences that seem to bring marked differences in course between centres. Most assume these cultural differences will turn out to be social factors, possibly related to family life, stigma or social exclusion (e.g. Warner, 2004), but there have been a range of other suggestions, including diet (too much refined sugar; Peet, 2004) or too little time outside in the sun (a lack of vitamin D; McGrath et al., 2004).

Exploration of potential causal factors

The findings above suggest a range of possible factors that contribute to risk, but none stand out as implicated strongly in first onset, which might trigger or provoke the condition in susceptible people. Although there is a widely held assumption that some kind of vulnerability–stress model explains the disorder, the quality of the stress involved remains largely speculative. More is known about suscepti-bility: the best predictor to date remains family history, and some role for genetic susceptibility is accepted. Yet this is a small part of the story. Something else is required, either physical or emotional injury. These are examined in turn below: genetic, organic and psycho-social factors that contribute to vulnerability.

Genetic evidence

Emil Kraepelin (1856–1926) is known to be one of the first psychiatrists to systematically sort the symptoms of his patients into groups, in search of mean-ingful distinctions so that their genetic origins could be studied. He expected to be able to demonstrate that what he termed dementia praecox (later labelled schizo-phrenia by Bleuler, and which he distinguished from manic-depressive illness) resulted from an inherited susceptibility.

A 1991 publication by Gottesman brought together progress made in this search, from more than 40 studies and from data collected over 60 years, to calcu-late the risk to individuals with a family member with a diagnosis of schizo-phrenia. His figures suggested that those whose genetic make-up is closer to the affected person have a greater risk of also being affected. That is, a member of the general population has a lifetime risk of developing schizophrenia of about 1 in 100 (or less), but if they have a second degree relative with the diagnosis (uncle/ aunt, niece/nephew) then their risk is 4–5%, for a sibling it rises to 9%, while for an identical twin, it is 48%. Data from Kestenbaum (1980) also showed risk to children of affected parents – 13% if one parent, 35–40% if both parents. Hence since the late twentieth century there has been a broad consensus that genetic, environmental and organic factors must be implicated in some way: that people inherit a susceptibility to develop a psychosis, which is likely to surface in the context of environmental stressors.

Genetic research has traditionally drawn its strongest evidence from twin studies: for instance, comparing rates in identical and non-identical twins; also studying twins reared by their biological parents or by adoptive parents, and twins separated and reared by different parents. These differing circumstances allow researchers to control for the possibility that higher rates of disorder are not due to the identical genetic profile of their identical twin, but explainable in terms of living with unusual behaviour of a twin with psychotic symptoms, or with particular character-istics of their birth parents. One of the more recent twin studies collating evidence from a large number of twins who had at any time in their life been treated for any diagnosed psychotic disorder, and had a same-sex twin (106MZ and 118DZ), again confirmed that diagnoses of schizophrenia, schizo-affective disorder and mania have a strong genetic component (Cardno et al., 1999).

But as identical twins still only stand a 48% chance of developing the disorder when their twin has a diagnosis, this means that something else must play a key role. In fact, as Gottesman (1991) acknowledges, nearly two thirds of people with a diagnosis of schizophrenia have no relative at all with the disorder. This must lead to there being some question that all people with this diagnosis carry a genetic vulnerability. Furthermore, a twin who does develop mental ill-health will not necessarily gain the same diagnosis, but may have other kinds of mental ill-health, which, as Warner (2004) concludes, may suggest that what is inherited is not a specific susceptibility to schizophrenia but an underlying biochemical or func-tional disturbance. Bentall (2004) and Joseph (2004) go further than this, and argue that the twin studies are open to challenge and that the certainty over genetic susceptibility should be questioned, as families willing to adopt children known to have a relative with a psychotic disorder should not be assumed to be comparable to other adoptive families.

Certainly the identification of precise genes and their mechanisms in studies that can be replicated has continued to elude biological psychiatry, despite exten-sive research, though the enthusiasm and confidence that they will soon be confirmed from the numerous suspects so far identified continue (Straub and Weinberger, 2006). Gottesman and Gould (2003) have suggested that genetic research might be more successful if it focused on endophenotypes rather than diagnosis, making a point not dissimilar to Bentall, in that they suggest decon-structing the diagnosis into components: in this case, components that are also genetic, and might more readily lead to clear-cut findings as they are each likely to be associated with a smaller number of genes than the diagnosis of schizo-phrenia. The endophenotypes for schizophrenia might include working memory and sensory motor gating (difficulty in filtering information from multiple sources), among others.

Burmeister and colleagues (2008), reviewing progress in psychiatric genetics to date, believe that this kind of shift is essential, and will lead to the eventual discovery of differing genetic contributions to susceptibility as well as the path-ways associated, and these will in turn reshape the current diagnostic labels we know today. 'We will probably soon recognize dozens of bipolar disorders and schizophrenias, just as there are now dozens of genetically defined forms of deaf-ness' (Burmeister et al., 2008: 538).

Organic evidence

Attempts to understand the disorders of thinking and perception that characterize the psychotic experience have, not surprisingly, been investigated in terms of possible differences in the brain. The development of CT (computed tomography) brain scans enabled researchers to see differences in, for instance, the size of the fluid-containing ventricles, or the width of the fissures between folds of brain tissue, and some differences have been noted in about a quarter of those with a diagnosis of schizophrenia (Warner, 2004). Research using newer scans ('functional imaging') enables researchers to literally see the activity of the brain as the person performs certain experimental mental tasks, and has shown hyperactivity in the temporal lobes, and the hippocampus, and low activity in the frontal lobe which may help explain memory problems and difficulty in screening out irrelevant stimuli respectively (see Warner, 2004).

How any such abnormalities arise has been most frequently investigated in relation to obstetric complications at birth, but viral infection of the mother during pregnancy, and child abuse, are other potential candidates. Jones and colleagues (1998) studied the North Finland 1966 birth cohort, checking their psychiatric records at age 28 against birth details. A higher proportion of the 76 people who were by age 28 diagnosed with schizophrenia were born both small and early (but this is only three of the 76, weighing under 2000 g, so not a major contributor), and those with schizophrenia were over-represented among the 125 babies experiencing perinatal brain damage (e.g. Apgar score 0 at one minute, admitted to neonatal care, convulsions). The most common negative outcome for survivors of such trauma (30%) is learning disability and/or cerebral palsy, but nearly 5% developed schizophrenia. They suggest that if this relationship were causal, it would account for 7% of cases of schizophrenia in the general population. (But again, looked at in terms of numbers, this is six of the 76 who developed schizophrenia, the other 70 had no significant birth difficulties.) In fact the most prominent risk factor appeared to be gender – two thirds of those with a diagnosis were male. One other difference of interest was noted, that mothers of babies who later developed schizophrenia were about twice as likely (22% compared to 13%) to describe themselves as depressed during the sixth or seventh month of the pregnancy (Jones et al., 1998).

An overview of the evidence on effects of perinatal problems by Cannon and colleagues (2002b) suggests there is an effect of all three: complications of pregnancy, abnormal foetal growth and development, and complications at delivery. However, the effects are 'vanishingly small', and through current epidemiological methods, little progress can be made with exploring these, given the sample sizes needed to study a small effect on a rare condition.

One of the brain functions that appears to be affected in many people diagnosed with schizophrenia is their ability to focus their attention on one thing at a time, and ignore irrelevant stimuli. This has been referred to as a deficit in 'sensory gating'. In an interesting aside, Warner (2004) suggests that the propensity for so many people with a schizophrenia diagnosis to smoke heavily is the possibility that it mitigates this problem, since sensory gating is linked to the function of the brain nicotine receptors. The super-sensitivity to stimuli leads to heightened levels of arousal, hence this also leads to suggestions that a high level of stress can overwhelm the person and lead to psychosis. Again, it has been suggested that the feeling that many people have when experiencing psychotic symptoms that they need to withdraw from others and from highly stimulating environments might be a protective response.

Interest in the biochemistry of psychotic symptoms first came to the fore in the 1950s, encouraged both by the efficacy of the newly introduced neuroleptic medication and by the discovery of similarities between the effects of amphetamines, and of hallucinatory drugs like LSD, and the positive symptoms of schizophrenia. No-one argues that there are not chemical changes in the brain associated with psychotic symptoms, as all mental states are reflected in biochemical activity, such that a comparison of those getting angry with those watching a love story on television would show biochemical differences. But the neurotransmitter dopamine has been a major focus of interest, due to the finding that the efficacy of the anti-psychotic drugs in damping positive symptoms appears to be in direct proportion to their effectiveness in blocking the ability of the dopamine receptors at the synapse to respond to dopamine (Warner, 2004). The dopamine hypothesis was initially that there was an overactivity of tracts of neurons where the mediator is dopamine, but later research suggests it is more likely to be a supersensitivity of dopamine receptors (Warner, 2004). Since dopamine is associated with the regulation of emotion, and helps in giving meaning and importance to events (also playing a role in movement, sleep, motivation and attention), and acute stress can lead to an increase in dopamine turnover, this could explain psychotic symptoms. Further refinements to the 'dopamine hypothesis' have been proposed, after many thousands of research papers in the past 20 years arising from these ideas (Howes and Kapur, 2009).

Cannabis

One other potential biological cause needs some consideration, and this is cannabis use in adolescents. There has been much debate on how far it may play a causal role in schizophrenia, as it is well established that people with the diagnosis have a raised rate of cannabis use. Warner (2000) reports that 89% of mental health service users in Boulder, Colorado used marijuana at some time in their lives, which he suggests is associated with being unemployed and lacking other daily activity. He believes that use prior to first onset is likely to be part of coping with feeling odd, lonely and unhappy in the months of pre-morbid symptoms before the first positive symptoms appear, rather than it being a causal factor. Arseneault and colleagues (2002) only partially support this interpretation in their examination of cannabis use among the Dunedin cohort – 1037 people born in Dunedin, New Zealand in 1972–4, followed up every two or three years to age 21, then again at 26. Those using cannabis by age 15 were four times more likely to have a diagnosis of 'schizophreniform' disorder at age 26, and though the difference was halved once the psychotic symptoms at age 11 were controlled for, the link remained. (This diagnosis means they include those with psychotic symptoms that have lasted more than a month, rather than the six months required for a schizophrenia diagnosis.) They recommended that 'psychologically vulnerable children' should be strongly discouraged from cannabis use, particularly in early teenage years (Arseneault et al., 2002).

Caspi and colleagues (2005) investigated this 'psychological vulnerability', drawing on data on the same cohort plus DNA samples (from blood tests), and demonstrated that there is a G × E (gene × environment) link between cannabis use and schizophrenia. They studied the gene, whose name abbreviates to COMT (catechol-O-methyltransferase), that plays a role in dopamine breakdown. Those cannabis users with the valine allele but not those with the methionine allele had a significantly raised risk of schizophreniform disorder, but only if their cannabis use started in early teenage years. However, Caspi and colleagues also noted that this does not mean that cannabis is a major public health risk, as 92% of cannabis users did not develop psychosis, and they do not claim that the Val allele is a major cause of psychosis. On its own it had no effect, and its effect even when combined with early cannabis use is modest – only one fifth of those with schizophreniform disorder were in fact Val homozygotes who used cannabis as a teenager.

Veen and colleagues (2004) examined age at first social or occupational difficulty, first psychotic episode and first negative symptoms among 133 patients in The Hague, and found that male patients and cannabis users were younger at each milestone than female patients and non-cannabis users. The same team studied a representative incident cohort of 181 people (Selten et al., 2007) and showed that those with continuous poor functioning over the next 30 months were more likely to be male, heavy cannabis users, whose first episode had an insidious onset. But gender and cannabis use were related, and it was male gender that was independently linked to poor outcome, not the cannabis use.

We know that men develop schizophrenia at an earlier age than women, and tend to have a worse outcome (at least in the West), and we know that young men often use cannabis. However, it seems that the causal role of cannabis is not as strong as might have been thought, and is limited to its use in early teenage years, by those with a particular genetic susceptibility (less than one in five of those developing a schizophreniform disorder; Caspi et al., 2005). Among those with established mental ill-health, Warner (2000) suggests that marijuana provides something to do with friends, relieves boredom, and can help them with depression, anxiety, insomnia and physical discomfort, which may explain its wide use, though at the same time it often worsens feelings of paranoia and hallucinations.

Psycho-social evidence: First onset

The 'vulnerability–stress' hypothesis is the one taken by the majority of the researchers in the field: that genetic and/or organic susceptibility becomes salient in the context of environmental stressors. The potential culprits here include family relationships; unusual communication styles; child maltreatment; or over-involved, critical and intrusive parenting; as well as life stress and social exclusion. Differing types of stress during pregnancy have been reported as connected with a raised risk of psychotic symptoms in the offspring, including maternal influenza A in the second trimester, exposure *in utero* to war, or flood disasters (Maki et al., 2005). For instance, Malaspina and colleagues (2008) linked birth records to Israel's Psychiatric Registry to examine the records of a cohort of 88,829 people born in Jerusalem in 1964–76, finding a raised rate of psychosis, particularly in females, in those in weeks 5–8 of gestation in Israel in June 1967, during the Arab–Israeli conflict. June 5–7 would have been the most stressful – the three days of bombardment in the six-day war. The risk was up to four times as high for female babies, and was particularly increased for babies of mothers who lived in the areas that received direct shelling.

Life events and family relationships, including critical comments and over-involvement on the part of parents, have been shown to play an important role in the *course* of psychotic disorder, as will be discussed below, but the evidence for this pre-dating the young person's mental ill-health is scant. Leff and Vaughn (1985) provided some thought-provoking case studies illustrating some unusual parent–child relationships that occur, and Doane et al. (1981) provided some tentative evidence that these pre-date ill-health. Communication oddities in the parent that have been considered over the years include conveying one meaning in spoken content, but another in tone of voice or facial expression (Bateson et al., 1956); raised rates of vagueness, irrelevance, interruptions and contradictory information (Singer and Wynne, 1966); and high levels of concern and protective-ness (Hirsch and Leff, 1975). The Hirsch and Leff study also noted raised rates of family disharmony in families where the child later gained a diagnosis of schizophrenia.

The focus on parents has also been prominent because the symptoms of schizo-phrenia typically emerge in very early adult life – Rajji and colleagues (2009) report the average age of onset of a first episode for 850 people drawn from a large number of studies reviewed as 23.7 years. But the probable genetic and organic features linked to susceptibility further complicate analysis of family relation-ships – whether odd interactions are as much a product of child characteristics as of parental behaviour. However, as many families will attest, the theorizing that they might be to blame for their son or daughter's psychosis has made the lives of many thousands of Western families more, not less, difficult. It has contributed to the stigma felt by the whole family, and sometimes denied them access to advice, information and support (Warner, 2004). In turn, the recognition of such effects has made discussing the role that family factors might play in the onset of psychosis almost 'taboo' (Read et al., 2004).

Despite these reservations, there has been a renewed interest in child maltreat-ment as a possible causal factor for mental ill-health of every kind. In relation to schizophrenia, the results are far from clear. For instance, in a study of child sexual abuse, Kendler and colleagues (2000) found it to be associated with all disorders studied, with highest odds ratios (ORs) for bulimia, and alcohol or other drug dependence, and not reduced by controlling for family circumstances or family psychopathology (Kendler et al., 2000). But the researchers did not measure or mention psychoses; nor do most other studies linking child abuse and adult mental health problems. The link is usually seen with the whole range of neurotic disorder, substance use, personality disorder, self-harm and suicide, and with earlier first admission, more time in seclusion, and more frequent hospitalizations. On the other hand, Read and colleagues (2004) draw together an impressive range of research to argue that the relationship between childhood trauma, particularly sexual abuse, and psychotic symptoms such as hallucinations is as strong as, or stronger than, between childhood trauma and other psychiatric diagnoses.

Goodman and her colleagues (1997) note the many difficulties associated with research in this area, but argue that where studies ask more detailed questions they tend to find higher rates, indicating that the majority of women with diagnoses of serious mental illness (including schizophrenia) have been subject to violent victimization (physical and/or sexual abuse) at some point in their lives, and a large proportion of these women are repeatedly victimized during their lifetime. This is not necessarily proof of a causal role, however, if those at risk of psychosis are at increased risk of abuse for other reasons, such as homelessness, substance use or poor judgement.

There is also the possibility that some symptoms are misdiagnosed as psychosis when a diagnosis of PTSD or dissociative disorder would be more appropriate (Goodman et al., 1997). This suggestion is supported by the high rate of delusions and/or hallucinations found among 40 women seeking support through sexual assault centres, student counselling or victim support, compared to a group with no known sexual assault and not seeking help (Kilcommons et al., 2008). H. Fisher et al. (2009) also found that among their control sample, with no diagnosed mental health condition, those who had experienced physical or sexual abuse had some psychotic-like symptoms. Read and colleagues (2003) show that of 200 consecutive referrals to a mental health team with a variety of diagnoses, hallucinations (but not other psychotic symptoms) were more common among the 92 people with a history of physical or sexual abuse at some point in their lives than among the 108 with no known abusive history (Read et al., 2003).

Goodman's suggestion that hallucinations are a common response to severe trauma, but may not in the longer term turn out to be appropriately diagnosed as a first episode of schizophrenia, may account for the differing findings of H. Fisher and colleagues (2009) and Spataro and colleagues (2004). The former team compared 181 people recently diagnosed with a first episode of psychosis with 246 general population controls in Nottingham and London, and demonstrated that women with psychosis, but not men, had almost double the rate of child sexual abuse before the age of 16 compared to controls (27% versus 16%), and more than double the rate of physical abuse (27% compared to 11%). For males there was no association.

By contrast, Spataro and colleagues (2004) found no association between child sexual abuse and schizophrenia for either men or women in one of the largest prospective studies to date of both male and female victims (1327 females, 285 males). They drew from the records of children born between 1950 and 1991 and examined for suspected sexual abuse, and confirmed as abused, by the Victorian

Institute of Forensic Medicine in Australia. Their records were then compared to the Victorian Psychiatric Care Register for evidence of treatment for mental ill-health between 1991 and 2000, again one of the world's largest psychiatric databases, recording all contacts with inpatient or community mental health teams – hence providing a fairly comprehensive set of data on psychoses, but probably only the most severe of the neurotic diagnoses. Hence both the abuse and the outcome measure were at the extreme end of the scale, as most of the abuse consisted of penetrative sex, and was confirmed from both individual report and medical examination at the time. However, they did not find a link between child-hood sex abuse and schizophrenia.

The damage to mental health from severe abuse is unquestionable, and leads to a threefold risk in becoming a recipient of adult mental health services (12.4% compared to age-matched population comparison of 3.6%; Spataro et al., 2004). But it appears to be a non-specific link from childhood abuse to a broad range of disorders. The harm is no less to men, as according to Spataro and colleagues (2004) it was in fact male rather than female child survivors that were most likely to be in contact with mental health services. However, abused women are more likely than abused men to experience hallucinations.

Is it possible to recognize a predisposition?

Welham and colleagues (2009: 603) have summarized key findings of 11 birth cohort studies from seven countries that have followed up a general population sample from birth or childhood and used schizophrenia diagnosis as an outcome variable. They conclude that the evidence is 'relatively consistent that, as a group, children who later develop schizophrenia have behavioural disturbances and psychopathology, intellectual and language deficits, and early motor delays'. For instance, the British cohort study of 5362 people born in one week in March 1946 found that 30 were diagnosed with schizophrenia between ages 16 and 43, and as a group they could be distinguished from the rest of the cohort in terms of learning to walk one to two months later, more often having speech problems, solitary play preferences at ages four and six, poorer education test scores at ages eight, 11 and 15, and less social confidence at 13 (Jones et al., 1994).

Cannon and colleagues (2002a), studying the Dunedin cohort in New Zealand, described above, found the same delay in walking (i.e. at 14.9 months rather than 13.6 months) among the 36 people (of 1037) with schizophreniform disorder (two or more psychotic symptoms, for one to six months only) at age 26, and poorer childhood motor skills, which were not evident in children who later developed other mental health problems (and were not related to obstetric history). There were also poorer skills in some tests of verbal comprehension and IQ. For example, receptive (but not expressive) language skills were below their peers by 0.2–0.6 of a standard deviation at ages three, five, seven and eight. By comparison, poor interpersonal skills and emotional problems in childhood were related to all three later psychiatric diagnoses studied (anxiety/depression and mania as well as schizophreniform disorder). Cannon and colleagues argue persuasively in favour of a neurodevelopmental model of schizophrenia; that is, that there is a genetic susceptibility, reflected in development of motor skills and receptive language ability, and influencing mother–child interactions, and that further studies of brain development will provide the greatest insights into this condition.

The prospective study of 87 high- and low-risk people from the New York high-risk project (Cornblatt et al., 1999) showed that the high-risk sample (that is, those with one or both parents with a diagnosis of schizophrenia) had significantly poorer capacity to maintain attention in tests repeated between ages 12 to 26 years than the comparison group, and that this is a stable, enduring marker of risk, as it does not vary with environmental factors in the way behavioural difficulties do, and hence could be used as part of any screening tool designed to identify risk of psychosis.

But these factors do not facilitate anything approaching a reliable means to predict whether any one person will develop a psychosis. The strongest predictive factor remains a first-degree relative with a similar problem and even then, unless this person is an identical twin, the odds are not very high, and those with a close relative with a similar disorder are in any event a small proportion of those who develop a psychosis. This does not mean that there are no preventive implications – as there are good reasons to suggest additional caution in childbirth plans and decisions for those with a raised genetic risk, and to ensure that all women with schizophrenia receive adequate prenatal care, with additional efforts to engage those with poor attendance. Medical records could be 'flagged' to indicate that where choices are made about delivery, these should minimize risk of a prolonged labour, foetal oxygen deprivation and early delivery. One might also propose paying extra attention to the child with raised genetic risk at school or home, to help improve any difficulties in receptive language skills, ability to maintain attention and risk of victimization.

The attention of research and practice has turned instead to those whose risk is much more obvious due to some emerging psychotic symptoms, in order to avert the onset of a full psychotic episode or to avert or postpone relapse in those already experiencing a first episode.

Is early intervention effective?

The possibility that a full acute episode of psychosis might be prevented by intervention at the earliest possible time has been a focus of considerable interest over the past 20 years, with evidence accumulating both that it does and that it does not work, and that it should and should not be instigated. The idea that intervention as soon as possible *after* onset might prevent an early relapse has received slightly longer research interest, and stronger support, evident in the development of 'Early Intervention Services' (and similar services in many European countries, the US, Canada and Australia), or services with other names with a similar remit.

The debate is as follows. The WHO study in 11 countries showed that outcome at 2 years is one of the best predictors of outcome at 15 years. The condition often seems to worsen rapidly, then plateau. Those with a long delay before starting treatment are more likely to have a poor outcome. Some assume that this may mean that untreated psychosis has some toxic effect through an unknown neurological or psychological mechanism that early treatment should reduce (Wyatt et al., 1997). Others place more emphasis on the long-term disruption that psychotic symptoms can bring to a young person's friendships, working life, education or family relationships at a critical point in their life (Birchwood et al., 1998). However, the opposing argument suggests that identifying people as vulnerable to psychosis and prescribing anti-psychotic medication are both in themselves likely to bring disadvantages, which cannot be justified if the person might not have developed a full psychotic episode without this intervention. Furthermore, whether such intervention is pre-onset or the early weeks post-onset, the intensive support recommended diverts much-needed resources away from mainstream psychiatry for people who should at this stage be helped in primary care (Pelosi and Birchwood, 2003).

Taking these issues in turn – does reducing the duration of untreated psychosis (DUP) improve the long-term course of symptoms? A review by Marshall and colleagues (2005) of 26 eligible first-episode cohort studies found that shorter DUP was linked to a more favourable outcome. They took DUP to mean the time between the first psychotic symptom and the beginning of anti-psychotic medication, and concluded that there should be some benefit to early intervention, though it might be a modest one, but that any harm resulting from lack of treatment appeared to occur in the very first weeks of psychotic symptoms. They claim that 'long DUP seemed to account for approximately 1 in 3 to 1 in 4 of those who did not achieve remission' (Marshall et al., 2005: 981), but that large-scale clinical randomized control trials to reduce DUP are needed to confirm that improved prognosis can be achieved in this way.

Bertelsen and colleagues (2009) describe one such study in Denmark, a large randomized study of 547 people followed up over five years and showing significant clinical benefits of intensive early intervention (involving assertive community treatment, family involvement and social skills training) at two years. But despite the intervention group continuing to show a better outcome in terms of days spent in hospital and likelihood of being in supported accommodation, the clinical benefits substantially diminished at five years. Gafoor and colleagues (2009) report very similar findings over five years in Lambeth, south London, with early benefits demonstrated through their randomized controlled study disappearing after five years. However, this same team conducted a cost–benefit analysis of their first 18 months, and were able to show that it was cost-effective in that the additional staffing cost of psychiatrists, psychologists, social workers and healthcare assistants were more than met by (though not significantly cheaper than) the savings in hospital admissions for the 71 people in the early intervention group, as compared to the 73 receiving standard care. If other improved outcomes were to be added, such as the higher number of the early intervention group in paid employment after 18 months (21 versus 13), then most would agree that this is a much better outcome.

Although the majority of studies show an overall modest benefit from early intervention to prevent a first episode of psychosis, the people who delay longest after first symptoms before seeking treatment are those with the most severe negative rather than positive symptoms (see e.g. Perkins et al., 2005). More severe negative symptoms are associated with poor prognosis, so this is a potential confounding variable. However, Marshall and colleagues (2005) controlled for 'pre-morbid functioning', and despite their reservations, Perkins and colleagues (2005) also concluded that their meta-analysis and review demonstrated an independent effect of early treatment on response to medication, symptom reduction and functional recovery from a first episode. They suggest it may also improve long-term prognosis, but the evidence for the effect on relapse rate is less clear, as they find three studies that demonstrated benefit and two that did not.

That psychotic symptoms disrupt the lives of those who experience them and those close to them is not in doubt. Many family members and mental health lobby groups wish to have appropriate help at the earliest opportunity, and describe the mounting risk of suicide, family stress, and compulsory treatment as the route into care when treatment is delayed (Rethink, 2002).

But should this intervention be directed at those with borderline symptoms as a prevention programme, or offered as early treatment to those with confirmed disorder? Morrison and his colleagues (2004) are among those who argue that intervention is justified in the pre-clinical phases (that is, with people at high risk of psychosis, with some symptoms just below what would lead to a confirmed diagnosis of psychosis) if what is offered is CBT rather than medication. In a small-scale randomized controlled trial, they demonstrated its potentially preventive benefits, with fewer of the experimental group moving on to full psychosis within the 12-month follow-up time (two of 35 compared to five of 23). Bechdolf and colleagues (2006) describe three randomized controlled interventions offering intensive support over 6 or 12 months to people at 'ultra-high risk' of schizophrenia (some psychotic symptoms but of short duration and insufficient in number to meet diagnostic criteria for schizophrenia, and/or experiencing some decline in mental health and having a first-degree relative with a psychotic disorder). They include teaching people skills to cope with positive and negative symptoms, such as distraction, reality testing, goal setting, problem solving, as well as cognitive restructuring, and show promising reductions (one third as many) in numbers progressing to a full psychotic disorder.

Warner (2003), however, judges the cost–benefit differently, whether the intervention is CBT or medication. He concludes that we do not yet have the evidence either that psychosis can be predicted with sufficient reliability or that the interventions make a sufficient difference to outcomes to justify the potential harm that can result for the much larger number incorrectly identified as likely to develop psychosis. That is, the disadvantages that derive from telling someone that they have a raised risk of a psychosis, and from taking anti-psychotic medication unnecessarily for a considerable period, are too high a price for those who would not have developed a psychosis.

Early intervention has a number of possible components. Rinaldi and colleagues (2010) argue that a good proportion of young people in a first episode of psychosis are already falling out of work or education by the time they come to the attention of services, and their own priority is to regain employment, complete their education, and recover the other features of an ordinary life. Yet this is not often part of the service. More common components of early intervention are psychological treatments, including CBT and 'psycho-education', and medication.

One might conclude that although the long-term clinical gains may be less than proponents hoped, the benefits in terms of social functioning are clear, and an intervention service that offers young people support as early as possible should be provided, if they seek help and want to be supported with symptoms that are interfering with their life. The role of the GP in making appropriate early referral is crucial here. The picture painted by Rethink of mounting family distress and difficulties sometimes reaching crisis point for all of them before help is provided is clearly not one to recommend. This early intervention can also be essential in gaining cooperation and engagement of the young person, particularly if the support is also determined by their own priorities, and includes help to get back into work or complete their education, provided in the least stigmatizing way possible. Services that so far demonstrate benefit include medication, CBT and family support (Bird et al., 2010). Bird and colleagues (2010) note that while family support and medication in the early months and years following diagnosis bring benefits at the time, in terms of reducing hospitalization for relapse, the benefits associated with CBT are less likely to reduce hospitalization, and do not become evident until about two years later, but they are then reflected in better control over both positive and negative symptoms. These components of support are discussed further below in relation to the longer term prognosis.

Psycho-social evidence: Course

Perhaps the most important change in understanding of the psychoses over the past 30–40 years is in the potential for recovery, and the role of social factors in this process. It is now much less common to find schizophrenia described as a long-term deteriorating and disabling condition. The recent overview of the WHO studies over the previous 25 years draws this more hopeful picture, with early recoveries found to be maintained in long-term follow-ups (Hopper et al., 2007). Menezes and colleagues (2006) have collated evidence from 37 prospective studies examining the outcome for 'first episode non-affective psychosis', a total of 4100 patients, and also concluded that the outcome 'may be more favourable than previously reported'. The more pessimistic figures that had often been quoted were that 20–50% might improve or recover, but the majority would follow a course of multiple episodes and increasing impairment. Menezes et al. (2006) suggest that this was often due to studies selecting samples in treatment for various periods of time, hence over-representing those who were not responding well to treatment – the 'chronic' patients. They collated data on first episodes, and found that a 'good' outcome was reported for 42% of the patients, an 'intermediate' outcome for 35%, and a 'poor' outcome in 27%. Variables associated with a 'good' outcome included receiving combination therapy (psycho-social and pharmacological), and living in a developing country. Recovery was not worse among longer follow-ups, suggesting that it is not a deteriorating condition.

Bertelsen et al. (2009) came to a similar conclusion from a five-year follow-up of 265 patients with first-episode psychosis in Denmark (though their recovery rates were not so high); that is, there was no decline in rates of recovery or increase in institutionalization over five years, hence no evidence that the condition deteriorates progressively. They found that men had a poorer prognosis, as did those with more symptoms or poor functioning prior to diagnosis. But at five years 18% were recovered – that is, free of symptoms and had a job or place on an educational programme, and were living independently. A further 27% were free of symptoms. This favourable outcome was already clear for this group at two-year follow-up, and of interest was the fact that only 29% of recovered patients were taking anti-psychotic medication at five years even though 70% had a diagnosis of schizophrenia.

The role of social factors in recovery has been known for a long time, and one might reasonably question the poor use of these significant discoveries over the decades since. In the 1950s the readjustment and readmission of male patients, mostly diagnosed with schizophrenia, discharged after two years of inpatient treatment from seven mental hospitals in south London between 1949 and 1956 was studied. This showed that readmission within 12 months was largely unrelated to age, or prior length of stay, but was associated with failing to find employment and with returning to live with parents or partners, rather than living in hostels or lodgings (Brown, Carstairs and Topping, 1958; also described in Harris, 2000). This was so even when symptoms were well controlled at discharge. The risk of relapse was greatest when the discharged patient was unemployed *and* living with parent or partner (each alone was less important), *and* the parent was also unemployed and at home most of every day. A second prospective study of 128 patients of any length of inpatient treatment for schizophrenia examined the role of what was assumed to be high emotional involvement, hostility and/or dominance in these situations. This confirmed its importance to rate of relapse and readmission, and showed further that there was something akin to a dose–response effect – when face-to-face contact was relatively low, risk of relapse was also lower (Brown et al., 1962).

Tension between unemployed family members spending lengthy periods of the day at home together is hardly unusual, but those susceptible to schizophrenia find such high levels of emotional arousal particularly difficult. The family's emotional involvement was later renamed 'expressed emotion' to reflect the evidence that it was not the dissatisfaction of the relative with the progress of their family member, but the way they expressed that dissatisfaction in critical comments that was important. These insights derive from the qualitative method for which the Brown team have become known, based on impressions developed by the interviewers after numerous and lengthy interviews with their subjects, usually tape recorded, then discussed by the research team, then rigorously tested in further study (Harris, 2000). Questionnaire methods and brief, single-interview methods would have been unlikely to reveal such qualitative detail, particularly in this case when it is tone of voice, volume, rate, pitch and expression as compared to that person's more usual speech that must be assessed. Care has been taken to avoid generalizing these findings concerning relapse to first onsets, as there is a circularity to the building of such tensions – the remaining symptoms of the individual leading to critical comments by the relative, which in turn worsen the symptoms and increase the criticism. That is, high expressed emotion may reflect very real problems that families are facing at home.

When this is the case, it appears that reducing the hours of face–to-face contact can help both parties. Brown and colleagues (1972) studied 102 discharged patients; Vaughn and Leff's replication in 1976 studied 128. They found 58% and 51% of their respective samples who returned to a high-EE (expressed emotion) home relapsed within nine months, compared to 16% and 13% respectively going to live in low-EE homes. Where the person and the high-EE relative were in face-to-face contact for more than 35 hours a week, relapse rates were even higher, at 79% and 67%, but if the individual stayed on their medication, these rates were nearly halved. By contrast, the medication had a much less important role in reducing relapse in low-EE households. Hence all three factors played a role, and people living with high-EE relatives, with over 35 hours a week face-to-face contact, and not taking their medication had the highest relapse rates.

Marom and colleagues (2005) show that expressed emotion, particularly critical comments, continues to be reflected in relapse rates after seven years. In a prospective study of 108 people treated in hospital in Israel for schizophrenia, whose closest relatives in the home (at the time of the admission) were rated from taped discussions as low- or high-EE households, they found an equal number of the two groups (just under two thirds) were readmitted at least once in the seven years. However, people living in the households high on critical comments relapsed more quickly, more frequently, and their hospital admissions lasted longer. As in the earliest studies by Brown and colleagues, they also found that medication was important to those in highly critical homes, but of little importance in low-EE homes.

In fact, Warner (2004) provides persuasive evidence that there is a subgroup of people with a good prognosis who will recover better *without* antipsychotic medication, as these drugs in fact increase dopamine production in response to blocked receptors, such that stopping the medication means the higher level of dopamine increases risk of relapse at this point, in a rebound effect. Unfortunately this good prognosis group are difficult to identify reliably, but are more likely to be those with an acute onset, functioning well before the crisis, living in a low-stress, low-EE environment, and in receipt of a supportive rehabilitation programme. Warner suggests short-term use of minor tranquillizers in such cases.

Expressed emotion that raises tensions in this way is defined by Leff (2000) as critical if the critical comments are conveyed in angry tones; as hostile if the critical comments are spontaneously expressed, and/or if directed at personal qualities rather than behaviour (hence likely to be experienced as rejecting); and as over-involved if the responses are over-emotional, over-protective, or involve excessive self-sacrifice, or over-identification with their family member. It might be associated with a sense of guilt and anxiety, a desire to make things better, or a wish to take over decision making, perhaps in the process undermining the person's confidence and skills. Researchers also assess the warmth in family relationships, again through facial expressions and tone of voice as well as by what is said, and assume this to be strengthened by a good level of insight on the part of the family into the difficulties and symptoms. For instance, their understanding that their family member may find it hard to rise in the morning due to the effects of their ill-health (or the medication) rather than due to laziness or selfishness is more likely to lead to a willingness to make appropriate allowances. Hence a number of 'psycho-education' interventions have followed, designed to lower-EE and improve family support, with powerful evidence that this has benefits on the course of disorder (Leff et al., 1985; Falloon et al., 1985; Hogarty et al., 1991). But again, changes to family tensions can be a result as much as a cause of improvements in symptoms.

The many studies that have followed have confirmed these overall findings, and Butzlaff and Hooley (1998) reviewed 27 of these and concluded that high EE roughly doubles the rate of relapse compared to living with low-EE relatives (65% versus 35%), the same effect size as Kavanagh (1992) calculated from a similar review – the median relapse rate was 48% for those living in high-EE households, compared to 21% of those in low-EE homes. Butzlaff and Hooley included some studies of EE in families of an individual with mood disorder or eating disorder and found an even stronger effect. Family homes could also be marital homes, with a partner rather than a parent, and partners were equally likely to be critical, but less likely to be over-involved (Leff, 2000). Butzlaff and Hooley (1998: 551) conclude that the suggestion that EE is an important factor in relapse no longer needs to be doubted, and the focus of enquiry now should be 'sophisticated research that will tell us why EE is associated with relapse in such a wide range of psychopathological conditions'. Their review shows that the effect of EE becomes clearer with samples of people who have been ill for longer.

Where the family home is low in expressed emotion, it appears that a relapse is often triggered by stress from other sources, such as upsetting life events (Leff and Vaughn, 1980). This was first shown in a study of 50 consecutive hospital admissions where the beginning of the episode could be accurately dated to within a week (Brown and Birley, 1968) by comparing the number of life events experienced within the previous three weeks with the number occurring to the same people in three three-week periods before this, and with those occurring in three weeks before interview of a comparison group of 325 people. The events were carefully defined as independent (unlikely to have been linked to pre-morbid symptoms of the individual) and likely for most people to have led to significant emotion (i.e. usually negative, but sometimes positive). This showed that 60% of the patients had experienced such an event in the three weeks preceding admission, compared to an average of 23% over the prior three three-week periods, and 19% of the comparison group (Brown and Birley, 1968). They argued that people who have a history of disorder diagnosed as schizophrenia have a high sensitivity to their social environment even when they have no apparent symptoms, such that an optimum balance between over-stimulation and under-stimulation needs to be sought – withdrawing from arousing circumstances, but avoiding extreme under-stimulation which can also increase arousal.

It is interesting to note, as observed by Birley and Goldberg since (Harris, 2000: 56), how unacceptable were such views at the time, as the first attempt to publish these findings in the *British Journal of Psychiatry* was declined on the grounds that it was too far-fetched an idea that schizophrenia could be brought on by psycho-social events.

Brown and Birley (1968), Birley and Hudson (1983) and Berkowitz and her colleagues (1984) provided some early accounts of the work that can be done with families to help them provide a structured and supportive environment that provides sufficient challenge for their relative's level of recovery. Numerous evaluations of family support have followed (see next chapter), and the evidence from good-quality randomized controlled trials has led to the clear recommendation from NICE (2010) (the UK body that commissions reviews of research evidence and guidance for health provision informed by this) that this should now be a routine part of clinical practice in order to help prevent relapse.

Other factors were also associated with recovery in some of the early research: again, men having poorer prognosis, and those with previous episodes, unskilled work status, no sexual relationships; perhaps suggesting a link with status, self-respect, or a sense of exclusion. Women, at least in the 1960s, might more easily explain, to themselves and others, being without work and at home. Warner (2004) has long argued this position: that the stigma and social exclusion of people with a diagnosis of schizophrenia in the Western world is a large part of the reason that recovery is not better than in many poorer parts of the world. The evidence he collates shows that the introduction of neuroleptics in the 1950s made relatively little difference overall to recovery rates over the decades, whereas the Great Depression of the 1920s and 1930s was reflected in a marked drop in complete recoveries. He suggests that one reason for the surprisingly good outcomes in some poor countries links to the ease (probably necessity) of gaining a useful working role in a subsistence agricultural economy, where people may then also feel less stigmatized and better accepted.

Birchwood and colleagues (2006) argue that the combined effect of stigma and unemployment in the West contributes to high levels of social anxiety and depression among people diagnosed with schizophrenia. The negative assumptions that are associated with the label mean that receiving the diagnosis can be considered the kind of humiliating and entrapping event that is clearly associated with onset of depression (see previous chapter). They and others (e.g. Gumley et al., 2006) suggest that this appraisal increases rate of relapse, recommending CBT to try to reduce negative beliefs. One might question whether support to find employment, further education, or other meaningful and rewarding activity might be expected to achieve this more readily.

Figure 6.1 provides an overview of some of the evidence relating to onset and course of schizophrenia.

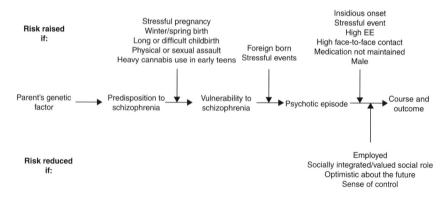

Figure 6.1 Evidence relating to onset and course of schizophrenia.

Summary and conclusion

There is some genetic susceptibility to schizophrenia, which can be increased by infection or psychological stress during pregnancy; lengthy, difficult childbirth; perinatal trauma; childhood maltreatment; physical or sexual assault, and cannabis use in early teenage years. Susceptibility can be reflected in behaviour from a very early age, in slight delays in walking, poor motor skills, some deficits in receptive language ability, and poorer capacity to maintain attention and to screen out irrelevant stimuli.

Other risk indicators include being male, brought up in a city, being a migrant, being socially isolated. But there is insufficient knowledge of how to prevent a first onset for there to be many pointers for targeted primary prevention, other than to:

- take extra care to ensure that pregnant women with a diagnosis of schizophrenia (or where the father is known to have such a diagnosis) receive good prenatal and perinatal care, and perhaps using a lower threshold of difficulty before deciding to deliver by Caesarean section
- campaign more vigorously against use of cannabis by young people under the age of 15 years.

The course of the disorder is worse if the first episode was preceded by a long period of negative symptoms that remained untreated. How well people are after two years of treatment is a good predictor of outcome many years later. Early intervention offering a range of psycho-social and pharmacological support helps to engage people with services and to reduce the stress of the individual and family, costs slightly less than standard care, and can help more young people into work or further education. It may do so at a cost of labelling people with a diagnosis and expectations that may carry negative consequences for their future. Hence secondary prevention includes:

- providing early intervention in the least stigmatizing way possible, carefully considering use of language and labels.

Most people recover; some completely, others sufficiently to lead active and satisfying lives even if experiencing some remaining symptoms. Recovery is sometimes better in low and middle income countries than in the West. Suicide is also more common in industrial nations. The negative associations of a diagnosis of schizophrenia are widely seen as contributing to poor longer term outcomes, through a sense of rejection, exclusion, low social status and discrimination. It is thought that these consequences may be more marked for men than for women, and for some immigrants, hence their worse prognosis. These assumptions prevalent in society need to be gradually reshaped to increase optimism about the lives of those diagnosed with schizophrenia. Strategies might include:

- anti-stigma campaigns
- improving the likelihood that people will gain employment and complete their education to the level they are capable of achieving
- offering CBT to challenge negative thinking
- psycho-education that provides people with insights and coping skills about what might help them to stay well, to recognize their own early warning signs of relapse, and to feel they have some control over their symptoms.

From the early stages of ill-health, and even when well, people remain highly sensitive to emotional arousal, hence there are clear implications for how families can best support them to remain well. An emotionally arousing life event will also sometimes trigger relapse. A warmly supportive, easy-going family home can markedly improve outcomes. If relationships remain strained, with high levels of expressed emotion, then it can help to reduce face-to-face contact and for the individual to stay on maintenance doses of neuroleptic medication (as it suppresses arousal). Hence it is important that:

- families are provided with support and helped to learn how best to develop a conducive home environment for all of them, and to manage particular difficulties
- there are supported housing options if the individual prefers not to live with their family
- the individual is taught self-management strategies through CBT or psycho-education, and supported to find work.

The recovery perspective advanced by service users themselves and more recently reflected in government policy should assist such developments, first by emphasizing optimism about the potential of recovery – a less negative assumption about its effects on one's future even if all symptoms do not fully resolve. Second, this perspective will bring greater involvement of service users in decisions about their care and delivery of some services, and should influence the types of support on offer.

7 Events, coping and support

That life events and stressful living circumstances play an important role in our mental health is well understood by all of us, and well supported by the evidence reviewed here. What has been debated in earlier chapters is what explains vulnerability or resilience in the face of such events and difficulties. This chapter explores what we know about how resilient people cope, and whether it is possible to teach those skills or develop those personal attributes in others to strengthen their resilience. Coping well is linked to the support received from those close to us, hence the second part of this exploration is of the qualities of such support, and whether there are implications for how supportive relationships can be strengthened, or developed; and conversely, whether there are implications for how relationships that undermine our ability to cope can be improved, or escaped. The importance of wider societal support – the role of the welfare state, neighbourhood, and social structures – is the subject of a later chapter.

The question to ask, given the evidence of the origins of mental ill-health discussed so far, is how is it that some people facing threatening events, maintain a sense of:

a   being respected, of dignity, being valued, and important
b   having control over their difficulties, and a positive future
c   being safe, protected from harm
d   adaptation to, and acceptance of loss
e   calm emotions?

This list can be seen as the outcomes that coping and support need to achieve.

The process of coping

Coping is a process that consists of 'cognitive and behavioural efforts to manage psychological stress' (Lazarus, 1993: 237), for which there are few clear generalizations about what is a 'good' coping response, and what is 'bad'. The effective strategy will depend on the person, the situation faced, its personal meaning to that individual, and the outcome sought. For instance, denial is often thought to be a poor coping response, particularly as urgent action is sometimes required (discovering a breast lump); in other circumstances (such as finding oneself permanently disabled after a car accident), it might buy time for the person to find smaller parts of the picture to which to adjust first (Adams and Lindemann, 1974).

But, as the definition suggests, coping has two major components, related to how we think about an event and what we do about it, or as Lazarus defines them, *emotion-focused coping* and *problem-focused coping*. In emotion-focused coping we either try to reduce the emotional impact of the stressor through reducing the mental attention given to it or try to recast the meaning; for example, the person did not intend the comment to be taken literally, or she was tired and flustered and not really angry with me. Western cultures tend to value the problem-focused more than the emotion-focused approach to coping; that is, they try to attack the problem directly, get information about it, try to change the event or our own relationship to it, such as our beliefs about it or commitment to it. However, this emphasis may be partly cultural, as Asian samples show a lower sense of control than British or American samples in studies of coping, and in these individual control seems less important to mental health (Sastry and Ross, 1998; O'Connor and Shimizu, 2002).

Coping with major trauma

Trauma of the level that commonly overwhelms our ability to cope, leaving many with what is now described as post-traumatic stress disorder (PTSD), includes experiences faced in war, natural disaster, violent assault, and other life-threatening situations. Summarizing the results of their examination of 284 papers published since 1980 that explored the rate of PTSD following natural disasters such as flood and hurricane and human-made disasters (mostly terrorist bombs), but excluding war, Neria and colleagues (2008) report linked PTSD rates in the months following ranging from 4% to 10% in the general population. Among those closest to the trauma they find much higher rates; for instance, as many as 44% of police involved in the Hillsborough football stadium disaster were reported to be experiencing symptoms of PTSD one to two years later. On average, they find that 30–40% of victims are left with PTSD symptoms, as are 10–20% of rescue workers, with magnitude of exposure to the event strongly linked to risk of PTSD, particularly in terms of threat to life, property destruction and number of fatalities.

Members of the military services on active duty around the world, as well as the civilians in war zones, face risk of death or serious injury on a daily basis, many experiencing horrors that they may never shake from their memory. Not surprisingly, those who come closest to death are often most traumatized. The symptoms now defined as PTSD include intense physiological arousal remaining long after the cause of terror has passed, a tendency to startle easily and sleep poorly, the regular intrusion to thoughts and dreams of the traumatic experience, momentary flashbacks along with the intense emotion and adrenalin of the event, and a tendency to avoid anything that is associated with the event, detaching emotionally, or constricting one's life to avoid places or activities that might be reminders.

Experience of violent assault is not confined to those in countries at war, of course. Crimes recorded by the police in the UK (Home Office, 2010) included 44,513 people who were victims of the 'most serious sexual crime' and nine times this number subject to 'violent assault with injury' in 2010. Kelly and colleagues (2005) drew on official crime survey data to show that 5% of British women over the age of 16 are raped at some point during their lifetime. As many rapes are not reported, these figures are an underestimate of attacks: figures from research in many European centres including the UK show higher rates than this (Regan and Kelly, 2003).

What lessons are there from studies of those coping with such events? During traumatic experience from which there is no escape, a person might dissociate (mentally distancing themselves from what is happening) instead of focusing on the threat (Herman, 1992). Subsequently they may avoid situations associated with it (sometimes without conscious recognition of doing so), reflecting the emotion- and problem-focused strategies described by Lazarus and Folkman (1984). But while these may have been key to survival at the time, their continued use when that specific risk of harm has passed prevents the integration of the event into conscious memory and the person reaching some sort of resolution. It can be a long and painful adaptation, which Herman (1992: 3) argues can only begin after the person feels safe enough to allow traumatic memories to resurface. The 'fundamental stages of recovery are establishing safety, reconstructing the trauma story, and restoring the connection between survivors and their community'. This process is, of course, the basis of modern psychotherapy.

Drawing on studies of those who did and did not develop PTSD despite sharing the same terrible experiences of war in Vietnam, Herman (1992) finds that the latter were distinguished by their task-oriented coping strategies (preparing themselves, avoiding unnecessary risks, their sociability, help given to others, even challenging orders that seemed ill-advised): a strong internal locus of control. These exceptional people focused their efforts on remaining calm, trying to see meaning in their situation, connecting with others, remembering their moral values. Iversen and colleagues (2008) demonstrate the same finding in reverse; that is, those who felt they were required to act above their level of competence and experience were more than three times as likely to be diagnosed with PTSD after deployment to Iraq from 2003. Spending more than a month in a 'forward area', witnessing a number of traumas to others and handling dead bodies were also strong risk factors.

Many background social factors also seem to contribute to this sense of being able to cope. For instance, those who were divorced, widowed or separated, and single people, had almost twice the rate of PTSD as married people; under 25-year-olds double the rate of those over 40; those with no educational qualifications had double the risk of others (Iversen et al., 2008). Having multiple childhood risk factors (agreement or disagreement indicating experience of a list of 16 childhood experiences such as truanting from school, closeness of family, being hit by a parent frequently) also substantially increased risk of PTSD – those with four or more having twice the rate of PTSD; six or more, three times the rate. Current protective factors included a good sense of morale in their unit, where they felt that their seniors cared about what they did or thought, and where they had a sense of comradeship with others. Together with background factors, this suggests that a sense of being cared for and protected throughout life builds resilience.

Trauma from child abuse: Effects on coping

Adults who as children experienced abuse that they had no power to prevent or escape may have learned that dissociating helped them cope, as did a strategy of complete surrender, neither of which helps them cope well with later difficulty. They may also be left with a legacy of anger and distrust, but at the same time blame themselves for past abuse, as this leaves room for some possibility of control over the situation, rather than blaming the abuser. Once past, deeply traumatic memories can be buried well away from active memory, inaccessible both to others and to themselves (Herman, 1992).

As Herman (1992: 110) describes it, the adult survivor of child abuse

> is left with fundamental problems in basic trust, autonomy, initiative. She approaches the tasks of early adulthood – establishing independence and intimacy – burdened by major impairments in self-care, in cognition and memory, in identity, and in the capacity to form stable relationships.

Adult relationships may be damaged by idealizing the person, creating inappropriately high expectations that cannot be realized, and then minor hurts can seem like major cruelty and rejection, leading to intense but unstable relationships. The adult survivor becomes at risk of further victimization, and can make poor judgements about risk – a problem borne out by data showing the significantly raised rate of rape among adult survivors of child sexual abuse (Diana Russell's study (1986), cited by Herman).

Preparing for frightening or distressing events

The exercise of 'anticipatory coping' for events that are known in advance was one of Caplan's central notions for primary prevention – anticipating the tension, envisaging possible responses, suggesting that 'When the experience arrives, the hazards will be attenuated because they have been made familiar by being anticipated' (Caplan, 1964: 84). Certainly this is one of the principles of the hospice movement, where staff appreciate that both fear and grief in the patient and his or her relatives can be reduced through anticipating the fact that they do not have much longer together and that this time can be used constructively to work through some of their anxieties.

Those who embark on stressful, life-threatening adventures on a regular basis learn to address their anxieties in advance. Studying novice and experienced parachutists, using physiological measures of anxiety (skin conductance), Epstein (1983) showed that novices became gradually more anxious as the day and moment of jumping approached, whereas the anxiety of the experienced parachut-ists peaked a day before the jump, then steadily reduced up to the moment of jumping. He argues that a graded 'stress inoculation' process, attending to moder-ately stressful cues and exploring and mastering their threat before allowing ourselves to explore more salient stimuli, is the natural healing process of the mind. For those failing to prepare themselves in this way, it can be taught, and is a process widely used in overcoming phobias and anxiety about impending surgery, and to assist readjustment to normal living habits following rape (see Meichenbaum and Jaremko, 1983). Otherwise the person may be reduced to falling back on an all-or-nothing strategy, in which awareness of the event is completely blocked out or is experienced in overwhelming intensity. Novice para-chutists who blocked out fear completely up to the moment of jumping were often overcome with an incapacitating anxiety such that not only did they not jump, but they decided to give up jumping forever.

Emotion- and problem-focused coping during and after threatening events

One of the effects of a violent confrontation, or other markedly challenging circumstances, is the 'fight or flight' response of the body, recognizable in the dry mouth and pounding heart. Frightening or angry thoughts and images maintain this rapid heart rate, whereas physical skills such as slow breathing can be used to try to lower it, reducing the automatic appraisal of the stressor as threatening. The person can then use a sequence of self-statements to change the perception of the stressor, and change the thoughts and images to be less anxiety provoking (Jaremko, 1983). Such 'cognitive restructuring' can be used to replace negative statements such as 'it's going to be terrible' with positive statements such as 'I'm sure I can manage' (Jaremko, 1983), or even statements that convert the threat into a challenge that promises achievement (Lazarus, 1976), such as 'I'll show them how well I can deal with this'.

In a prospective study with 205 family members of a relative dying at home (most from cancer, and provided with hospice support), Davis and colleagues (1998) found that people strived to *make sense* of the death, with non-threatening explanations (it's God's will, old age, or the result of lifestyle, for instance). That is, they explained the loss to themselves as an understandable, even justifiable event, rather than a random and inexplicable one. Secondly, they tried to *find benefit* in the situation, for instance reappraising their own priorities in life, changing their own risk behaviour, deciding to value relationships more. Those with a generally optimistic approach to life were more likely to be able to see a benefit in their loss, whereas those with a religious belief, and those whose relative was quite old, were more likely to be able to make sense of their loss. Making sense of loss was most important in the first six months, whereas seeing some benefit in the loss was more important in relation to adjustment at 13 and 18 months.

Pearlin and colleagues (1981) described the coping strategies of the 88 of 2000 Chicago residents they interviewed who had been made redundant or fired from work in the four years between first interview and follow-up. Those who had fewer symptoms of depression were more likely to cope by comparing their lot with those in a worse economic position, or with times in their own past when things had been worse. Other positive coping strategies included demeaning the value of money and monetary success, seeing current hardship as the forerunner of an easier future, or devaluing the importance of the troubling aspects of an event and magnifying the good features – such as being glad to no longer work for the unpleasant boss, emphasizing too the great opportunity to reappraise the jobs to be sought in future (Pearlin et al., 1981).

A religious belief can help with managing the meaning of events, particularly those with an emphasis on forgiveness, of dealing with anger, discouraging the pursuit of material wealth. Many religions use parables to help people see their difficulties in a different context: providing hope; recasting difficulties as less important, as manageable, or which their God will be working with them to overcome. Great political and religious leaders have long recognized and used these insights. Stone (1998) begins his history of psychiatry textbook with four powerful stories derived from Christianity, Buddhism and Hinduism that empha-size standing together in love to face a shared sorrow; that tragedy, often greater than our own, is commonplace; that addressing a problem immediately rather than complaining about it and ruminating on it brings rapid relief; and that a good life is one free of anger, lust and greed. As he reminds us, 'Psychiatry was Religion before it was Psychiatry' (Stone, 1998: xi), and the essence of talking therapies has changed little in three millennia.

Resources that assist coping

Optimism

There is growing evidence that optimism and related concepts associated with positive mental health are powerful factors in recovery from physical ill-health of many types, and in adapting to the news of a life-threatening diagnosis; hence some of these issues are revisited in Chapter 8. Also gaining ground in mental health is the 'recovery' perspective, with a much greater focus on hope, choice, and meaning – the discovery of purpose and direction – for those coping with existing serious mental ill-health (see Jacobsen and Curtis, 2000).

The key to the benefits of optimism, according to Segerstrom (2006: 8), lies in how it makes people behave in the face of life difficulties. 'Very optimistic people believe that more good things will happen than bad, and that things will go their way, that the future is positive.' But crucially, optimists 'believe their goals are achievable. They don't give up easily.' In other words, 'optimistic beliefs work to make optimists' lives better because they cause optimistic people to behave in particular ways' (p. 10). In the face of obstacles, or very distressing life events, optimistic people cope better because they 'attack their problems head-on', seeking advice, staying focused, using problem-focussed strategies. When the event has happened and there is nothing to be done to change it, they are more likely to accept the situation, using emotion-focused strategies (talking through emotions, trying to think about it in a different way) to reduce its threat (Segerstrom, 2006). While partly an inherited personality characteristic, optimism can also be developed from experience, and may potentially be taught. Segerstrom describes experiments dividing students into those rated as optimists and those as pessimists, which found that optimists persisted in trying to solve a set of difficult and impossible anagrams for longer than pessimists (11.5 compared to 9.5 minutes). Other experiments showed that optimistic and pessimistic expectations could be fostered by how the task was set up and explained, which was then reflected in perseverance with the task, confirming both that expecting to succeed makes you work harder to achieve it, and that this expectation can be shaped by experience.

Cognitive therapy – better coping styles can be taught

The brief 'talking treatments' falling under the umbrella of the cognitive behavioural therapies are essentially structured techniques for teaching people a more optimistic coping style. For instance, 'solution-focused' therapy explores a person's future hopes and the resources they have for achieving these rather than examining current problems and their causes, and helps a person think how they could move towards their aspirations. Once a happier future scenario is envisaged, the person explores the times when they have found courage to do what is needed to move forward (Iveson, 2002). Another common approach is one in which the individual examines their explanations for everyday events (someone passing them in the street without acknowledging them, potentially seen as ignoring them, but could also be considered likely to be absorbed in their own worries), and the emotions and bodily sensations arising from the two explanations, and then the likely action resulting (go home and avoid the person, or go home and ring them up to ask how they are) (RCPsych, 2010). The therapy can involve diary keeping and rehearsing the approach as homework exercises between meetings, and aims to break the 'vicious circle' that develops from this negative thinking; that is, withdrawing from contacts, assuming others think badly of them, and thereby finding more evidence to support their negative self-perceptions.

Such talking treatments are now widely offered, with evidence to support their effectiveness in managing anxiety disorders and obsessive compulsive disorder (O'Kearney et al., 2006; Hunot et al., 2007; McManus et al., 2008), helping those with psychotic thoughts to find less distressing explanations for them (Morrison, 2004), treating acute depression (Butler et al., 2006; Meyer and Scott, 2008), PTSD, bulimia nervosa and many other diagnoses (Butler et al., 2006). Helping a person achieve an enduring change to the way they interpret everyday events and difficulties can be more effective than medication in terms of preventing relapse or recurrence (Bockting et al., 2005). Butler and colleagues (2006: 28) review 16 meta-analyses of the effectiveness of CBT and conclude that 'In the cases of depression and panic, there appears to be robust and convergent meta-analytic evidence that CT produces vastly superior long-term persistence of effects, with relapse rates half those of pharmacotherapy'.

One problem that it is assumed CBT can help is a person's tendency to interpret quite minor setbacks as well as more serious events in terms of a negative perception of themselves. A friend failing to turn up for a date may reawaken deep-seated fears of abandonment. Instead of thinking that she probably missed the bus, negative assumptions spring to mind, which spiral toward a grossly exaggerated interpretation of the event (sometimes described as 'catastrophizing'): 'She didn't want to meet me tonight – I'm not good company – why would anyone want to spend time with me? – I'm stupid and boring . . .'

Teasdale and colleagues (2001) suggest that this is how CBT works in preventing relapse. That is, rather than succeeding in changing the content of negative thoughts, it reduces the person's tendency to catastrophize. The immature all-or-nothing responses at the extreme end of the scale – 'totally agree' or 'totally disagree' – absolute, judgemental, dichotomous thinking style, is moderated as the person learns to challenge their own negative thinking. That is, they learn to have a second thought, and shift their negative view to a less extreme one, but do not usually arrive at a fundamentally different explanation. They found it to reduce relapse but not to bring a change to depressive symptoms at 20 weeks. The 80 patients receiving 16 weekly cognitive therapy (CT) sessions had a cumulative relapse rate of 29% compared to 47% of the 78 control group subjects after 68 weeks. All patients in both groups also received medication. This kind of extreme thinking was strongly linked to relapse in both groups – 44% of the whole sample with any extreme ratings relapsed, compared to 17% with none – providing a helpful perspective on the style of thinking of those with chronic depression, and suggesting it may be possible to target CT referrals through GPs screening patients on such a questionnaire.

Intervention to help people develop more benign interpretations of stressful events was argued by Caplan to be most effective during the crisis period. Crisis theory, as he formulated it in 1964, suggests that when facing major difficulties and life crises people are particularly vulnerable, but also more open to advice and support, and to examining possible changes to their lives or behaviour than they might be at other times.

Positive thinking – developing one's own skills

The recently developed field of 'positive psychology' is also enabling people to reappraise their strengths and aiming to help people improve their own happiness and their satisfaction with life in terms of engaging in activities that use their strengths, and give their lives meaning. The research on the effectiveness of such strategies is in early stages of development, and the methods used in many are open to criticism, though their authors write persuasively about the benefits. A meta-analysis of 51 studies designed to improve positive emotions, cognitions, and behaviours selected by Sin and Lyubomirsky (2009) included studies of variable quality and with comparison groups but few controlling for placebo effects. Interventions included positive writing, engaging in enjoyable activities, mindfulness, gratitude, replaying positive memories. The authors argue that the evidence is sufficient to include these in clinical practice, with improvement in symptoms of depression or measures of wellbeing occurring in roughly twice as many people as in the comparison groups. Intervention samples gained most if they were depressed, had self-selected to receive positive therapies, if they worked harder at developing the skills, and were older.

One of the studies included in the above review is based on use of a measure of a person's 'character strengths and virtues' (CSV), a lengthy self-completion questionnaire developed by Peterson and Seligman (2004) and intended 'to do for psychological wellbeing what the *Diagnostic and Statistical Manual of Mental Disorders (DSM)* of the American Psychiatric Association (1994) does for the psychological disorders that disable human beings'. The CSV describes and classifies six virtues and 24 character strengths 'that enable human thriving' (Seligman et al., 2005: 411), such as the virtue of wisdom (with character strengths in curiosity, creativity, open-mindedness and love of learning), or courage, humanity or temperance (forgiveness, modesty, prudence). They argue that this list of virtues and strengths finds a strong level of endorsement across cultures and countries.

This was evaluated in a randomized control trial undertaken through the internet, on those logging in to their positive psychology website. Hence the sample was likely to be biased towards those wanting to improve their mental health, who were motivated sufficiently to complete lengthy questionnaires, and easily able to use a computer. Respondents were randomly allocated to one of six exercises for a week, one of which was writing about their early memories each night, and used as the placebo control. The other five tasks were (1) a gratitude visit – write and deliver in person a letter of gratitude to someone who had been especially kind to them; (2) three good things – each night think of, write down and explain three things that went well that day; (3) you at your best – reflect on a time you were at your best, review this story each day, reflecting on strengths identified; (4) use signature strengths – complete the CSV and plan to use one of the top five identified in a new way on each day; (5) identify signature strengths through completing the CSV, note the top five. There were 411 people completing one of these tasks for a week, as well as the online questionnaires at each follow-up date to six months. Tasks 2 and 4 led to positive and significant benefits that lasted six months, as compared to those completing the placebo task, and measured on both a scale of positive wellbeing and a separate assessment of depressive symptoms. The gratitude visit created a greater beneficial effect than all other tasks, but the effects lasted only a month.

Psychotherapeutic support

Recovery from major trauma starts with establishing safety, feeling protected, after which the person needs to strengthen the sense that they have control over their lives. Herman (1992) argues that this means listening to the person's story, enabling them to come to their own solutions, rather than offering advice and practical help. This process can start immediately following the event; for instance, there are implications for medical examinations of a rape victim that might otherwise be experienced as a further trauma – asking the person's permission, ensuring as much choice and control as possible, including how best to live and what treatment and what legal action to pursue, if any. For those escaping abusive relationships, it means establishing a home and income that are independent of the abuser. Feeling safe can be helped by attention to basic health needs – sleep, diet, exercise, control of self-destructive behaviours, which should be followed by helping to rebuild a positive sense of self. But close others face a difficult task in providing support, as a traumatized person is likely to be short-tempered, argumentative, solitary, but also feeling neglected. Once able to acknowledge their trauma, they then need to mourn that which has been lost. The community can at times play a role in this: ceremonies, monuments, special holidays and parades are very important in assuring war veterans that their efforts are recognized, that the public remember the sacrifice of so many (Herman, 1992).

Vickerman and Margolin (2009) review 20 studies of therapeutic approaches for rape survivors, which suggest that CBT can reduce the rate of PTSD by about half by the end of treatment sessions, though as many as one in three rape victims continued to live with these symptoms. Herman (1992) discusses the value of group therapy, emphasizing the importance of ensuring that participants are at the same stage of adaptation, and that the focus of the group work is informed by this. A 'first stage' group will focus on current life circumstances, self-care, learning skills such as those taught in CBT, building a sense of safety. By contrast, people ready to remember, revisit and mourn their traumatic experience must be in a closed time-limited group with strong group cohesion, where participants set themselves clear goals. People who have made good progress, and have been able to integrate the traumatic memories with their life story, are ready then to look to the future, and plan a life in which they regain 'a sense of belonging somewhere, being part of something good', as one post-treatment war veteran expressed it (see Herman, 1992: 232).

But brief interventions with traumatized people can also do more harm than good if not well planned, as Roberts and colleagues (2009) conclude in their systematic review of psychological interventions to prevent PTSD following a disaster, in the form of either single-session or multiple-session debriefing. Herman herself cautions that programmes 'that promote the rapid uncovering of traumatic memories without providing an adequate context for reintegration are therapeutically irresponsible and potentially dangerous, for they leave the patient without the resources to cope with the memories uncovered' (Herman, 1992: 184). She explains how the timing and process must address feelings of safety *before* revisiting painful memories, and must be determined by the person himself or herself. Hence interventions in the very early days after a trauma should be of an educational format, providing an exchange of information, a focus on self-care and self-protection.

Therapeutic and preventive intervention that focuses on psychological coping can, then, help people to enhance their sense of control, improve adaptation to loss, and help people learn methods to improve their wellbeing and stay calm. Other outcomes listed earlier – a sense of self-respect, of being valued, of safety and of having a positive future – will more likely derive from the support of close others.

Support from close others: Does it help us cope with adversity?

Earlier chapters have demonstrated the crucial protective importance of close supportive relationships in depression, and in relapse of psychosis. Many studies of coping with specific life events also demonstrate this relationship. However, the effects of well-meaning advice from close others are not always experienced as positive (Bolger and colleagues, 2000), and findings on the role of support are complex. The published work is extensive – several thousand papers since the late 1960s – although the methodology in many is not sufficiently sophisticated to clarify its role, what exactly it provides and when, with wide-ranging definitions and measures of support.

While most confirm that perceived availability of social support is protective, some of the research designed to demonstrate what this looks like in practice fails to find the expected effects (see Bolger et al., 2000). Even the number of people to whom we think we can turn is far from a straightforward story – numbers seem to be important only to men. For instance, a follow-up over 18 months of a stratified sub-sample of 2406 respondents in the 2000 National Morbidity Study in the UK found that having fewer than three friends at time 1 predicted poorer mental health at time 2 in men but not women (Brugha et al., 2005). This finding was not explained by differences in their perception of the support available, but was linked to actual numbers. Stansfeld and colleagues (2003), in their follow-up of a large cohort of British civil servants, also found men but not women seeming to be protected from common mental health problems five years later if they reported a confiding relationship at time 1. But for both men and women, negative interactions and perceived inadequacy of support from the person identified at time 1 as their closest 'other' predicted depression at follow-up (Stansfeld et al., 2003).

Hence some of the conflicting evidence about the value of support seems likely to derive from the negative role these same social contacts can play. Those who can protect us best can also harm us most. For instance, the close other – the parent or spouse – crucial to the sense of love, esteem and value of the individual treated for psychosis, who reacts with hostility, overt criticism and an over-involvement in his or her relative's everyday life, significantly increases their risk of relapse (see Leff et al., 1985; Falloon et al., 1985; and Chapter 6). Yet if they are able to stay calm and uncritical, help their relative too to stay calm, and provide warmth and affection together with practical assistance in helping them to improve their social competence and negative symptoms, their support can be very important in reducing risk of relapse.

So too in risk of depression. Brown and colleagues (1986a) showed that a woman whose core relationship with her partner was characterized by negative interactions (coldness, discord, tension, indifference) was three times more likely to become depressed following a major event or marked long-term difficulty compared to a woman with a better relationship with her partner.

Thus although close others can strengthen our ability to cope, their significance is more often linked to their role in undermining it. A further complication is that the severe events and difficulties most frequently implicated in depression, capable of making us feel humiliated and trapped, often involve those very rela- tionships on which we depend for support – our core ties (Brown et al., 1995). These issues are discussed below.

So what is social support?

Reviewers often draw on a distinction made many years ago by House (1981) in what can potentially be provided: functional support (tangible help such as money, services), information (including advice), and emotional support, described by Gottlieb (1983: 19) as 'an expression of reliable alliance with the respondents and a genuine concern for their wellbeing'. Those adopting this perspective see social support as something recognizable, emphasizing that the supporter must be present or accessible during stressful episodes. Others, following Cobb (1976), conceive of support more as something that arises in the eye of the beholder; that is, it is anything that influences the person to believe that he or she is the recipient of positive affect, any information 'leading the subject to believe that he is cared for and loved . . . esteemed and valued' (Cobb, 1976: 300).

Similarly, Weiss (1982) emphasizes the sense of comfort and security and of being valued that can come from close others, while functional support and infor- mation can come from a wide range of relationships – the general practitioner, the priest, senior staff at work. But he reminds us they are not only important in helping us cope with adversity. Investments in the welfare of others through parenting or caring roles provide a rationale for continued striving, a sense of continuity, and an opportunity to relive and master unsatisfactory experiences in one's own childhood. Friendships can be important in so far as they reflect atti- tudes and behaviour that inform, support and strengthen one's own identity and beliefs, and reassurance of self-worth in their acceptance.

Two sorts of evidence confirm the importance of support: evidence that those with support are protected, and evidence that those without it are vulnerable. In relation to a clinical level of mental ill-health, the evidence is primarily linked to the negative aspects, as indicated above – of discordant or highly critical relation- ships and single parenthood, and partners who 'let you down'.

If expected support does not materialize, vulnerability is increased

Women with seemingly good close relationships are more vulnerable to depres- sion when the support they were expecting from the persons in question is not forthcoming. The longitudinal study by Brown and colleagues (1986a) found that a surprising number of women judged to have a supportive marital relationship at first interview became depressed after a crisis in the following year (17%, not greatly fewer than those without – 24%). When the lives of the women were examined in detail, it transpired that in the majority of these cases support had not been forthcoming *during* the crisis. The kind of situation involved might be an event such as the arrest of a child, when instead of supporting and reassuring the mother, the partner instead blamed her for the child's behaviour – perhaps for working away from home too often. Married/cohabiting women were more likely to be 'let down' in this way, and when this occurred other forms of support were rarely able to mitigate the depressive response. Their rate of depression (37%) was higher than the rate among single women or married women whose prior unsupportive relationship had not led them to expect much support in the face of difficulties (24%). By contrast, if their partner provided the expected support, they had a very low rate of depression following severe life events (4%). Single women, and women who did not expect support from their partner, had a reduced risk of depression if they had named another person as very close, or as a 'true friend' (Brown et al., 1986a).

A similar point was made by Herman (1992), drawing an illustration from case studies of the treatment of war veterans reported by Kardiner and Spiegel (1947). For instance, the experience of a man and his ordinary navy peers who were left in the water clinging to a raft, while officers in the relative safety of a lifeboat were rescued several hours before them, was experienced as particularly traumatic. The realization that he was expendable, that the support he was expecting was not forthcoming, affected his mental health and subsequent relationships far more than the pain, the time in the water and loss of life around him.

If visible and unreciprocated, it may be unhelpful

Yet the concept of support might be more subtle still. Bolger and colleagues (2000) suggest that when the recipient is very aware of being given support, it can in fact reduce their sense of self-efficacy through the process of acknowledging that they need help. There is effectively a cost to the self-esteem of the recipient in admitting being in difficulty. They propose that support is most effective if it is provided without being seen to be sought, nor acknowledged as received. They find some evidence for this suggestion by studying support provided and received by couples when one is preparing to take the New York State Bar exam. 'Invisible support' – diary rating by the providers that they gave support, but no diary rating by the recipient that they received it – was effective in reducing symptoms of 'anticipatory depression and discouragement' over the 32-day period, which was not the case in the other possible combinations (given and received, not given and not received, not given but received): that is, practical help without saying it is being done to help, or provided skilfully enough that it avoids drawing any attention to the person's distress or to any possible failings of competence. This is of course, as they acknowledge, 'the essence of good parenting, good mentoring, and good friendships, and being a good clinician or social worker' (Bolger et al., 2000: 959). Similarly, advice offered in the presence of others, while intended to be constructive, can feel humiliating, a comment on failings, as compared to observations made obliquely to the whole group about what 'some people' have found to be useful.

Many studies of people coping with chronic illness have also found that tangible help can sometimes 'backfire'. Abraido-Lanza (2004) summarizes the evidence and notes how a balance has to be found between enabling someone to accept help and undermining their sense of competence. However, where cultural expectations are that, for instance, it is the role of a daughter to provide such support, as she found it to be with Latina women with chronic arthritis, there is no cost to self-esteem when they do so. Similarly, support to men over 65 by their partner was only beneficial in terms of their health and mortality five years later if part of a reciprocal emotionally supportive relationship; that is, the man provided emotional support to, as well as received it from, his partner (S.L. Brown et al., 2003).

Hence, it appears that believing that there is support available from another person who cares about us, and believing we are loved, esteemed and valued as we cope with stressful events and long-term difficulties, is protective against depression. But finding that the presumed support is not available after all then increases risk further than if no support was expected. Equally, when the close other positively undermines our sense of being able to cope, through critical comments, hostility, coldness or indifference, or even very visible well-intentioned support, the risk of mental ill-health following a life event is increased.

Can intervention address poor support and reduce vulnerability?

One of the implications for primary prevention is to help people avoid entering into, or staying in, abusive relationships. Another is to find new sources of support for those vulnerable in other ways and lacking good support. Benefit is unlikely to be demonstrable without existing vulnerability and current social problems or adverse life events. Three examples follow: the role befriending might play in strengthening the support available to women vulnerable to depression; psychoeducation and family support to change negative aspects of close relationships of those vulnerable to schizophrenia; support to adolescents with prior experience of abuse or neglect to help them avoid involvement in abusive intimate relationships in adulthood. Evidence from randomized control trials is presented.

Improving social support: The role of befriending

A systematic review and meta-analysis of befriending projects by Mead and colleagues (2010) found a significant but modest beneficial outcome on depression. Their analysis included interventions that offered non-directive one-to-one emotional support by unpaid volunteers or paid workers (but free to the individual), who were able to offer information and practical help as well as emotional support. All 24 eligible studies identified were randomized controlled trials, but eight offered their friendship over the telephone rather than face to face. The studies were diverse: those befriended were carers, pregnant women, post-natal women, people with chronic physical illness, schizophrenia, depression or prostate cancer, or people who were recently bereaved. Friendship was time-limited, varying from a few weeks to one year, with a median length of intervention of weekly one-hour meetings for three months. The review does not elaborate on the types and length of intervention that seemed most effective.

The results of the study by Harris (2008) are more positive. This befriending intervention was carefully targeted at a group of pregnant women considered to be particularly vulnerable to depression (from a measure rating self-worth, negativity in core relationships, childhood adversity). From week 30 of the pregnancy through to nine months post-partum, a random half of the 71 women were provided with one-to-one befriending and group sessions of psycho-education through a London befriending charity called Newpin. The other half formed a wait list control, to be offered the service 12 months later. Crucially, benefit was assessed in relation to coping with life events. Among those who experienced a severe event during the year (characterized by humiliation, entrapment or loss), 80% of control group women became depressed, as compared to 30% of those partici-pating in the Newpin befriending project.

Befrienders were not just a sympathetic listener, however; they sometimes provided practical help to their Newpin friend, exchanging babysitting, helping with writing letters to the Council, and encouraging and supporting them when close relatives were undermining their confidence – acting as a true friend might do (Harris, 2008).

Harris and colleagues (1999a) also show that befriending can bring remission in a chronic depression. The 86 north London chronically depressed women randomly allocated to befriending support or control group for 12 months showed a significant difference in recovery rates between groups, with 65% of the former, compared to 39% of the latter, becoming substantially less depressed after one year. The focus was on friendship, engaging in activities together, offering prac-tical support for current difficulties, for a minimum of one hour each week. Their analysis of differences in those who recovered and those who did not showed that lack of remission was to a large extent explained by poor coping – denial or help-lessness as assessed at baseline interview, and the occurrence of further stressful experience during the year. By contrast, the occurrence of a 'fresh start event' was an important predictor of recovery. These experiences explained recovery equally for befriended and non-befriended women, hence the value of the befriending came to the fore only for those women experiencing more adversity during the year (Harris et al., 1999b).

Improving family social support for psychosis

The role of emotional arousal in risk of relapse in schizophrenia, and the part critical comments and over-involvement by close others can play in this, were discussed in the previous chapter. Early studies evaluating attempts to change the level of 'expressed emotion' by family members showed marked benefits. The small-scale but carefully controlled trial by Leff and colleagues, who followed up the sample for two years (Leff et al., 1985), was one of the first. They showed they could reduce relapse rates at nine months among those whose families received four educational sessions about schizophrenia in their home alongside nine months of fortnightly support group meetings with other family carers. However, by two years, there were also two suicides in the family supported group, raising concerns about the emphasis on reducing family contact in the high-EE families. It encouraged other researchers such as Falloon and colleagues (1985) and Hogarty and colleagues (1991) to place more emphasis on the positive role that families could play and included skills training for the individuals themselves. The latter study found that this combination was particularly effective after 12 months in reducing relapse (rates were 20% relapsing in 12 months with one, 40% with neither, 0% with both – 103 subjects in total). Significant differences remained after two years, though not as marked, suggesting that the intervention is particularly important in the 'stabilization phase'.

However, the studies since then have varied the methods, length and frequency of intervention, members of the family involved, training of therapists, and setting, and have led to heterogeneous findings. Some have found almost no effect, such that a Cochrane review of 53 randomized or quasi-randomized controlled trials, updated to 2008 (Pharoah et al., 2010), gave a lukewarm endorsement to family intervention. They found an effect, but not a very powerful one, in reducing expressed emotion by family members, improving medication compliance, and reducing relapse and hospital use at 12 months, drawing on studies from China, Australia, Europe and the USA. Overall, seven families needed to receive the intervention to prevent one relapse.

These findings contrast with those from NICE (2010: 300), whose review of 32 RCTs conducted between 1978 and 2008 led it to conclude that 'there was robust and consistent evidence for the efficacy of family intervention. When compared with standard care or any other control, there was a reduction in the risk of relapse with numbers needed to treat of 4.' There were also benefits to severity of symptoms for up to two years, and in reductions in hospital admission during the intervention. Some reasons for the difference between the reviews may be linked to the focus by Pharoah on studies with the most rigorous designs, not necessarily the best intervention processes. Hence one of the better studies, according to their ratings, was one conducted in Italy by Carrà and colleagues (2007) in which families were randomly allocated to join a weekly information group (IG), or to this plus family support meetings (IG + SG), against those receiving treatment as usual. Equal numbers (nearly 40% of each group) had high-EE homes at the start of the intervention, which achieved a significant reduction, with all 10 of the IG + SG high-EE families changing, half the IG families, and none of the control group. But the intervention produced only marginal reductions in relapse at 12 months, and no effects on admission to hospital at 12 or 24 months or in employment rates. However, only one person from the family home was targeted, and the individual with schizophrenia received only standard care. This is quite different from the family work in other studies that involves as many of the family as possible, including the patient, and is able to help them resolve issues of conflict between them.

A related issue that may explain some disappointing results is the circular process linking critical comments and over-involvement by relatives. That is, when a person is becoming unwell, their symptoms of psychosis increasing, the criticism of family members may also rise. This issue was discussed by Kanter and colleagues (1987), and most recently revisited in a reflective discussion by Kuipers and colleagues (2010). A follow-up over nine years of parental EE by Lenior and colleagues (2002) among families participating in a 15-month family programme suggests that emotional over-involvement is reduced by family intervention, but tends to increase again after about 34 months. Critical comments were less affected by their intervention, but more closely related to the severity of the disorder, suggesting an effect in the opposite direction – the individual influencing parental or partner behaviour.

As Kuipers and colleagues (2010) conclude, it suggests that there may need to be greater engagement with the differing situations and challenges of individual families. Family intervention is designed to help where EE is high, which often links with family sense of 'burden', their assumptions that the individual is in control of their behaviour, and feelings that their relative is 'to blame' for some negative events (Kuipers et al., 2010). An exacerbation of symptoms might thus reinforce such views and increase their criticism and over-involvement. Kuipers et al. describe three broad groups and their somewhat differing needs for support. The first are those where family relationships were previously warm and strong, where they recognize that the ill-health is the cause of the troubling behaviour, are receptive to outside efforts to help, are less likely to give up other roles to care full-time, are low EE and, while unlikely to be depressed, will still often be experiencing a good deal of stress and greatly value information, support and respite. The second group are those who tend toward over-protectiveness, feel guilty, blame themselves (so are most often parents), feel a strong sense of loss, and might devote themselves full-time to caring for their family member. In their case, information might not succeed in changing their concern, and intervention might be more productive if focused on helping the individual to gain employment or further education, or engage in other positive adult roles, and the relative too to re-establish social contact and activity outside the home – a life of their own.

The third and most common response is criticism and hostility to the individual, common where prior relationships were also poor, and the individual may have had a troubled adolescence, drug or alcohol misuse, and may be seen by the relative as to blame for their current difficulties rather than experiencing a mental illness. Hence a long untreated phase of psychosis may have occurred, with perhaps a dramatic incident leading to a first admission to hospital. Carers will not usually blame themselves, but may be angry, depressed, and feel helpless and stigmatized. They may be rejecting towards their family member, and not engage well with services, but if they do engage they are more likely to be receptive to information from other family carers than from service providers directly. Information can be very helpful to them if it enables them to understand that the psychotic symptoms are influencing the behaviour and beliefs of their family member – they are not simply badly behaved. An important focus of intervention for this group is the carers' own depression, pessimism and their relationship with the individual, as well as practical help with social difficulties, respite and ongoing emotional support.

Kuipers and colleagues (2010) reiterate the important role a supportive relationship can play in the course of psychosis, but note the complexity of family dynamics, past history and the difficulties experienced by each family member that shape this. They suggest that carers merit the attention of clinicians in their own right, but as the NICE (2010) review concludes, and the Carrà and colleagues (2007) study shows, the service user must also be part of the intervention. It seems likely that many studies have failed to address such complexity sufficiently to demonstrate the benefits that most expect to see, and some have demonstrated, from family work.

Avoiding abusive relationships

Early teenage years are typically the first steps towards establishing romantic relationships, hence the primary prevention of intimate partner violence and abuse needs to start from here. However, researchers in the US report that violence and abuse in relationships in mid-adolescence are often already well established – physical aggression, intimidation, coercion, or forced sex being part of 10–20% of relationships at a conservative estimate; far more than this if the definition is extended to include verbal and psychological abuse (Wolfe et al., 2003). Interviews with 1353 young people aged 13–17 years from eight schools by the NSPCC and Bristol University in the UK found the same. One in four girls (the same proportion as adult women) and one in five boys reported some form of physical abuse from their partner, and nearly three times as many experienced emotional abuse, such as 'being constantly checked up on' (Barter et al., 2009). Wolfe and colleagues note the association between adolescent dating violence and other risk factors for mental ill-health such as substance abuse and unsafe sex; the established link between experience of child maltreatment and current aggression in partnerships; and the poorer problem solving abilities of those with a maltreatment history; hence the importance of preventive intervention with this group.

A number of dating violence prevention programmes have been evaluated, usually assessing changes to attitude rather than behaviour, and without comparison groups. Three with a more rigorous evaluation are the *Youth Relationships Project, Safe Dates* and *FourthR*. The first of these (by Wolfe and colleagues, 2003) targeted high–risk young people – 14–16-year-old (mostly Caucasian) recipients of Youth and Child Protective Services (CPS) in Canada. These were 191 young people who had grown up in violent and abusive homes, 60% of whom were now living outside the family. Those who had criminal convictions (person, not property), developmental delays or were being treated for a mental health condition were excluded. The 18-session Youth Relationships Project included interactive videos, conflict resolution and communication skills, community visits to useful resources and relevant agencies, aiming to develop healthy, non-violent relationships through better recognition of abuse, the gender power relationships that support it, and their options if they experienced it. The mixed sex groups of six to ten young people who followed the programme were interviewed at periods over two years, and showed a greater decline in likelihood of involvement as victim or perpetrator in abusive relationships, as compared to the control group. The intervention group did not rate their relationship skills more highly than controls at the end of the programme, nor report less victimization, but did report perpetrating less emotional abuse. There were also significant improvements to the level of trauma symptoms in the intervention group compared to controls.

By contrast, Safe Dates is a school-based programme for all 14-year-olds – a play performed by students and 10 taught sessions of 45 minutes over a three-month period, finishing with a poster competition. Fourteen schools in North Carolina were involved in the research: half as participants, half as controls (Foshee et al., 2005). It aims to change gender role norms, violence norms and conflict management skills, and to raise awareness about when and how to seek help. Students completed questionnaires four times over the following three years, including ratings on frequency over the last year of a range of actions or experience with someone they had a date with (relating to bullying, intimidation, violence, forced sex), and opinions on when violence might be justified, and gender role expectations. The programme resulted in significantly less perpetration of abuse – psychological, moderate physical and sexual – and significantly less victimization in relation to moderate physical violence at all follow-up points, and a borderline significance in reduction of sexual victimization. More serious violence was not affected by the programme, nor was psychological victimization. The positive effects appeared to be mediated by changes to gender role norms, dating violence norms, and awareness of community services rather than improvements to conflict management.

Wolfe and colleagues (2003) debate the advantages and disadvantages of their targeted community-based approach as against the more common model of a universal school-based programme – the improved safety of participation of the former, the reduced stigma of the latter, and the difficulties in either approach of assessing actual behaviour in intimate relationships. They have recently reported the results of a two-year follow-up of their own universal violence prevention programme FourthR (Crooks et al., 2011). This suggests that the most high-risk children in fact benefit the most from a universal scheme. Ten Canadian schools delivered 21 75-minute lessons to 14-year-olds, with a focus on skill development through role play, some in gender segregated groups, while 10 delivered the standard school health and relationships programme. The focus was personal safety and injury prevention, healthy growth and sexuality, and substance use and abuse. Parents were kept informed of the content, and a student steering group oversaw developments.

Being violent at age 14 was a strong predictor of violence at 16; others were being male, experiencing child maltreatment, and attending a school where the whole student group rated the school low in sense of personal safety. Schools differed markedly on rates of delinquency, from 2% to 32%, and this variation was not due to the intervention. However, there was a significant interaction effect of experience of child maltreatment and intervention. That is, the more numerous were the damaging early experiences, the greater was the effect of the intervention on violent behaviour. Each additional form of child maltreatment increased the young person's risk of delinquency by 46% in control group schools, but had negligible effects in intervention schools. Youth reared in safe and predictable environments with the foundation for healthy non-violent relationships showed minimal difference in delinquency rate between conditions.

Both strategies may be needed – universal and targeted. The troubled history of those who go on to develop abusive adult relationships shown by these studies, and the consequences for their own mental health and that of their partner and children, mean that even modest success will have important long-term benefits. These include reducing the raised risk of physical abuse during pregnancy (with associated effects on intra-uterine growth and perinatal complications), and later child maltreatment. The prevalence of childhood abuse is increasingly recognized as substantially higher than suggested by official data – as high as 22% in a US national survey cited by Crooks et al. (2011). They argue that maltreated young people do not simply re-enact what they know, but have come to see relationships as between coercer and coerced, with emotions of fear, anger and mistrust, in which they struggle to regulate their own emotions and behaviour (Wolfe, 2006). They will benefit both from a 'safe' school environment and from programmes that help them develop the skills they need in negotiating the many challenges they face at this crucial stage in their lives.

Self-help

Finally, it should be noted that mutual help, so often emphasized as a crucial part of preventive programmes, is being fostered through both organized schemes such as the UK 'expert patient' programme, where those with similar health problems can meet and exchange information on best coping strategies, and through the worldwide web (Phillips, 2010). Numerous voluntary sector organizations and some individuals have also set up information websites, chat rooms and blogs, and these are widely used. They can help people feel less alone with the problems they face, reappraise their difficulties, give and receive heartfelt support, and find important information that can help with specific difficulties. For instance, over half of the women failing to conceive a child search the internet for information; many also exchange information and support in online chat rooms (Weissman et al., 2000). Evaluation of this type of provision is at early stages of development, but will no doubt bring important insights with time. The cost-effectiveness of the method is likely to lead to a rapid increase in these.

Conclusion

Those who seem resilient in the face of stressful experience in adult life are unlikely to have experienced severely traumatic events before, in either childhood or adulthood, and are more likely to have support in their lives now – someone who cares about them, who seems likely to be a good resource in times of trouble, who won't let them down, or draw attention to their need for support. They have effective coping skills. They prepare themselves in advance for predicted terrors, use problem-focused coping to avoid unnecessary risk, reflect on action that might help, have a strong locus of control, focus on staying calm, look for meaning in their situation and the opportunity behind the threat, compare themselves with others with greater problems, have optimistic personalities and connect with others, staying sociable.

Those who do not already have such good fortune can be helped to strengthen their resilience. They can be taught to re-evaluate life events through a more optimistic lens, to recognize their own strengths and plan to use them, to catch their tendency to negative thinking and try to moderate it. They are going to be more receptive to these offers of help when facing a crisis. But effective coping is undermined by negative relationships with those whose opinions the person might otherwise have valued. Examples of preventive interventions have shown benefits both for family work with those treated for schizophrenia who live with relatives to address such problems, and through befriending projects with those vulnerable to depression, particularly if these interventions also help an individual see the possibility of a 'fresh start'.

Hence helping people to move out of damaging relationships, or to find a new source of self-esteem, or to intervene to try to improve family relationships and destructive communication styles, can bring preventive benefit if targeted on those facing stressful life events or difficulties, particularly if they already have some symptoms of mental ill-health. The process of providing such help can easily undermine the individual's sense of control if not sufficiently skilful. To influence the extent of violence and intimidation in close relationships in young people setting out in life, there are promising indications for school-based programmes that aim to change the accepted gender role and dating violence norms of teenage behaviour.

8 Mind and body

In our renewed interest in the links between mind and body – a holistic approach to wellbeing – evident from a good deal of media coverage, as well as that by mental health support organizations, we are to some extent revisiting the thoughts on mental health of our forefathers. Porter's (1987) fascinating history of psychiatry in the past three centuries reminds us how for a long period, the source of the problems of the mind were seen to lie in the body (principally the heart or abdomen – the intestines), and therefore the solutions too (bleeding, enemas). Of course the links between nervousness and the workings of the intestines have long been recognized, though more commonly in the opposite direction – mind affecting body. Certain foods were thought to be damaging or beneficial to the mind; for example, Cheyne, writing between 1724 and 1743, believed that heavy eating was linked to heavy spirits, and depression sometimes the result of too much rich food. Cheyne's cure was milk and seeds.

Later, as the role of the spinal cord in linking the brain with the body was understood, the roles of the heart and the intestines were demoted. It was apparently William Cullen in 1769 who argued that all mental diseases are mediated through the nerves, and crucially he is the author of the term 'neurosis' to refer to those diseases of the nervous system without cause in the organs, deriving from the nervous system itself. Pupils of Cullen then argued that mania was a state of over-excitation of the nerves, melancholy under-excitement – hence mania needed sedatives (e.g. opium); melancholy needed stimulants (e.g. alcohol). Body and mind were for centuries seen as part of a continuum, and mild bodily disorder could give rise to particular types of mood, while more severe bodily dysfunction would be linked with insanity.

Porter also argues that, far from this being due to medical dominance, it was what ordinary people wished to believe. Then, as is often true now, many people would rather receive a somatic explanation for their ill-health than a psychological, imaginary or demonic one. They did not wish to be exposed to any dishonour, reproach or guilt by being in any way to blame, wanting an explanation that was morally, spiritually and medically acceptable. The 'somatisation of such disorders involved far more than the tactful stratagems of fashionable physicians. Sufferers themselves strove to attribute their own palpitations, tetchiness, morbid delusions, or mood swings to organic malady' (Porter, 1987: 56). 'In such circumstances, sympathetic doctors and patients tended to concur in a diagnosis that made such conditions "real" by basing them in the body, and "natural" so as to minimize personal responsibility, guilt and shame' (Porter, 1987: 57). Goldberg (1992) has argued that this is often true today, noting how videotapes of discussions in general practice often show a level of collusion to keep the focus as 'non-psychological' as possible. While this means that much depression in primary care goes undetected, patients are often satisfied with such consultations, as the physical examination shows their problems are taken seriously, they may receive analgesics or anti-inflammatory drugs or antacids that can provide some sympto-matic relief, and a psychiatric label or the need for either of them to engage with distressing personal circumstances is avoided.

Porter (1987) explains how once the key role of the brainstem was recognized, and the connection between the body parts and the brain seen as some way akin to electrical impulses, the possibility of mania and melancholy to become a specialist field for nerve and brain experts, later known as neurologists, emerged. These specialists then had to decide how much of the bodily responses could be actively controlled by the mind, and how much was unconscious and automatic. Clearly some bodily actions – blushing, sexual responsiveness – fell between the two, and speech defects and obsessive behaviour were also seen to fall in this category. Porter explains that this all helpfully continued to somatize mental processes, and had implications for maintaining health – people needed to keep these nerves in good health, strung neither too loosely nor too tight – and it gave a new language and thinking to inform the mind–body debate, mental disorders became real diseases, and language was now about nervous disorder, not disorders due to vapors, or the spleen. By the late nineteenth century neurophysiology was fully established.

Links between the health of the body and the health of the brain are regaining their place in mental health debates in the West. While Chinese medicine did not lose its emphasis on the need for an equilibrium between the person and their environment, Western medicine has for some time been far less holistic, often searching for the physical causal agent that is disrupting the efficiency of an other-wise smooth-running machine (Lovallo, 2005). Since the late 1960s, however, 'bio-behavioural medicine' has featured more strongly, and in the 1970s the speciality of health psychology emerged. It is now understood that, for instance, keeping calm will lower blood pressure, recognized that it might be possible that a positive attitude will speed recovery from physical disorder, that what we eat may affect our behaviour, that stress affects everything.

This chapter touches on just a few of these complex and often contentious issues, showing first the strong relationship between physical and mental ill-health, then describing the principles of a bio-behavioural model of the effects of stressful experience, essentially the biological mechanisms linked to the coping and support processes described in the previous chapter. Some evidence is then discussed that ill-health can be reduced by

a   mental strategies such as building positive expectations, or calming emotions through meditation
b   physical health promotion strategies such as a healthy diet, or exercise.

Mental and physical ill-health often coexist

Raised rates of depression are commonly found in surveys of people with diabetes, arthritis, HIV, cancer, stroke, multiple sclerosis, coronary heart disease, and many other types of physical disorder (van Straten et al., 2010). The UK National Psychiatric Morbidity Survey found that 7% of those without a chronic illness had significant psychiatric morbidity on the CIS-r, compared to 20% of those with one of the 11 named conditions, and 35% of those with more than one (Cooke et al., 2007). Taking the figures the other way around from the earlier UK survey, they found that 58% of their population sample of 8575 adults who had a neurotic disorder also had a longstanding physical complaint, compared to 38% of people with no mental disorder (Singleton et al., 2001). The prevalence of musculo-skeletal disorders, digestive disorders, respiratory problems, genito-urinary problems and skin problems were all double among those with a neurotic disorder compared to those without. People with a 'probable psychosis' had raised rates of heart and circulatory system problems and nervous system complaints. By contrast, those misusing drugs or alcohol did not have raised rates of physical disorder, though the authors speculate that this may have been due in part to their younger age (Singleton et al., 2001).

A large-scale cross-national WHO survey in 17 countries of the coexistence of somatic and psychiatric ill-health confirms this picture (Scott et al., 2009) – the majority of people with chronic physical conditions and pain do not have depression or anxiety, but a disproportionate number do. They also found that mental disorder tended to be more disabling than physical disorder, and the disabling effects for those with both was greater than would be predicted from adding the effects of each. They speculate on what biological, behavioural or psychological processes may explain these results – perhaps an underlying shared patho-physiology through the autonomic nervous system and neuro-endocrine system. Or it could be the effect of one disorder on the other – some of the biological effects of depression making the development of diabetes more likely, and then the emergence of diabetes worsening the depression through its effects on life-style changes required. A third possibility is that depressive symptoms may mean the person takes less care of their physical health, adheres less well to medication regimes, leads a less healthy lifestyle, and has a lower expectation of being able to cope. Finally, it may simply be that once the physical disorder reaches a severe level, the mental health problems are a natural result. The full analysis of their results leads them to argue that many of the psycho-social factors linked to mental ill-health, such as childhood adversity and adolescent depression, also raise the probability of chronic physical disorder such as asthma, hypertension, diabetes and arthritis (Von Korff et al., 2009).

Stegmann and colleagues (2010) interviewed a large sub-sample from the WHO study, to explore the role of functional disability – assessed on number of days completely unable, or able with great difficulty, to work or perform normal activities in the past 30 days. Arthritis was the most prevalent of the chronic disorders assessed, and was also the disorder most strongly associated with depression (doubling risk). Arthritis, heart disease and stomach/duodenal ulcers were the three disorders with the strongest effect on functional disability (OR of 2.2, 2.3 and 2.0 respectively for days out of role, whereas no other disorder had an OR higher than 1.5), hence they argue that functional disability is likely to contribute substantially to the link between depression and painful chronic conditions and heart disease. By contrast, allergies and diabetes did not seem to be independently linked to depression, but linked via their association with other long-term conditions.

While the explanations may still be contested, the evidence of the existence of a link between mental and physical ill-health is increasing. For instance, in relation to diabetes and dementia, Velayudhan and colleagues (2010) prospectively followed up 103 primary care patients aged over 65 years, who were identified, and confirmed through further testing, as having a mild cognitive impairment. Of those they successfully followed up for four years, 19 developed dementia. Comparing those with (16%) and without (84%) diabetes, they found that the former were three times more likely to be in the group that developed dementia during the follow-up period.

A prospective 10-year study of 388 people being treated for depression and 404 matched community controls showed that the former group experienced a significantly higher number of both severe and trivial physical disorders during this period (Holahan et al., 2010). It also seems that depression lasts longer among those with long-term physical ill-health (Huijbregts et al., 2010), and the course of physical disorder can be worsened by the depression (Hermanns, 2010).

A bio-behavioural model: Stress, social support and immunity

Prominent among most explanations of the association of mental and physical ill-health is the role of life events and long-term stressful experience, and the effects of associated stress hormones. The negative consequences of stressful life experience for physical as well as mental ill-health are well established (see for example Brown and Harris, 1989); so too the role of negative emotions. For instance, Everson and colleagues (1996) have shown that negative emotions (particularly a sense of hopelessness) put people at much higher risk of death from all causes, including violent death and injury. A cohort of 2428 men in Finland completed questionnaires relating to a sense of hopelessness about the future, grouped according to their low, medium or high scores, and showing that six years later scores related in a dose–response fashion to likelihood of death.

Lovallo (2005) attempts a synthesis of the bodily and mental processes, starting with a description of the nervous system and the hierarchical system of processing stressful experience, the top being the cortex and the limbic system, through the hypothalamus, the brainstem, the autonomic systems, to the normally self-regulating tissues of the bodily organs. Although there is a two-way communication between these, higher levels can override the lower levels. For instance, the need for the heart to pump more quickly as the person is planning a sprint derives from higher level decisions, and though the level of blood circulating is perfectly adequate for the present resting state according to all lower level information feedback, the cerebral cortex is the area where conscious decisions can be made that something different is required of the organs, and is the first-level explanation of how the mind affects the body.

Lovallo discusses four stages in our response to stress, two as proposed by the cognitive model of Lazarus and Folkman (1984): that we first evaluate events for their threat value, and second we consider our available coping options; his additions emphasize our emotional response to that evaluation, and associated physiological effects in terms of immune system function and blood pressure increase. Our pre-existing beliefs and our commitment to action contribute substantially to this process (see Figure 8.1). Coping involves thoughts, emotions and action, and both our thoughts about the coping options, and our initial appraisal of the threat of the event, influence the autonomic, endocrine and immune system responses.

Figure 8.1 illustrates some of the many potential contributors to the biological processing of stressful experience: our socio-cultural environment and past history helping to shape how we think about the stressor and what we do. For instance, an appraisal of the significance of a burglary will include judgements about likely police response, being insured, being able to take time off work to repair the locks, as well as prior experience – numbers of previous times it has happened, fear of personal harm, and what has been lost. The social and personal context affects cognitive appraisal; our appraisal affects our emotional and behavioural responses; our responses, particularly emotional responses, affect our physical and mental

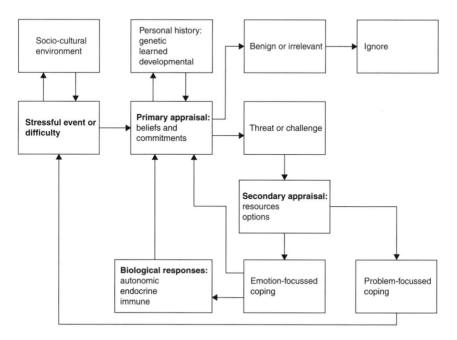

Figure 8.1 Expanded model of the stress response process, adapted (with permission) from Lovallo (2005) and Lazarus and Folkman (1984).

health. While social scientists might define stress in terms of environmental demands that exceed a person's perceived ability to cope, a biologist might define it as a stimulus that activates the hypothalamic–pituitary–adrenal (HPA) axis and/ or the sympathetic nervous system (SNS) to enable a person to adapt physiologically to deal with the threat. Behavioural medicine integrates these approaches and is 'the study of how sociocultural and mind–brain processes can influence the health of an individual' (Lovallo, 2005: 25).

Hence stress results in a response from the immune, endocrine and cardiovascular systems, and while short-term stress has no adverse effects on immunity, stress that is long lasting, triggering continued low-level immune responses, can interfere with the primary role of the immune system – as a response to the presence of antigen. Many people know too well from experience that stress can allow a latent herpes simplex virus to resurface, which is a commonly chosen outcome by stress researchers (see Martin, 1998; Lovallo, 2005). Cohen and colleagues (1998) demonstrated the effects of stress on catching a cold – people volunteering to take part in their study of the common cold were more likely to develop symptoms in response to nose drops containing the virus if they were coping with stressful experiences that had been going on some time, of which unemployment or underemployment (work-related difficulties) and difficulties with relatives or friends lasting more than a month were most potent (see Figure 8.2).

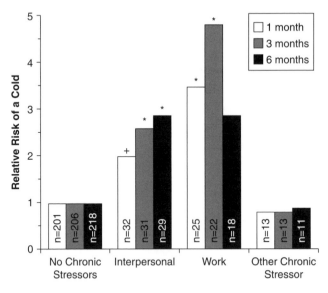

Figure 8.2 Relative risks (odds ratio adjusted for standard controls) of developing a cold, contrasting persons with interpersonal, work, and other chronic stressors with those with no chronic stressors. The odds ratios are derived from separate analyses using the 'at least one month', 'at least 3 months' and 'at least 6 months' criteria for chronic stressors. Sample sizes are indicated inside each bar. * $p < 0.05$, + $p < 0.15$. From Cohen et al. (1998) (used with permission).

In other words, there seem to be a number of interactions between the immune system and stress-related mechanisms, so much so that Lovallo argues they are expressions of the same bio-behavioural process. So our state of health and immune function affects our emotions and behaviour, and vice versa – our emotions and cognitions affect the immune system (see Figure 8.1). Lovallo points out that traditional Western medicine would not have considered this possibility before these bio-behavioural models became more acceptable. The two-way direction of the arrows between the social environment and events, and between personal history and the appraisal process, also contrasts with the traditional medical model illustrated in Figure 4.1.

The study of the effects of stress on the way the central nervous system, endocrine and immune systems interact has been named psycho-neuroimmunology (PNI). PNI research has developed rapidly over the past two decades, establishing clearly that chronic stress has negative effects on immunity. Evidence comes from humans and animals given infections or vaccines in experimental studies, or in naturalistic comparisons of those living (or not living) in stressful circumstances such as caring for a seriously ill partner, and of humans already carrying a latent infection. For instance, people with HIV progressed more rapidly to AIDS when they had a high number of stressful events or low social support, and people with latent herpes virus were more likely to suffer a re-emergence of the virus under a variety of stressful conditions, from examination preparation to caring for a relative with dementia (see Glaser and Kiecolt-Glaser, 2005, for a review). The same stressful situations have been shown to link to slower healing from minor skin wounds. Hence, one important preventive implication that arises is for the recovery of surgical patients. Pre-surgical intervention that helps reduce the stress and anxiety of the experience has been found from a large number of studies to provide benefits in terms of fewer post-operative complications, better treatment compliance, and less pain (Kiecolt-Glaser et al., 1998), though presumably changes to all other contributors to stress and support apart from the surgery itself would be even more beneficial.

Glaser and Kiecolt-Glaser (2005) explain how stress-related immune disregulation might be a core mechanism behind a diverse range of health outcomes, emphasizing the role of inflammation. One of the secondary effects of the 'stress' hormones once the immune system is activated is the production of cytokines, some of which have a pro-inflammatory and some an anti-inflammatory action to promote or moderate the immune response. Although inflammation is an essential immune response to injury, continuous chronic low-grade inflammation in response to chronic stress represents a disregulation of the system. To take just one pro-inflammatory cytokine that is frequently explored in its link to stress and depression – interleukin-6 (IL-6) – this also plays an important role in cardiovascular disease through its role in promoting the production of C-reactive protein (CRP). In fact raised levels of IL-6 and CRP play a pathogenic role in a range of diseases associated with aging, including arthritis, osteoporosis and congestive heart failure, suggesting that the role of chronic stress and depression in physical disorder is more important in old age (see Kiecolt-Glaser et al., 2002). Both physical and mental stressors increase its production, as do depression, anxiety and disturbed sleep.

IL-6 is also raised in carers of a family member with dementia. Anisman and colleagues (2008) suggest that inflammatory effects of stress may also explain the comorbidity of depression with degenerative disorders such as Alzheimer's and Parkinson's diseases as well as cardiovascular pathology. In addition, existing depression has been found to be a significant risk factor for both Alzheimer's and Parkinson's diseases, and both anxiety and depression to increase the likelihood that mild cognitive impairment will progress to Alzheimer's disease (see Anisman et al., 2008). The active treatment of anxiety and depression in those with mild cognitive impairment or dementia is an obvious recommendation arising.

Stressful experience and dampened immunity do not necessarily lead to either mental or physical ill-health, of course. A further complication is that stress can produce symptoms and no pathology, as Creed (2000) illustrates. Among his evidence is some of his own research from the 1980s with young women undergoing appendectomy, an operation that not infrequently revealed a normal appendix, despite there being no other physical symptoms to explain the abdominal pain. Drawing from interviews with the patients before surgery (hence 'blind' to outcome), he found that 60% of those who turned out to have no inflammation in the appendix had experienced a severely threatening life event in the nine months leading up to surgery, compared to 25% of those with confirmed appendicitis and 20% of the healthy comparison group. He noted other studies with similar findings relating to various diagnoses for which the symptoms were stomach pain – irritable bowel syndrome, peptic ulcer, colitis – and noted that 'The commonest difficulties in all these groups concerned close relationships' (Creed, 2000: 277). This link with symptoms of physical disorder held whether or not the women were also depressed.

Events related to personal relationships also feature in many types of confirmed pathology. In a prospective study of psycho-social risk factors and dementia among a random sample of 70-year-olds followed up until they were 79, Persson and Skoog (1996) were able to compare the 38 who by this time had been diagnosed with dementia with the 326 other people in the sample on 18 lifetime and recent events in their lives collected at time 1. Death of a parent before age 16, arduous manual work for a large part of their adult life, physical illness in their partner or serious illness in a child after the age of 65 made independent contributions to risk of dementia, and risks increased for those with more than one of these. Twenty per cent of people with three or more of the risk factors developed dementia, compared to 3% with none, 8% with one or two. They note that such findings need replication before further conclusions could be drawn. However, there is much evidence to support the role of close relationships in all kinds of ill-health. To take one example, the existence of a good level of perceived support among 298 people successfully treated for a recent cardiac problem with angioplasty was seen by Helgeson (2003) to mediate the perceived control, positive expectations of the future and positive views of self that appeared to explain significantly lower risk of further cardiac events over the following four years. Furthermore, the reviews by Kiecolt-Glaser and colleagues (2002) confirm that the chronic stress linked to disruption of immune responses via inflammatory processes is most often associated with close relationships – raised in discordant relationships, low in close supportive relationships – arguing that the link between social relationships and immune function is one of the most robust findings of psycho-neuroimmunology.

If emotional responses to chronic stress raise blood pressure and reduce immunity, and there is a two-way process between experience and health, should we presume that raised blood pressure and reduced immunity may make us feel stressed or affect our behaviour? There are two other important implications of pursuing this integration between biology, thinking and emotion. First that many physical as well as mental disorders might be improved through psychological means: behavioural and cognitive therapies, for instance. Second that if stressful events produce negative outcomes for physical and mental health, then there may be scope for positive events and positive emotions to produce positive outcomes. Cohen and colleagues (2003) show that this may well be the case in a repeat of their experiment using the cold virus and measuring positive emotional style.

Further, might physical health and fitness affect emotions, thinking and mental health, and might this also be a two-way process? We know for instance that one of the consequences of depression is that depressed people get less sleep, take less exercise, eat less healthy food, smoke more, drink more alcohol and use more drugs, and all of these behaviours contribute to lowered health and immunity (Martin, 1998).

Exploring the evidence in relation to positive expectations, however, is fraught with difficulty given the challenges in disentangling which factors bring the necessary effects.

Mind affecting body

The placebo effect

Meditation or exercise might well be justified by the bio-behavioural model above, but there is already very strong evidence that positive expectation is a large component of why any treatment works. The 'placebo effect' is one of the best known and clearest examples of how the mind can heal the body. The expectation that a pill, exercise or other intervention such as meditation might improve health is often enough on its own to generate some benefit. Hence experimental studies to test the benefits of an active compound or other treatment must control for positive expectations on the part of both those taking it and those providing it created by participation in the experiment itself. A comparison group is required of those who take an inactive substance or an assumed ineffective therapy that is physically indistinguishable from the active compound by recipient and provider, so that neither knows which are receiving the active treatment – a so-called 'double blind' control trial.

Placebo effects can in some cases be as great as the active medication for up to a third of participants (e.g. Benson and McCallie, 1979, discuss effects on angina, cited by Lovallo, 2005: 18), and have been known to last for up to a year. As Lovallo notes, these are impressive benefits for an inactive compound. Others have argued, however, that on average the effect size of a placebo is relatively small: one calculation by a review of a review is that it is about 0.14, something in the order of one third as effective as an anti-inflammatory drug on painful arthritis but greater than the effect of cardiac patient education on exercise (Hunsley and Westmacott, 2007). However, as noted below, many factors influence the strength of its effect.

Martin (1998) notes the research that has shown that placebo medicines work better if their psychological importance is increased by injecting them rather than swallowing them, and that in tablet form, colour, size and shape make a difference. Such information is important for pharmaceutical companies, of course. As Kaptchuk and colleagues (2008) have shown, its effects also come through the traditional clinician–patient relationship. In a large prospective study with patients with painful irritable bowel syndrome, they compared sham acupuncture (needles inserted but into non-valid acupuncture sites) with sham acupuncture plus warm, friendly discussions with the acupuncturist before the insertion of needles. The latter brought much greater improvement (to symptom severity and quality of life at three weeks) as compared with the former, which in turn resulted in more improvement than that experienced by the waiting list control group. The discussions followed a script, avoiding any recognized therapy, but asking about lifestyle, symptoms, meaning, and offering sympathy and encouragement that the treatment (sham acupuncture) should work (Kaptchuk et al., 2008). This suggests that it is not just being offered a ritualized type of treatment with a positive expectation that it will work that creates a placebo effect, but also the interaction with the therapist.

The more powerful and convincing the proponent of the method, the more likely and the more powerful will be the placebo effect. Our socio-cultural background will also contribute to these expectations. In the West, we know there are strict controls on the development, licensing and supply of new medication, and we believe that doctors choose from those available the one presumed to have the most benefit for our particular condition. Our trust in our doctors is very important to their ability to help us.

To emphasize this point, a study by Benedetti and colleagues in 2003 provoked great interest, when they used hospitalized patients to investigate the effects of medication given (or discontinued) for post-operative pain, anxiety or Parkinson's symptoms in open and hidden conditions. That is, there was no placebo, just a comparison between medication given face to face by the doctor, and that given intravenously by machine without the knowledge of the patient or the physical presence of the doctor. The difference in the effectiveness of the medication was significant, though it varied by drug in the extent of the difference. (Effects were measured over a few hours only, by patient diary and electronic sensors of hand movements (for Parkinson's).) The results suggest that the term 'placebo effect' can be misleading, as it is not the placebo that brings the effect, but the expectations created by the treatment process.

In other words, not only is a placebo made more effective by a positive doctor–patient interaction, the colour, shape and brand name of the pill, or the ceremony of the treatment process, but so too is the power of the active treatment. Similarly, any negative expectations created during the treatment process can have adverse effects. Screening people and telling them they are at raised risk of a disorder, or that they have high blood pressure, can increase resting blood pressure when tested later, and increase responsiveness to mild stress (faster heart rate, higher adrenaline levels) as compared to hypertensive people not so informed (Martin, 1998). This is also true for those told their pain relief medication is about to be reduced. They experience a greater, more rapid increase in pain than when the reduction is done without informing them (Benedetti et al., 2003; see above).

One additional complication is that there are also likely to be some unconscious conditioned responses to some treatments. Those going for a therapy that has made them physically sick will know how the queasiness can begin just before the next dose is delivered. Animal experiments have demonstrated the 'conditioned response' more powerfully. Lovallo describes a study of rats given an immuno-suppressant drug, and at the same time a saccharine drink – a novel taste for the rat. At a later time, after the immune system recovered, the rat was given a saccharine drink again, but no drug, resulting in a similar suppression of the immune system (Ader and Cohen, 1993, cited in Lovallo, 2005: 19). Some tentative evidence of such conditioned effects has been found in humans, but studies in this field are few (Kiecolt-Glaser et al., 2002b).

Positive thinking and meditation

Hence we know that positive expectations can be therapeutic, that these are established by the treatment process itself, that our interactions with clinicians or close others can strengthen or weaken those expectations, and that most medical treatments use the double blind randomized control trial to try to control for these effects; hence the challenge in separating the various sources of positive expectation for those aiming to evaluate interventions intended to enhance these effects.

In addition, the bio-behavioural model suggests that it may be possible to exercise some conscious self-control over these expectations, or our emotion-focused coping with all types of stress including that associated with pain and physical ill-health, through hypnosis, relaxation, exercise, prayer or meditation. While not often framed in terms of building optimism, they do provide methods to reduce pessimism and anxiety, or to reduce the attention given to the potential negative outcomes. 'Mindfulness' falls into the latter category, and is claimed to be helpful to a person with depression in teaching them strategies to diminish the significance of their negative thoughts, and their tendency to dwell on them (rumination). Mindfulness meditation is an ancient Buddhist practice, aimed at reducing anguish (Ramel et al., 2004), which Jon Kabat-Zinn developed and brought into his medical practice at the Massachusetts Stress Reduction Clinic as a treatment for chronic pain and stress-related disorders. It is 'about paying attention to your own inner experience by quieting the mind' (Kabat-Zinn, 2005: 23).

Participants are instructed to attend to a bodily sensation, or breathing, and to notice thoughts and feelings that arise, but without becoming absorbed in their content. For instance, the thought, 'I am useless at this' would be noted as a judgemental thought, but not pursued. Ramel and colleagues (2004) evaluated a course delivered in the way advised by Kabat-Zinn – eight weeks of two-hour weekly sessions, one half-day of meditation, and daily 'homework' of 30 or 45 minutes' meditation, run for 23 people with a history of depression. They found some limited benefit in reducing rumination, though their subjects did not comply well with the requested homework tasks. Davidson, with Kabat-Zinn and colleagues (2003), evaluated a similar programme but also measuring brain activity and immune function of the trained group compared to a randomized wait list control group, tested before and after the eight weeks, and four months later, and were able to show significant differences, including antibody response to a flu vaccine.

However, much of the research in this field is unsophisticated in methodology, or small scale, with before and after measures, and any control groups included are simply those that do not receive the meditation training. Hofmann and colleagues (2010) found 39 studies evaluating the benefits of mindfulness in coping in the acute phase of a range of conditions, including cancer, anxiety and depression, showing consistently clear but modest effect sizes pre- and post-training that were maintained in three to six month follow-ups. Most studies did not have comparison groups; none were randomized controls. Ledesma and Kumano (2009) also reached cautiously positive conclusions from examining 10 studies of the use of mindfulness training to assist the psycho-social adjustment of cancer patients. But only three studies had randomized controls, and all control group subjects knew they were not receiving the intervention.

A religious faith can be a resource for emotion-focused coping: the calm atmosphere of the church, silent prayer or meditation, perhaps lowering physiological stress responses, the services perhaps helping to foster a sense of hope, love and forgiveness (Cornah, 2006). Some religions actively discourage negative emotions such as anger or fear. Martin (1998) discusses meditation and prayer along with techniques for relaxation and argues that these techniques can relieve pain as well as distress, and if used to achieve a deep sense of relaxation will bring a fall in blood pressure, pulse rate and breathing rate – the opposite of what happens in response to stress. By linking these skills with a stimulus, such as a mantra, imagined scene or music, the stimulus can act like a trigger for a conditioned response to bring the benefits more easily with repetition. Martin draws on several studies, including one with medical students preparing for an important examination (repeated with a sample of older people), which showed that those taught a hypnotic relaxation technique over a one-month period had a higher proportion of helper T-lymphocytes (which play a key role in attacking antigens inside cells) in their blood than those who did not relax (see Martin, 1998).

Body affecting mind

Exercise

Similar claims are made about the psychological benefits of exercise, and again, there is evidence to support them. While physical improvement to muscle tone, cardiac function, weight and immunity are well established, so too is the fact that exercise can bring improvements in self-esteem, mood and sleep, and these in turn can contribute to effectiveness at work and in sexual relationships and to feelings of being in control. The exercise should be regular and not too intensive, as excessive physical exercise can produce negative effects (Martin, 1998).

The physical benefits of regular moderate exercise derive in part from its effects in lowering blood pressure, improving levels of HDL cholesterol (the 'protective' cholesterol), reducing insulin resistance and improving glucose metabolism, improving endothelial function and, in turn, blood circulation. Lack of exercise contributes substantially to chronic diseases, particularly coronary heart disease, colon cancer, diabetes, stroke and breast cancer (DH, 2004). But the mental health effects are more complex. Reviews by Donaghy (2007), Wipfli and colleagues (2008) and the DH (2004) find more evidence for its therapeutic value, than its preventive potential. They discuss likely benefits as including various psychological, social and physiological factors, and show that studies that used another therapy as one of their comparison groups often found that an exercise programme provided equal benefits (including CT, group meditation, group therapy, medication; see Donaghy, 2007). Wipfli and colleagues (2008) make the same claim from their review of the benefits of exercise for the treatment of anxiety, finding that it can sometimes have greater effects than more traditional anxiety reduction treatments. But the prospective studies identified by these reviewers found that those who exercised were less depressed, and as such provide little insight into the likely role of the exercise, as in almost all cases the many possible alternative explanations that one can easily imagine for such results could not be ruled out by the study designs. The conclusions to date appear to support the suggestion that exercise helps people feel better about themselves, is potentially an important component of treatment, but plays a limited role in prevention (DH, 2004).

The type of evidence for the role of exercise in the prevention of depression is also found in relation to dementia; that is, mainly from prospective cohort studies. A systematic review by Hamer and Chida (2009) found 16 such studies involving a total of 163,797 people in whom exercise habits had been assessed. Of these, 3219 had developed dementia during the follow-up period (Alzheimer's, other dementias, or Parkinson's disease), which was from 5 to 21 years later. They judged five of the dementia/Alzheimer's studies to be of good quality, and both Parkinson's studies, concluding from these that regular moderate exercise (the most active subgroup as compared to the least active) reduces risk of Alzheimer's disease by 45%, and has a lesser effect on other dementias (28%) and Parkinson's (18%). Their speculation on process is primarily in terms of physiological effects: vascular health improves oxygen supply to the brain (through lower blood pressure, lower lipids, lower weight, inflammatory markers and endothelial function); possibly also through reducing amyloid β plaques; or increasing neurotrophic factors; or that the anti-inflammatory effects of exercise are important.

Mental health service users surveyed by national MIND in the UK, along with the general public, felt that exercise benefited their mental health, but preferred walking to lift their mood rather than aerobic exercise (Baker, 2001). However, as a therapy for depression, Dunn and colleagues (2005) argue that its effectiveness is increased by higher levels of energy expenditure (though it seemed unimportant whether people exercise three times or five times a week). Their four treatment groups and one control group were a randomized controlled design, but showed some of the challenges in this type of research, as it was clear that the placebo subjects quickly knew they were the control group, and several dropped out immediately. The Department of Health in the UK recommends (the public health dose) 'a total of at least 30 minutes a day of at least moderate intensity physical activity on five or more days of the week' (DH, 2004: iii). The US adds to this an energy expenditure requirement of 17.5 kcal/kg per week. Given the positive service user view, clear physical benefits and low cost, general practitioners have been encouraged to consider exercise 'prescriptions' alongside, or instead of, prescribing medication for common mental health conditions (DH, 2004).

An intriguing experiment by Crum and Langer (2007) suggests that the benefit from exercising is primarily due to its placebo effects on one's 'mindset'. They studied 84 mostly Hispanic women working as room attendants in seven hotels in the US, who cleaned an average of 15 rooms a day, working 32–40 hours a week. All completed the same assessments, including body-mass index (BMI), waist–hip ratio (WHR), blood pressure (BP) and lifestyle questionnaires, and were told they were participating in a study designed to improve their health and happiness. Despite far exceeding the recommended levels of exercise in their physically demanding employment, two-thirds of them initially responded that they did not exercise regularly, and more than one in three that they did not exercise at all. Women working in four of the hotels were given information to explain that their work is good exercise, and posters were put in the staff lounge to this effect. Four weeks later, the informed group adjusted their perception of the amount of exercise they got, though not reporting any actual change to their lifestyle, workload or exercise, either in work or out. They had also lost an average of two pounds in weight, lowered their systolic BP by 10 points, and body-fat, BMI and WHR were also significantly improved compared to the control group. The researchers suggest that greater attention should be given to helping people change their mindset.

Diet

Finally – does what we eat affect our cognitive functioning or emotional response to stress? Certainly our Western diet has changed dramatically over the past 50 years or so, with a sharp rise in consumption of processed food, and food high in sugar, trans fats, saturated fats, omega 6 fatty acids and chemical additives, and a reduced intake of omega 3, unprocessed grains, nuts, fruit, vegetables and legumes. The change in farming methods and use of pesticides is also changing the nutritional content of what we eat. For instance, according to data presented by Crawford (2007), compared to a chicken eaten in 1870, those we eat today have twice as many calories, five times as much fat, and about three quarters the amount of protein.

Drawing on the National Food Survey by the UK government, and its more recent equivalents, Van de Weyer (2006) traces the weekly consumption of food since 1942. These show a 34% reduction in consumption of vegetables (apparently less than 15% of us now manage to eat our recommended five portions a day), and a 59% reduction in our fish consumption. We eat half as many eggs, and use much less milk, and increasingly (particularly younger people) buy ready prepared meals. We eat on average 44 kg of sugar each per year, which is too much, but less than we consumed in the early 1960s when the figure was 53 kg. Similar data is available from many other countries, also revealing a marked increase in consumption of meat and alcohol across the Western world.

Concerns raised relate not only to the rapidly rising prevalence of obesity and diabetes, but also to potential effects on early brain development, violence in children and adults, and the health of the aging brain. For instance, food additives and specific food intolerance have been linked to children's hyperactivity; low intake of vitamin B to aging and brain shrinkage; a high ratio of omega 6 to omega 3 in the diet to inflammatory disorders and depression; and a range of dietary factors to offending and violence. Early campaigners such as Michael Crawford warned 30 years ago that the dramatic rise in heart disease in the West would soon be followed by a rise in mental ill-health, as the nutrients required for a healthy brain are the same as those needed for a healthy heart (Lang, 2006), and many argue that this is what is now happening (e.g. Hallahan and Garland, 2005).

For instance, Richardson (2007) explains the significance of the changed balance of omegas 6 and 3. Both of these essential fatty acids (linoleic acid (LA) – omega 6; alpha-linolenic acid (ALA) – omega 3) are major parts of the structure and function of the brain (and the structure of the eye), essential for the fluidity of cell membranes, for signalling, and for brain growth and connectivity. It has been estimated that our diet hundreds of years ago would have provided us with close to a 1:1 ratio of omega 3 (derived mainly from oily fish) to omega 6 (consumed in soy and numerous other now common food types), but that the Western diet now provides anything from 1:10 to 1:20 (Crawford et al., 2009). They cannot be manufactured by the body, but must be consumed in food. The conversion of omega 3 into the highly unsaturated fatty acids (HUFAs) required by the brain can be blocked both by excessive consumption of other fats – omega 6, saturated fats, hydrogenated fats and trans fatty acids – or by a lack of other contributors to its synthesis such as zinc, magnesium and manganese, and vitamins A, B3, B6 and C. Hormones released in response to stress can also impede the synthesis of the essential fatty acids, while alcohol and smoking can reduce them in the body (Richardson, 2007).

International comparison data has been presented by Hibbeln et al. (2006), showing that people in Iceland and Japan have markedly higher intakes of omega 3 than almost all other countries, and very significantly lower rates of death from coronary heart disease, stroke and homicide, and strikingly low rates of major depression, post-partum depression and bipolar disorder. They are convinced that these two facts are linked, and suggest that the Western world needs not only to increase fish consumption, but also to significantly decrease consumption of omega 6 (for example, using less soybean and sunflower oil). They have conducted numerous studies showing benefits of higher levels of fish consumption to the brain at all life stages. Starting with the developing foetus, they draw on a cohort study of over 14,000 pregnant women in SW England and the children born to them in 1992, and the questionnaire responses collected about fish and seafood consumption at 32 weeks' gestation (Hibbeln et al., 2007). The performance and behaviour of the children was then assessed through school and health check data over ensuing years. Comparing three groups – children of mothers who did not eat any seafood or fish, those who ate 1–340 g per week, and those who ate more than this – showed that the third group had superior performance (the greatest difference being to verbal IQ at age 8, OR 1.48 highest to lowest fish consumption group) with those eating the least fish having the lowest scores. The consumption of fish was also significantly associated with measures of disadvantage (education and housing) and other confounding variables like smoking and breast feeding, and although these were controlled statistically with regression analyses, it is less easy to see the effects of these than if data on comparable subgroups had been presented, where like could be compared with like.

However, further support comes from a similar cohort study in Denmark by Oken and colleagues (2008). They followed up 25,446 children and repeated the questions about maternal fish intake during pregnancy with mothers. They also showed child development benefits at age 18 months of the highest versus the lowest quintile of fish consumption by the mothers, a finding that held both among those breast feeding for a lengthy period and those who breastfed for a very short time or not at all.

Among adults, the evidence of benefit of high intake of omega 3 is good in relation to depression, schizophrenia and aggressive behaviour. Freeman, Hibbeln and colleagues (2006) find that seven of the eight randomized control trials they examined showed a benefit of supplements for depression; Harbottle and Schonfelder (2008) find 10 good-quality randomized control trials (including two tryptophan studies, four omega 3 studies and one zinc study), noting the largely positive findings on depression, but remaining cautious about the quality of the evidence. A recent double blind randomized placebo control trial in Vienna, with young people (aged 13–25) at ultra-high risk for psychosis (defined numbers and types of psychotic symptoms), found that supplements of omega 3 helped prevent transition to a full psychotic episode – only two of the 40 omega 3 treated group developed a full psychosis within 12 months, compared to 11 of 40 in the control group (Amminger et al., 2010). This is an important finding, with just four people needing to be treated to prevent one transition to psychosis – a similar level of effectiveness to anti-psychotic medication – and must warrant further study.

Other positive reports include a double blind RCT of the benefits of supplements of polyunsaturated fatty acids (PUFAs), vitamins and minerals to young (18–21-year-old) male prisoners, in terms of reduced aggressive behaviour over nine months (Gesch et al., 2002). Personal testimony of teachers of disturbed children is also persuasive in describing the substantial improvements in behaviour of children involved in an omega 3 trial (see minutes of the meeting of 18 April, Associate Parliamentary Food and Health Forum, 2007).

In fact, data from numerous surveys and cohort studies supports the benefit to mental functioning of higher levels of fish consumption. Unfortunately, the attempts to confirm that supplements are beneficial to children through double blind randomized control trials has not always produced the expected results. Although Richardson (2006) concludes that evidence from five randomized control trials is persuasive that omega 3 supplements from good-quality fish oil improve reading, spelling, memory and ADHD symptoms in children, these were fairly small-scale: the follow-ups were by this date only for a few months, and they did not all demonstrate an effect. A much larger randomized double blind control trial on children in Australia and Indonesia found very little benefit for omega 3 supplements, though a small but significant benefit to memory and verbal learning was achieved through the supplement of multiple micronutrients over a one year period (effect size 0.23, NEMO Study group, 2007). A recent double blind RCT in England with 450 8–10-year-olds found almost no effects on cognitive tests of various types, or from teacher and parent questionnaires, from a 16-week programme of omega 3 and 6 supplements (Kirby et al., 2010).

In old age, there are again some indications that fish consumption might be protective against cognitive decline and dementia. Issa (2006) conducted a systematic review of the effects of omega 3 on incidence and treatment of dementia, finding one poor-quality randomized control trial but four good-quality cohort studies that all found a trend in favour of the higher omega 3 group in terms of either reducing dementia risk or improving cognitive function. One interesting example is the study in France (Barberger-Gateau et al., 2002) of 1674 'free living' people aged over 68 years, which found that only one of the 19 who ate fish every day developed dementia in the seven-year follow-up period, compared to one in nine of the 1122 people who ate fish once a week, one in seven of the 240 who ate fish 'sometimes', and one in 3.5 of those who never ate fish (i.e. 10 of 35). However, as the careful review by Freeman, Hibbeln and colleagues for the US showed in 2006, some of the benefits of fish-eating groups might be confounded by the association between education and fish consumption.

There are clearly a large number of researchers who are convinced of the importance to mental health of omega 3, vitamin B12 and zinc (and many other micronutrients besides), particularly in relation to dementia and depression. The range of differing types of evidence is convincing. The evidence linking an even larger range of nutrients and additives to externalizing behaviour is also accumulating. However, as reviewers frequently note, the quality of the evidence has not been considered sufficient to allow firm guidance to be issued. The authors of the Cochrane Review (Lim et al., 2006) relating to the value of omega 3 to prevention of dementia came to the same conclusion – that the RCT evidence to support a general recommendation for supplementing omega 3 for children or older people is not yet strong enough. However, the potential benefit to particular groups showing early signs of mental ill-health or dementia, along with potential benefits to physical health, low cost if targeted, and little risk of harm, could easily justify dietary recommendations to practitioners, in schools, hospital wards, in primary care and in prisons, that they should at least be considering this factor in planning how best to help those for whom they have concerns, and perhaps before prescribing medication.

Where there appears to be least disagreement is in recommending the Mediterranean diet over the northern European and American diets. It is a diet high in vegetables, fruits, legumes, cereals, fish and a moderate amount of red wine during a meal, as opposed to a diet high in red and processed meat and dairy produce, and many argue it is the combination of healthy ingredients, not their individual effects, that is most important. A meta-analysis by Sofi and colleagues (2008) of 12 prospective studies (the longest being 18 years), which controlled for confounding variables such as age, smoking, physical activity, body-mass index, and which rated adherence to the main components of the Mediterranean diet, showed numerous benefits. These included lower mortality, coronary heart disease and cancer, the strongest benefits of all being to Parkinson's disease and Alzheimer's disease, which were both 13% lower among those adhering to the Mediterranean-type diet. Unfortunately, they did not include in their review data on the functional mental illnesses such as depression and schizophrenia, or on outcomes for children.

Conclusions

Physical and mental ill-health often go together. Severe life events and major life stress that are associated with a great deal of worry over long periods are a large part of the explanation for this. Difficulties centred on close relationships and work difficulties are particularly likely to characterize such stress. These raise blood pressure and provoke an immune system response, involving, for instance, pro-inflammatory cytokines such as IL-6. These inflammatory processes in turn are implicated in depression and anxiety, but also in coronary heart disease, arthritis, dementia and many other chronic conditions. These problems are visible in, for instance, carers of close others needing constant attention such as a child with a disability or a parent with dementia, who so often develop auto-immune conditions as well as mental ill-health. Painful and/or life-threatening chronic conditions also appear to contribute to depression through the limitations they bring to lifestyle.

Given the lowered immunity that comes with old age, the comorbidity of mental and physical ill-health increases with age. Arthritis doubles risk of depression; it appears that dementia is more likely if one is depressed, even more so if one is diabetic. Depression will worsen the progression of many physical conditions including dementia. Hence depression, anxiety and pain should be addressed as early as possible to prevent additional disorders developing.

Conversely, positive expectations about recovery improve prognosis, and these can be strengthened through good clinician–patient relationships, an active treatment process that inspires confidence, and good support from close others. Patients and the health services benefit if any anxieties of those about to undergo medical treatment are reduced. The individual might also benefit from learning techniques to control negative thoughts, to lower blood pressure. It is possible that exercise programmes can achieve as much as some psychological therapies and medication regimes, and that the benefits of all these approaches derive not from the nature of the intervention itself, but from their 'placebo effect' in changing the person's mindset.

Finally, a lengthy review of the evidence on diet was provided, as research in this area is extensive, by numerous research teams who are clearly convinced that what we eat plays an important role in the functioning of the brain. The dietary component that has received most attention is omega 3, and the strongest evidence of its importance comes from studies of fish consumption in pregnancy in relation to the brain development of the foetus, of its importance in alleviating symptoms of mental ill-health, and in old age as potentially preventive of dementia. Supplements did not seem important for the average child or adult. Much research exists on the role played by numerous vitamins and minerals, but these were not covered here.

Help to stay positive and calm is clearly beneficial to both physical and mental health. It seems likely that through meditation, prayer, taking exercise, eating well and thinking positively a person can improve their own mindset, their wellbeing, their risk of mental and physical ill-health, and recovery from established ill-health. Important contributors to help us achieve this when unwell are those in a position to provide care and support – the clinician, and close others.

9 Childhood

Secure foundations

> A secure base for the child plays a similar role to that of the officer commanding a military base from which an expeditionary force sets out and to which it can retreat, should it meet with a setback. Much of the time the role of the base is a waiting one but it is none the less vital for that. For it is only when the officer commanding the expeditionary force is confident his base is secure that he dare press forward and take risks.
>
> (Bowlby, 1988: 11)

Starting this review as Geoffrey Rose advises, the first question to ask is: in the developed world, where most people have enough to eat, and in countries where there is no war – in which of these countries do children seem most content? What does a 'normal' or an averagely happy childhood home look like there, and what is normal practice in controlling child behaviour? Common sense tells us that an adequate childhood must include affection from a parent or parents, protection from harm, and learning skills and behaviour that ensure not only survival, but also compliance with group norms and expectations in order to attract support rather than antagonism from others. In basic, evolutionary terms, it should be the time we learn skills that will enable us, in time, to earn a living, attract a good partner, assuming we want one, and rear our own well-adjusted children able to do the same (assuming we want them). The last of these will be more easily accomplished with more than one adult per household to ensure that the child is protected and the resources are found to sustain them, particularly when a child is too young to be left alone.

Such population comparisons give us some clues about what matters, and enable us to reflect on what common sense tells us, and what John Bowlby taught us over 50 years ago (see Bowlby, 1988) – that a young child needs to develop a secure bond with his or her parent-figure, from whom he or she can confidently expect to receive care and protection from harm. We assume that the factors that threaten the child's security in that sense are those that will to a great extent determine their mental health, as was concluded in earlier chapters looking at adult mental ill-health, which noted the important role of mother's mental ill-health, maltreatment in childhood and discordant family homes. This chapter revisits these from the point of view of the child's mental heath, to see what more can be learned about the mechanisms linking risk factors and disorder, and if and how and why it may translate into adult mental ill-health.

Most children grow up to be well-adjusted, well-behaved citizens, including the majority of those with marked early difficulty. Their resilience will be explored in later sections of this chapter, in order to learn from them how it might be possible to help others to be similarly resilient. To what extent is resilience explained by characteristics of the child, the family situation, the presence of other caring family members, or simple good luck in other aspects of life? Follow-up studies of troubled children as adults throw further light on this.

Between-population comparisons in childhood experience: Some statistics

One of the most comprehensive attempts to compare the lives of children and young people across the rich countries of the Western world is the UNICEF 'Report Card' (2007) showing comparable data under six headings for 21 of the OECD countries. Much of the data on family life and risk behaviour is drawn from a WHO survey, Health Behaviour in School-age Children (HBSC), under-taken regularly in the same way across the OECD counties, which select cluster samples of 1500 children at each of ages 11, 13 and 15. Northern European coun-tries claim the top four places in the overall ratings: children in the Netherlands, Sweden, Denmark and Finland have the best childhood environment, while the UK and US have the worst (see Table 9.1). For instance, 'health and risk behav-iour' covers diet and exercise (where the US is worst), smoking, cannabis and alcohol use, and early sexual activity (where the UK is worst). Data on violence (fighting and being bullied) completes the measure. One in three British children aged 11, 13 and 15 report having been drunk more than twice, compared to less than one in 10 in France and Italy; 38% of British children reported having sex before age 15, the next highest countries (Sweden, Finland and Germany) falling over 10 percentage points below the UK (the remainder lie between 15% and 25%). But whereas a large proportion of the UK's sexually active women aged 15–19 years give birth, third highest after the US and New Zealand, half as many sexually active young German women and one third as many Swedish and Finnish teens do so (lowest numbers are in Japan, the Netherlands and Switzerland).

The UNICEF (2007) authors reflect on the high rates of teen births in the UK and US, suggesting that it is a particularly important indicator of overall child wellbeing. Given that these countries have a relatively high (though not the highest) proportion of young people not in employment, education or training, and a poor rating on 'family and peer relationships' (proportion living with a lone parent, or in a step-family, eating meals with the family, spending time talking with them, and having kind and helpful friends), they comment:

> To a young person with little sense of current wellbeing – unhappy and perhaps mistreated at home, miserable and under-achieving at school, and

Table 9.1 UNICEF shows that high overall levels of child wellbeing are achieved by the Netherlands and Sweden, while the US and the UK have low ranking (1 ranks the best-performing country)

Dimensions of child wellbeing	Average ranking position (for all six dimensions)	Material wellbeing	Health and safety	Educational wellbeing	Family and peer relationships	Behaviors and risks	Subjective wellbeing
Netherlands	4.2	10	2	6	3	3	1
Sweden	5.0	1	1	5	15	1	7
Denmark	7.2	4	4	8	9	6	12
Finland	7.5	3	3	4	17	7	11
Spain	8.0	12	6	15	8	5	2
Switzerland	8.3	5	9	14	4	12	6
Norway	8.7	2	8	11	10	13	8
Italy	10.0	14	5	20	1	10	10
Ireland	10.2	19	19	7	7	4	5
Belgium	10.7	7	16	1	5	19	16
Germany	11.2	13	11	10	13	11	9
Canada	11.8	6	13	2	18	17	15
Greece	11.8	15	18	16	11	8	3
Poland	12.3	21	15	3	14	2	19
Czech Republic	12.5	11	10	9	19	9	17
France	13.0	9	7	18	14	12	18
Portugal	13.7	16	14	21	2	15	14
Austria	13.8	8	20	19	16	16	4
Hungary	14.5	20	17	13	6	18	13
United States	18.0	17	21	12	20	20	–
United Kingdom	18.2	18	12	17	21	21	20

Source: UNICEF (2007) Child poverty in perspective: An overview of child wellbeing in rich countries, *Innocenti Report Card 7*, UNICEF Innocenti Research Centre, Florence.

with only an unskilled and low-paid job to look forward to – having a baby to love and be loved by, with a small income from benefits and a home of her own, may seem a more attractive option than the alternatives. A teenager doing well at school and looking forward to an interesting and well-paid career, and who is surrounded by family and friends who have similarly high expectations, is likely to feel that giving birth would de-rail both present well-being and future hopes.

(UNICEF, 2007: 31)

Although marriage has been declining across all countries of the OECD, falling most steeply between 1970 and 1990, couple families are still the norm. Across the 22 countries on which data is shown, over 80% of children aged 0–14 years live with at least one of their parents, and his or her partner, possibly other adults too (OECD, 2009). This proportion is highest in Italy (90%), and lowest in Estonia, the UK and the US (70–75%). Most children have one or more siblings/step-siblings; countries with the highest proportion of single-child households are Bulgaria (37%) and Portugal (35%). The divorce rate has increased too, but the length of time people are married before divorcing has remained largely unchanged, at an average of 12 years (OECD Family Database, 2008). Poverty in households with children is about 12% across the 30 member countries, but considerably higher among single-parent households than couple families in all countries, though the Nordic countries have the lowest rates of child poverty in all family types. It is also higher, of course, amongst unemployed households.

Other data confirms the positive picture of childhood in the Netherlands. Using the Strengths and Difficulties Questionnaire (SDQ) to assess the mental health of 12–18-year-olds across 13 European countries, Ravens-Sieberer and colleagues (2008) found children in the Netherlands to be among the least troubled (but also German and Swiss children, which does not fully match with ranking in the UNICEF table), while the UK again came bottom of the table. Young people aged 15–16 in the Netherlands have the lowest rate of self-harm, Australia the highest, among seven countries studied by Madge and colleagues (2008) (England, Ireland and Norway being intermediate between the two). Self-harm and suicide show strong gender differences, the former being twice as high in girls as in boys; the latter (in 15–19-year-olds) three times as high in boys as in girls (though rare overall). Suicide rates are lowest in southern Europe – Greece, Spain, Portugal, Italy – and in the UK (OECD, 2009).

Differing rates of mental ill-health: Some possible explanations

Benjet and colleagues (2009) report very high rates of childhood disorder in Mexico City (a total of 25% reaching criteria for one or more disorders on the CIDI), which they speculate as being due to social changes in internal migration into cities (diminishing family links), increased divorce, more mothers taking paid employment, more children engaged in money-raising activities. This follows their discovery of a higher rate among those dropping out of school early and/or those taking on burdensome adult responsibilities (working, married or with children). Poverty is an important part of the context here, as OECD data shows Mexico at the bottom of the tables, alongside Turkey, of up to 30 countries measured on average child income, child poverty, children without the basic school necessities, average educational achievement of 15-year-olds, child and infant mortality, and teen births (OECD, 2009).

Ravens-Sieberer and colleagues (2008) found that parental mental ill-health distinguished between samples of children with and without disorder in nearly all countries, and, along with the availability of wider sources of social support, was the main explanation for differing rates of ill-health between countries. Social support was assessed using a brief measure (Brevik and Dalgard, 1996) of numbers of people available to offer a sense of security and support, and the emotional and instrumental support they provided. Family climate and socio-economic status were also assessed, and when several risk factors occurred simultaneously, the prevalence of mental ill-health in children increased markedly.

Meltzer and colleagues (2003) confirm the association of childhood disorder with parental mental ill-health in the UK, in a detailed and careful analysis. A sample of over 10,000 children aged 5 to 15 years was drawn from the Child Benefit Records database and either the child (if over 11 years) and/or a parent was interviewed, obtaining questionnaire data also from teachers. A total of one child in 10 (more of them boys) were considered to have a clinically significant mental health problem. Those with disorder were more likely to be in a low social class, living with unemployed parents, and with step-siblings. Almost half of them were judged to have special educational needs, three times as many as children with no mental disorder. Their family life showed many difficulties in addition to a raised rate of parental mental ill-health – unhealthy family functioning (e.g. not talking to each other, bad feelings between them), child more likely to be punished frequently, and family relationships and health were in turn affected by the child's difficulties (e.g. relationships with partner, other children, or other family members, and causing tiredness, anxiety and embarrassment to the parent) (listed in Table 9.2).

A second cross-sectional survey five years later found much the same picture (ONS, 2005). Both also discuss some features of family life that indicate how problems in the family affect all the family to some extent, parents blaming their marital problems on their child's behaviour, children also seeming to have more problems where parents had difficulties. For instance, Meltzer et al. (2003) found that more than one in five teenagers (13–15 years) with disorder had a parent who had been in trouble with the police. These adolescents were also particularly likely to have mental health problems after a break-up with their own boyfriend or girlfriend.

The diagnostic groupings frequently used in studies of child mental health categorize troubled young children as having an 'emotional disorder' such as depression, anxiety or obsessions, or a 'conduct disorder' characterized by awkward, troublesome, aggressive and antisocial behaviour (ONS, 2005). Less common

Table 9.2 Summary of factors associated with raised rates of mental ill-health in children

It is more likely that:

- *the child* has special educational needs; has dropped out of school early; is working or has children of their own before the age of 18; and if considered to have a conduct disorder or hyperkinetic disorder is male
- *the family* has a parent with mental ill-health; and/or with no qualifications
- *social circumstances of the household* are relatively poor; low in SES, with neither parent in work; living in social housing
- *the make-up and social dynamics of family relationships* provide low social support, the child lives with lone parent due to separation, divorce or widowhood; family includes step-siblings, where the child is frequently punished, and family relationships are affected by each other's difficulties.

Drawn from Ravens-Sieberer et al. (2008); Meltzer et al. (2003); ONS (2005); Benjet et al. (2009).

diagnostic labels for children include hyperactivity (that is, problems of attention and over-activity), autism and eating disorder. They found that of these young people aged five to 15 years:

- 5% had a clinically significant conduct disorder
- 4% had an emotional disorder
- 1% were rated as hyperactive, using the ICD-10 criteria.

Together these studies provide a good deal of information on four main groups of factors associated with raised rates of childhood disorders: characteristics of the child, the family, the social circumstances of the household, and the social dynamics of family relationships (see Table 9.2). They are a long catalogue of obvious social disadvantages.

Unpicking which social difficulties are associated with onset, and which result from other problems (such as living in social housing, often associated with unemployment rather than with child mental health directly), helps us explore what might be most useful in terms of prevention. So too will an examination of the problems with greatest long-term significance for the child, as compared to problems that might resolve relatively swiftly without intervention or lasting harm.

Longitudinal data: persistent disorder

Here the follow-up after three years of the first UK sample of 5- to 15-year-olds proves particularly helpful, allowing analysis of the persistence of disorder (ONS, 2003a). They were then, of course, aged 8 to 18 years, and many had moved from primary to secondary school or from school to work, and some from the parents' home. Many had experienced a number of the social risk factors between time 1 and time 2, such as parental separation or loss of family income; for others the social difficulties apparent at time 1 might have continued, or improved.

Meltzer and his colleagues (ONS, 2003a) were able to examine those children who developed emotional, conduct or hyperkinetic disorder between times 1 and 2, those whose difficulties diminished and those whose difficulties remained the same, and contrast the circumstances and experiences of the three groups. They included all of those with, and one third of those without, a disorder at time 1, who could be traced, achieving full information on over 80% of both samples (slightly more of those without than those with disorder).

Three out of four young people with *emotional* disorders at time 1 no longer had clinically significant problems at time 2. Those who did had experienced a large number of stressful events in the interim, and the child frequently experienced physical health problems. But the factor that was independently and significantly related to continued emotional disorder in the child (after regression analysis to control for correlations between factors) was continued emotional disorder in the parent: i.e. the parent, usually mother, scored above the cut-off on the GHQ both at time 1 and at time 2, indicating her own chronic mental ill-health. Other social factors were non-significant.

By contrast, *conduct* disorder was both more likely to continue throughout the three years (in 43% of children with conduct disorder at time 1), and its continuance was correlated with a large number of factors linked to social disadvantage – low family income, living in rented housing, parents separated or divorced. They were also more likely to have special educational needs, and a mother with continued mental ill-health, family difficulties (discord or poor relationships), and the child frequently shouted at. After logistical regression analysis controlling for associations between variables, the three factors emerging as independently linked to continued conduct disorder were:

- the child having special educational needs
- a mother with chronic mental ill-health
- being frequently shouted at.

Longitudinal data: new onsets

Those children who did not have any disorder at time 1, but developed an emotional disorder by time 2 (4% of the sample), compared to those who had no disorder at either point, were more likely to be older, have a physical illness, have a special educational need, have recently experienced family separation, be living with step-siblings, and with low-income, unemployed parents, in fact – almost all social factors were negatively associated with developing an emotional disorder. However, if logistical regression controlled for their association, one with another, three factors again emerge more clearly as having an independent relationship with onset of emotional disorder in children:

- older age
- physical illness
- number of stressful life events.

Stressful life events were events such as parental separation, loss of employment, court appearance, close family member admitted to hospital with serious illness or died, ending of close friendship. Physical illness included developmental problems such as speech difficulty as well as health problems such as asthma and migraine.

A similar proportion of the sample developed a conduct disorder between time 1 and time 2 (4%). Again, almost all family, household and individual disadvantages were associated with a raised likelihood of developing a conduct disorder. Those that emerged as independent of other factors were:

- being male
- having special educational needs
- having step-children in the family
- having a mother with chronic mental ill-health (ONS, 2003a).

Having experienced any mental disorder in childhood significantly increased the chance that the child would at some point have experienced school exclusion, that they would leave school at the earliest opportunity, and, more often than other children, with few or no qualifications (ONS, 2003a).

To recap on what has been described here so far: the evidence confirms the central importance to the child of his mother, her chronic mental ill-health being the greatest threat to his mental health, but also vice versa. Given the findings of previous chapters showing how her own mental health is related to adverse events and difficulties, and her coping with these to the support from a close other, her self-esteem, and her own experience of childhood adversity, many of the other factors emerging as risks to the child seem most likely to be affecting the child via the effect on the mother. However, special educational needs, physical ill-health, stressful events, being frequently shouted at, and the coexistence of step-siblings also threaten the child's mental health.

Changes over time

There is worrying evidence from both the UK and the US that these disorders are increasing (Kessler and Walters, 1998, Collishaw et al., 2004). In the UK, Collishaw analysed data from two ongoing prospective cohort studies that followed up over 14,000 children born in 1958 and over 7000 children born in 1970 at the age of 16, and a sample of over 800 young people who were aged 15 years old from a national survey in 1999. The parents of all these children had been asked a series of questions, using almost identical questionnaires, items including stealing, fighting, bullying, disobedience, restlessness, worries, misery, fearfulness of new situations. Care was taken to ensure that the minor differences in questions were not important by checking their rating on another separate sample.

They found that conduct problems increased significantly for both boys and girls, from 1974 to 1986 and from 1986 to 1999, so that numbers falling above the cut-off to be described as having a conduct disorder doubled over the 25 years.

Emotional problems increased slightly, but only between 1986 and 1999, and hyperactivity decreased somewhat in boys between 1974 and 1986, but otherwise showed little change. The increases in conduct problems were consistent across social classes, family type, and whether the family were home owners or not, for both boys and girls, and were strongest on measures of stealing, lying and disobedience rather than aggression. Speculating on the meaning of such uniform changes, Collishaw and colleagues (2004: 1360), believe that it is unlikely that raised rates of single parenthood or divorce can be blamed, and that it may turn out to be more to do with broad societal changes such as expectations relating to educational achievement and love relationships, changes to youth culture, drug use, media or social cohesion.

The following sections explore the insights gained from studies into the main threats to the child's wellbeing identified so far: parental mental ill-health, parental separation or family discord, child maltreatment, and physical ill-health and special educational needs in the child. The last two issues are discussed below in terms of their links with parenting problems that have resulted in children being 'in care'.

Threats to security

(i) Parental mental ill-health

Depression is common among parents – much more so than among couples without children – and in most instances does not come to the attention of services. Foreman (1998) reflects on the frequency of the coexistence of maternal and child mental ill-health, with one in three mothers of children referred for help with emotional or behavioural disorder also having a psychiatric condition, usually depression, and depressed mothers having three to five times the rates of disorder in their children compared to the average for non-depressed mothers. Possible mediators suggested include the effects of the depression on the parent's responsiveness to the child, less effective action to prevent harm to the child, and less warmth. If this contributes to child misbehaviour, it may produce humiliation and frustration in the parent, and affect her intimate relationships adversely (Foreman, 1998).

In some families, parental mental ill-health can lead to a role reversal. Aldridge and Becker (2003) draw on data from a survey of 18–24-year-olds by a national children's charity in the UK to estimate that over 1% of them had regularly cared for a family member through their childhood with problems related to mental health or drug or alcohol misuse.

Two studies suggest that most mothers even with serious mental ill-health can provide adequate parenting as long as there is good support from a partner. Nursing staff judged 70–80% of mothers of a newborn baby admitted to inpatient psychiatric care as coping well (Abel and colleagues, 2003; Howard and colleagues, 2004). The main worries of staff related to women whose partner also had mental ill-health, or where the relationship between the parents seemed poor, and they suggest that partners should be included as needing support and treatment in their own right, as well as help with their parenting skills. Kim-Cohen and colleagues (2006) argue on the basis of results from their twin study that the mother herself should be considered a considerably higher risk to her child where depression coexists with antisocial behaviour.

All too often, however, there are other problems, invariably linked to the cause of the mother's mental ill-health, and it is the combination of several of these that can pose the greatest threat to the child, not only of maltreatment but, in numerous cases each year, of child death. In particular, the combination of maternal mental ill-health, substance misuse and domestic violence can prove lethal to the child, as Brandon and colleagues (2008: 9) find. They review the 161 'serious case reviews' held in the UK from 2003 to 2005, as required each two years by the government to discover whether improved practices by statutory agencies could have done more to prevent the deaths. They recommend that these three risk factors where occurring in combination should be a priority for assessment and intervention. The largest group of child deaths occurred to those under the age of one at the time, many of these with 'shaken baby syndrome' which can kill, and can leave the child who survives with disabilities such as blindness or learning difficulty. The difficulties for professionals in supporting them were evident from case notes showing that roughly one in three families had moved home frequently. A similar proportion lived in poor material circumstances; very few were seen as having 'supportive family links'.

There are also tragic cases, however, where the child had featured in a parent's psychotic delusions, which may be impossible to foresee, and was asphyxiated, drowned or poisoned. Friedman and Resnick (2007) describe some examples, distinguishing these rare cases from the more common deaths by 'battery' which usually follow a lengthy period of abuse, where the parent is more likely to be depressed than psychotic.

Falkov (1995) recommended three protective strategies with a parent with mental ill-health. First, that mental health professionals employed to work with adults be reminded to be alert to, and educated about, the needs of, and potential risk to, any children in the home, and to consider the extent to which parenting capacity was adversely affected, noting also that a child in the home with health needs of their own, or with demanding behaviour or a difficult temperament, is more likely to be at risk of serious harm. Second, those same workers should discuss with the parent how their mental ill-health is affecting their ability to be a good parent, and far from jeopardizing their therapeutic relationship with the service user, Falkov argues that an open discussion should alleviate fear, reducing stigma by recognizing the person in their parenting role. Third, a psychological history of a parent with mental ill-health should include full details about any previous overdoses, self-harm or suicidal thoughts.

(ii) Parental discord and separation

Separation and divorce need not have any deleterious consequences for children, as Hetherington (2003: 217) concludes after a lifetime of longitudinal research on the marriage, divorce and remarriage of more than 1400 families. In fact for many children and parents divorce is an escape from 'an unhappy, conflictual or abusive family situation' and presents an opportunity to 'build new, more fulfilling relationships, and an opportunity for personal growth'. While initially most children will be distressed, angry and resentful, difficulties diminish over the course of the next year or two in most cases.

On the other hand, for some children the effects last, and children of divorced parents in America are more than twice as likely as children of non-divorced couples to show marked emotional and behavioural problems (20–25% compared to 10%), reflected particularly in aggressive, non-compliant behaviour and poorer classroom conduct and academic achievement. Such negative consequences were more likely if the separation followed a good deal of family conflict, the most damaging being that which involved or was focused on the child, and was physically violent, threatening or abusive. Effects that continue into adolescence lead to a higher rate of dropping out of school, unintended pregnancy, substance misuse, unemployment, and involvement with antisocial peers, which in turn affect average educational and socio-economic attainment and marital relationships (Hetherington, 2003).

These problems, and the high rates of separation and divorce in the US, have led to a proliferation of educational programmes attached to family courts there to help children adjust to changes and stresses of the divorce, including the conflict between parents. Pollett (2009) identified 42 programmes offered in 152 counties in 2001, two of which have been subject to controlled evaluation studies and report benefits to behaviour in school, self-confidence, and even physical symptoms. (Some states or counties have made attendance a legal requirement, some at the discretion of the judge, though over half have no legal mandate for it to be provided.) While suggesting that more research is needed into the best approach, Pollett draws on conclusions by researchers to date that effective programmes are those that help parents to reduce the destructive conflict that their children are exposed to and drawn into, and that help children learn skills to cope with pressures to side with one parent over the other, and to feel a sense of responsibility for their problems. However, the New Beginnings Program is one with the best evidence to date (involving 11 group sessions, two individual sessions) and this shows that intervention with the residential parent alone is effective in reducing a wide range of child problems, and direct work with children does not increase the benefit (see Wolchik et al., 2005).

Children find it most difficult when the conflict between parents continues after the divorce, as Moxnes (2003) shows from interviews with children of separating parents. Insufficient income for weekly bills, moving away from friends, home and school, and lack of involvement in any decisions also made the change more distressing. When family disharmony becomes violent, many violent incidents will be witnessed by the children, some of whom will try to protect their parent or mediate. Typically domestic violence continues for many years before the parents separate (NCH, 1994), and risk of child abuse increases by a factor of three to nine in homes where adult partners hit each other (Moffitt and Caspi, 1998). The review by Cleaver and colleagues (1999), also drawing on use of Childline, a free UK telephone helpline for children to ring at any time of day or night, provides ample illustration of this. They argue for more intervention in the lives of families where intimate partner violence is suspected, suggesting voluntary befriending schemes for mothers, key workers to co-ordinate family support, direct support for children, better information sharing and collaborative work between agencies, and improved information and training for front-line staff (Cleaver et al., 1999: 43).

(iii) Child maltreatment

WHO (2002) reports major inter-country differences not only in what is considered abuse (with some countries not legislating against forced marriage or genital mutilation), but also in practices widely agreed to be abusive. A definition drafted after consultation with 58 countries in 1999 is cited as:

> Child abuse or maltreatment constitutes all forms of physical and/or emotional ill-treatment, sexual abuse, neglect or negligent treatment or commercial or other exploitation, resulting in actual or potential harm to the child's health, survival, development or dignity in the context of a relationship of responsibility, trust or power.
>
> (WHO, 1999)

Country differences between acceptable levels of chastisement, however, are marked, and test such a definition of abuse. The WHO report in 2002 cites research data from parental interviews suggesting that up to two thirds of parents in Korea have whipped their children, and nearly half of Romanian parents beat their children 'regularly'. A careful comparative study (WorldSafe) in Chile, Egypt, India, the Philippines, and replicated in the USA, shows that moderate physical punishment such as smacking the child on the buttocks with the hand is common in all five countries, though more so in the Philippines (75% report having done this in the past six months) and India (58%) than in the USA (47%) (see WHO, 2002: 63). Parents in all five countries most frequently used non-physical methods of chastisement, explaining why the behaviour was wrong, but shouting at children was also commonplace. Shouting is also the most frequently used control in the UK, where about 45% of families also admit to having at some point smacked their child with their hand (ONS, 2000). WHO (2002) reported that corporal punishment was at this time still legal in the family home in all but 11 countries,[1] and in schools was then permitted in at least 65 countries, despite the passing of the UN Convention on the Rights of the Child which requires states to protect children from all forms of physical and mental violence while in the care of their parents or others. Sweden was the first country to prohibit all forms of corporal punishment in 1979.

But child maltreatment is not usually defined in terms of what is considered 'normal' chastisement. It is the experience of not being loved, valued and safe from physical harm from one's primary carers, or uncommonly harsh chastisement. The components measured in one well-validated tool, the CECA (Child Experience of Care and Abuse), include affection, indifference, companionship, concern, rejection, intrusiveness, role reversal, antipathy and lax control, as well as physical and sexual abuse. *All* of these aspects of mothering affect child and adult mental health, whereas only physical abuse by fathers is as significant in the lives of young women (Brown et al., 2007a). This team show from regression analyses that three central factors emerge as having independent effects on adult depression, based on their detailed interviews of 198 sister pairs in adulthood in London:

- affection by mother (expression of warmth, spending prolonged time together)
- rejection by mother (cold, children just a nuisance, wish they'd never been born)
- physical abuse by father (usually repeated assaults, though one very violent act counts).

A 'moderate' rating of difficulty (scale is 'none', 'moderate', or 'severe') in just one of the three is unrelated to adult depression in their analyses, but anything higher (two 'moderates' or one or more 'severe') markedly increases risk of adult depression – with over half (53%) of those with raised scores experiencing a period of depression in adult life lasting over one year, compared to just 7% of those with none (or just one moderate rating).

Other use of this measure suggests that between 20% and 25% of the UK population have experienced such child maltreatment (Brown et al., 2007a). Cawson et al. (2000) report a similar figure, but possibly higher: 26% of a national random probability sample of 2869 British young people aged 18–24 reported experience of some family violence. Although more than three quarters strongly agreed with the statement that they grew up in warm and loving homes (and over half (56%) were still living with their parents), Cawson et al. argued that there were clear indications that they underplayed the abusive nature of some of the experiences they described.

Sexual abuse is much less common than other types of maltreatment (about 10% of substantiated reports of abuse; NSPCC, 2007), but there are many more longitudinal studies of its effects. Consequences for mental health of all types of maltreatment have been noted in earlier chapters and in numerous studies not covered. For instance, a birth cohort of 1000 young people studied to age 25 in New Zealand estimated that child sexual abuse accounted for 13% of the mental health problems experienced by the cohort, and another 5% were linked to physical abuse (Fergusson et al., 2008). Schilling and colleagues (2007) showed that the adverse effects of childhood sexual abuse on depression during their senior year of high school and in the following two years were mediated by choices and experiences in relationships, education and employment. Collishaw and colleagues, following up their Isle of Wight sample at ages 15 and 45, concluded that their findings 'suggest that child abuse is not only linked to adult psychiatric disorder per se, but also to the severity and persistence of disorder across the lifespan' (Collishaw et al., 2007: 225). Brown and Moran (1994) came to similar conclusions following up depressed women in London. Draper and colleagues (2008) found that childhood physical or sexual abuse was more common in those with current poor mental health in their survey of people over age 60 in Australia, suggesting the effects can last a lifetime.

Factors associated with raised rates of physical violence towards children across numerous developed and developing countries include young age, lack of education, single parenthood, overcrowding, stress, social isolation and low income. WHO (2002) also note that the two forms of violence – between partners, and between parents and children – show an association in studies in China, Colombia, Egypt, India, Mexico, the Philippines, South Africa and the United States. The countries with the lowest rates of child death from maltreatment also have very low rates of adult deaths from assault, while those at the top of the league also have high adult deaths from assault (UNICEF, 2003). Spain, Greece, Italy, Ireland and Norway have an exceptionally low incidence of child maltreatment deaths, while five countries – Belgium, the Czech Republic, New Zealand, Hungary and France – have rates four to six times as high, and the US, Mexico and Portugal have rates 10 to 15 times as high.

Abuse that leads to physical harm or death is most likely to occur before the age of one year. Three-quarters of the estimated 1760 US children dying as a consequence of maltreatment in 2007 were under three years of age (US DHHS, 2009). Neglect accounted for 60% of substantiated maltreatment and one third of deaths. Abuse is most commonly perpetrated by the birth parent, more often the mother than the father, although child sexual abuse in particular occurs in a variety of settings, including daycare (US DHHS, 2009). But abuse is not just physical or sexual, and the more subtle aspects of abuse represented by psychological abuse (such as degrading the child, corrupting or terrorizing), lack of affection, and particularly rejection can play an equally important role, and are inevitably also associated with the more overt types of abuse (Brown et al., 2007). This accounts for the low rate of physical abuse by mothers as an independent contributor to the harm experienced as detected in surveys – as it is important mainly when part of wider abusive experience. It also calls into question the value of so many studies that focus exclusively on physical or sexual abuse without considering other types of maltreatment, including lack of affection and rejection.

Detecting abuse and intervening is a core social work task, but a small proportion of the total will be substantiated and officially registered. Previous admissions to accident and emergency services, and contact with the police linked to violent family conflicts, will help detection (Brandon et al., 2008). Abuse of a sibling is another obvious indicator, one study finding that 60% of the siblings of an abused child also experienced abuse, though not necessarily to the same degree (Brown et al., 2007). Intervention in the lives of families with multiple problems, who may not welcome it, can be challenging for professionals. Many of the children in the serious case reviews described by Brandon et al. (2008: 11) had been known to agencies for several years, and their histories 'were complex, confusing, and often overwhelming for practitioners'. They argue that it can lead to a sense of helplessness in practitioners, who might then be tempted to put aside knowledge of the past, and simply focus on the present child and present circumstances, to 'start again', rather than using past history to inform current action, with some disastrous consequences. Teenagers too can become 'hard to help' after years of rejection, loss or maltreatment, evidenced in truanting from school, misusing drugs, harming themselves and running away.

(iv) Substitute care, educational disadvantage, physical ill-heath

One population with particularly high rates of neglect and abuse is, of course, those children removed from their parental home into the care of the state, placed in institutional care, foster homes, or at home under supervision. The coexistence of special educational needs, physical ill-health, and child neglect or abuse is painfully apparent in these young people, along with their high rate of childhood emotional and behavioural problems. (These coexisting problems are no coincidence, of course; as earlier discussions make clear, they each share links with chronic stress, maternal depression, lack of affection and rejection.)

For instance, a national survey of 'looked-after children' in the UK in 2002 (which was not fully representative, as fewer than half of the selected young people were able to be interviewed), found that 45% of the 1039 final sample had a mental disorder, slightly fewer than this if living with foster parents or at home, many more than this if in residential care. Compared with national survey data by the same ONS team on children in private households, twice as many 11–15-year-olds, and nearly four times as many 5–10-year-olds, had an emotional disorder; seven times as many of all ages had a conduct disorder, five to seven times as many a hyperkinetic disorder (ONS, 2003b). Pecora and colleagues (2009) were able to make a similar comparison in the US between 14–17-year-olds in foster care and young people of the same age studied in the National Co-morbidity Survey (NCS), and also documented their markedly worse mental health.

Two thirds of the UK sample had at least one physical health problem (ONS, 2003b). Those that were much more common in looked-after children compared to children in private households included problems with sight, speech or language, bedwetting, soiling pants or co-ordination. These were all even more prevalent among those looked-after children who also had a mental disorder.

Educational difficulties were commonplace, as many as 60% of children being described by their teachers as having some or marked difficulty with reading, maths or spelling. Two thirds of the sample were considered to have special educational needs. In all their indicators of poor educational achievement, rates were doubled among those with a mental disorder compared to those without (ONS, 2003b). Not surprisingly given the catalogue of challenges facing them, exam success by looked-after children is low. In the UK in 2008, 14% of looked-after children achieved five A*–C grades at GCSE (the UK measure of a good level of exam passes at age 16), compared to 65.3% for all children, and narrowing this gap has become a priority for the government (DCSF, 2009). Perhaps, as UNICEF (2007) suggested, these restrictions to opportunity explain some of the high incidence of teenage parenting – two and a half times as common as among their peers (Social Exclusion Unit, 1999).

Pecora and colleagues in the US are able to provide data on longer term consequences for mental health. Their sample of 1087 foster care leavers aged 20–51 years, and 3547 people from the general population matched on age, gender and ethnicity, again drawn from the NCS data set, seems to show a very worrying level of mental disorder, higher even than for young people still in care, leading the researchers to comment that in many cases youth are not helped by the current services approach, and it is unlikely that improvements in children's mental health services will have much effect unless foster care systems become more thera-peutic (Pecora et al., 2009: 141). In particular, the rate of PTSD was five times as high as the general population – as high as rates found for Vietnam war veterans (Figure 9.1).

Living in out-of-home care is associated with fewer problems if some stability is achieved. Rates of mental disorder among young people in the UK sample dropped with each additional year that they had been in their current placement (from 49% of those placed less than a year before to 31% of those in the current placement for five years or more). However, placement failure rates are unfortu-nately high, and each failure and move compounds the young person's difficulty. Fisher and colleagues (2009) describe how the Oregon programme providing multidimensional treatment foster care (MTFC) support to foster parents taking pre-school children with multiple prior placement failure can considerably reduce subsequent placement failure. Foster parents receive 12 hours' intensive training and ongoing supervision over a period of six to nine months, including a daily

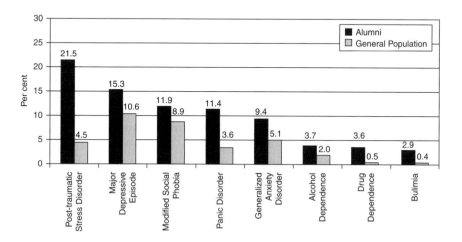

Figure 9.1 12 Month mental health diagnosis among Casey National Study alumni and the general population. From Pecora et al. (2009) (used with permission).

'checking in' phone call, a crisis response, respite, and treatment for the child. Further examples of this type of intensive help are given in the following chapter: an expensive but important intervention, given the evidence reviewed in this chapter.

While stability and continuity in care can reduce the young person's problems, they all too frequently leave the relative security of their foster home or other care home at the earliest possible time, at age 16–18 years (Stein, 2006), whereas most of their peers stay at home well into their 20s. For many, this is a final event, with no option to return when problems arise. This has been a focus of research and recent policy development given the loneliness, unemployment, poverty, early parenthood and 'drift' that is significantly more often the experience of the early adult life of care leavers (Stein and Wade, 2000; Wade, 2008). Stein (2006) finds that care leavers can be divided into three groups. First are those 'moving on', with a secure attachment, a stable care history, some educational success, and a gradual and planned move from care to independence, able to make good use of the help they have been offered and maintaining some contact with one or more past carer.

The second group are the 'survivors', with more instability, few qualifications, further problems after leaving care, periods of homelessness, unemployment and casual work, often leaving care with little planning. Stein argues that professional services and mentoring (including peer mentoring, and mentoring by older care leavers) can help this group, and this needs to take an early focus on finding and maintaining accommodation. The third group he describes as 'victims' – those with the most damaging pre-care family experiences, for which care has not been able to compensate. Their difficulties will have led to many unsuccessful place- ments, and disruptions to friendships and education associated with these moves. They have emotional and behavioural difficulties, probably do not have a relation- ship with a member of their family, leave care early, often following a final place- ment breakdown, then continue to have trouble maintaining accommodation, employment and mental health. They will need much more extensive help throughout life, but will lack support, frequently alienating those who offer help.

These threats to the child's security are closely interrelated, and some of the implications for prevention have been discussed – vigilance for and treatment for depression and other types of mental ill-health in mothers; support for parenting difficulties, particularly where children have physical ill-health or educational needs; educational programmes with the main residential parent when families are separating; vigilance and appropriate intervention for child abuse and neglect, most urgently when parental mental ill-health is combined with domestic violence or substance misuse, or personality disorder; intensive foster care support for foster parents taking children whose placements have failed before. Given the relatively low rates of substantiated abuse in the UK in comparison with other countries, but the high levels detected in surveys, and the poor rating of child wellbeing, it may be that it is the lack of affection and rejection that is prominent, perhaps due more to mental ill-health of the parent, low social support and stress of the home situation. If not, then much abuse is being missed.

What is now also clear is that part of the link between child maltreatment and later mental ill-health is the marked increase in behaviour problems in the maltreated child (Jaffee et al., 2004; Brown et al., 2007). That is, the effects of the maltreatment on behaviour can in turn lead to an increase in adverse experience, to a propensity to cause trouble for themselves and others, and to the likelihood of further interpersonal problems.

In turn these experiences not only perpetuate any depression occurring, but can increase the probability that through deficient supportive relationships they re-create similar problems with their own family in the future (Hammen, 2010).

Childhood adversity and the young person's resources when becoming a parent

Although the vast majority of maltreated children will become average or good parents to their own children, more will have difficulty in doing so in comparison to those not maltreated. Dixon and colleagues estimate it to be 17 times more likely that abused young people will in turn abuse their own child, as compared to a non-abused parent. In their sample of 4351 families with new babies visited by the health visiting service, there were 135 parents who had been physically or sexually abused as a child. Of the 27 babies referred for maltreatment by the age of 13 months, 9 were from the abused parent group, i.e. 6.7% of their children, compared to 0.4% of the non-abused group. Studying the circumstances of the families, and modelling the role of contributing factors, they noted that abused parents (APs) were more likely to be under 21, have a history of mental ill-health, and live with a violent partner, and together these increased their probability of poor parenting styles. They conclude that 'prevention may be enhanced in AP families by the promotion of "positive parenting" in addition to providing additional support to young parents, tackling mental illness/depression and domestic violence problems' (Dixon et al., 2005: 67).

(i) Teenage parents

One of the consequences of childhood adversity is a much greater chance that the young person will become a parent at a young age, often before they have much in place to support them. Delaying childbirth and having fewer children has been a notable development across OECD countries since the 1970s. In 2005 in the UK, the average age of the first time-mother was 29.8 years (only in New Zealand do they postpone childbearing for longer – to age 30), and in 22 other OECD countries it was over 27 years (OECD, 2010). This makes teenage childbearing all the more atypical. The E-risk study of a sample of same-sex twins born in the UK in 1994–5 was used by Moffitt and colleagues (2002) to compare mothers who gave birth to their first child (not necessarily the twins) before the age of 20 and those whose first baby was born after they were 20. The two samples of 562 and 554 mothers were 18 and 28 years old on average respectively at first birth, and aged 30 and 36 on average at time of interview. They were markedly different, with the young mothers being multiply disadvantaged. The largest differences (effect size) between the two groups were (in order): living in council housing (55% versus 9%); university educated (2% compared to 23%); earning less than £10,000 (31% versus 5%); number of public benefits received; breadwinner in manual employment. There were also significant differences in both mother's and biological father's mental health, and the young mothers were significantly more likely to be living with a partner who was not the biological father of the child through the child's first five years of life. The children of young mothers were more likely to be living with step-siblings, and to be in need of special education services.

While the authors stress that a large proportion of young mothers do not experience each disadvantage, a disproportionate number face marked difficulties 'in multiple life domains: education and literacy, employment and finances, neighbourhood and housing, mental health and substance abuse, lack of support from their children's fathers, and in their children's health and wellbeing'. They conclude that 'Young maternal age at first birth is an easy to-measure marker that reliably signals elevated rates of a variety of health, social, cognitive and behavioural problems in both women and children' and that 'contemporary interventions are needed to prevent teen childbearing and to assist young women who do become mothers' (Moffit et al., 2002: 739–40).

(ii) Care leavers as parents

Further evidence to support these suggestions comes from studies of young parents raised 'in care'. Comparing 80 young women in their twenties who had lived in one of two children's homes in the early 1960s with a group of similar aged women who had not been raised 'in care', Quinton and colleagues (1984) showed that twice as many of the former group had become pregnant and given birth by the follow-up interview, two fifths of the care group but none of the comparison group before age 19. Fewer of the care group were living with the father of their child, and one fifth of their children had been taken into care. Up to one third of the care group had experienced some form of transient or permanent parenting breakdown with at least one of their children.

There were also substantial group differences in the quality of parenting, and a wide range of other social problems, as well as partner difficulties and likelihood of experiencing mental ill-health. This finding is in accord with the studies by Harris and colleagues (1987, 1990; Brown et al., 2008b) who show that poor support in childhood (abusive or neglectful) increases the chance the young person will form an adult partnership offering poor support, sometimes replicating the violence and humiliation of their own childhood, meaning that their vulnerability continues.

Of course, as in all these studies, these are statistical associations, not general rules, so there were also a substantial number of 'good' parents among the 'in care' groups (31%), and the examination of the reasons why this group did well gives some helpful clues for a consideration of prevention (Quinton and Rutter, 1984a, 1984b).

First, positive school experiences were found to be important. They were rated as positive if the subject had two or more of: examination success; a positive assessment of school work or relationships with peers; or a clearly positive recall of at least three aspects of school life. Forty-three per cent of the ex-care girls without positive experiences, compared to 6% of those with positive experiences, had poor social functioning in adult life. The relationship also held for parenting. However, positive school experiences were not related to outcome among the comparison sample, presumably because they had other more important sources of self-esteem (Quinton and Rutter, 1984a, 1984b).

Second was the importance of decisions made and the support available after leaving care. Those who returned to live within discordant family situations were much more likely to become pregnant than those who stayed in institutional care until independent, or who returned to harmonious family situations (93%, 51%, 30% respectively). There was some suggestion that those most likely to return to discordant homes were those who had experienced more early disruptions in parenting before being taken into care, and they were more likely to become pregnant, move in with a partner or marry for negative reasons; that is, to escape this home situation. Unfortunately, care leavers were also more likely than the comparison group to find themselves living with a partner with problems, or without a partner at all.

Those care leavers living with a partner who seemed relatively free of problems, and with whom they experienced a seemingly harmonious relationship, had more often planned their marriage or cohabitation. The researchers defined planning as having known the partner for at least six months before moving in together, and doing so for positive rather than negative (needing to escape an unhappy home, or motivated primarily by unintended pregnancy) reasons. Girls who reported positive experiences at school were more likely to be 'planners', suggesting that:

- young people with a marked lack of support from family should be a priority for school-based intervention to find positive, rewarding experiences to confirm their own competence and value.

They also concluded that if by planning or chance, the young woman ended up with a supportive untroubled partner, she was no more likely to experience problems in parenting than women in the comparison group, meaning that

- interventions that support young people lacking good family support in making decisions about relationships might bring benefit
- interventions that assist pregnant care leavers or others from troubled backgrounds to find supportive living arrangements for themselves and their child and avoid a return to families or partners where violence has been suspected are recommended.

Their conclusions mirror earlier discussions, that childhood experiences led to disadvantage for the young women in two ways – through increasing chances of experiencing further social disadvantage, and through decreasing their resources to cope with difficulties, including the difficulties of childcare.

What factors contribute to resilience?

(a) Genes

The inherited qualities of each child will moderate the effects of environment, but will also shape that environment. Recent years have seen a marked increase in interest, and sophistication, in methods of studying gene–environment interaction. One type of interplay lies in the child's appraisal of their environment. Some children are more susceptible to stressful experience than others even in the same family home; for instance, one more liable to blame themselves, another with more self-confidence or more intelligence perhaps able to see other causes for the magnitude of the angry outburst from a parent. A second example is the child's effect on the environment, and on events. One might respond to an angry parent by acting out, and challenging the parent, while another might sulk or cry, so that the former receives further angry responses, while the latter behaviour might serve to defuse the situation, meaning siblings can have marked differences in their relationships with their parents (see Dunn and Plomin, 1990). Similarly, many life events are far from chance occurrences, and the impetuous, active toddler is more likely than the slower moving, careful sibling to have an accident, and living with a parent with a drink or drug problem and poor supervision of his or her toddlers might be more risky for one than another.

Some of the differing accounts given by siblings of parental rules, expectations, chores, closeness and ability to participate in family decisions are provided by Dunn and Plomin (1990), as well as their experience of how strict, proud, fun, or sensitive their parents were towards them as compared to their sibling, suggesting that children have a non-shared as well as a shared environment in the home as well as outside it. By way of illustration, they cite writer Edith Sitwell's descriptions of her mother as unloving, egotistical and cruel, while the writings of her brothers Osbert and Sacheverell describe her as a figure of affection, beauty and romance (Dunn and Plomin, 1990: 63). This is recognized too by parents studied, two thirds of whom admit loving, and treating, one child differently from another. Children are not able to compare their treatment easily with that of children in other families; their main comparison is the treatment by their parents of their siblings, and a sense that one is not the preferred child can feel threatening. (How familiar is the cry of 'It's not fair!'.)

A new area of research into gene–environment interactions is the potential biochemical change to the genome resulting from environment. Adverse early experience during sensitive stages of development can produce a stable alteration in the infant's response to stress that lasts well beyond the period of maternal care (see Meaney, 2010), and epigenetic modification of genes that encode parts of the stress response contributes to such enduring effects. Much of the research is on rats, nurturant and neglectful parenting defined by the frequency and diligence of the licking and grooming behaviour of the mother in the days following birth. Pups briefly separated from mothers by the experimenters receive extra licking and grooming on their return, and become stress-resistant. Those separated for longer periods are often ignored on their return. Such pups, and those born to neglectful mothers, become more stress-reactive. Epigenetic modifications of gene expression appear also to be heritable, affecting the quality of care that pups provide to their own offspring.

Weder and Kaufman (2011) argue that such effects are not necessarily permanent, and that the pessimism about long-term effects from early childhood trauma may be misplaced. They review evidence that ideal 'foster care' and environmental enrichment, even outside the sensitive period of early childhood, can reverse such effects. Indeed, such effects were shown in Meaney's influential rat studies: where rats from low-nurturant mothers were taken in by high licking and grooming foster mothers, they became stress-resistant adults.

The implications of these findings are that early childhood intervention to enhance environmental influences will be most effective before neural circuits become well established and more difficult to change, and at the relevant sensitive period for particular types of cognitive development (Fox et al., 2010). Hence intensive language support would be most effective at age 16–18 months, and the negative effects on intelligence of being in an institution from birth might best be countered by a high-quality foster placement before the age of two years (Fox et al., 2010). Later in life, personal characteristics that increase vulnerability will be much less open to change.

(b) Other caring relationships

A number of studies show that other relationships can protect. For instance, among the Isle of Wight children followed up at age 45 years by Collishaw and colleagues (2007), roughly 10% had experienced child maltreatment, and showed the same profile of multiple disadvantage in family relationships and poor child, adolescent and adult mental health. But a proportion of the abused group did not show these mental health problems. It was found that 'relationships with parents, friends and partners were potent predictors of adult resilience' (Collishaw et al., 2007: 224), i.e. having normal peer relationships in adolescence, reporting either parent as caring; and in adulthood, the quality of adult friendships, and the stability of a love relationship. They argue that maltreated children remain suspicious in relationships, with negative expectations, and it is not just a chance encounter with a supportive person that makes the difference, to make them resilient, but a learning process from a number of relationships (with a parent figure, peer, and love partner) through which they learn the competencies necessary to benefit from and maintain supportive relationships, and personality plays a role in this.

Hetherington's follow-ups of children experiencing parental divorce also showed that almost all of the most competent, successful, well-adjusted adults had 'a caring, involved adult in their lives – usually a parent, but sometimes a grandparent, step-parent, teacher or neighbour', and as the children grew older, friendships with peers grew in importance (Hetherington, 2003: 224). Werner's cohort study (summarized in Werner, 1995) of all 698 children born on the Hawaiian island of Kauai in 1955 confirmed the importance of both inherited characteristics and a caring adult in fostering resilience. About 30% of the Japanese, Hawaiian and Filipino families were considered high risk, due to their poverty, discordant home circumstances or parental mental ill-health, and two out of three children experiencing four or more such risk factors had learning or behavioural problems by age 10, or had pregnancies, delinquency or mental ill-health by age 18 (Werner, 1995). But one in three did not. These resilient children had several advantages.

First, they had personal qualities – alert and intelligent, so able to appraise threats well, but also affectionate, good-natured, easy children. But their key asset was their capacity to elicit care and support from a nurturant family member, perhaps a sibling or grandparent. 'Resilient children seem to be especially adept at recruiting such surrogate parents. In turn, they themselves are often called upon to take care of younger siblings and to practice acts of "required helpfulness" for members of their family who are ill or incapacitated' (Werner, 1995: 82). Second, they benefited from a same-sex role model – a firm male who upholds rules, but can also express emotion; a female providing reliable support but also independent, perhaps in work. These were further strengthened by teachers who took an interest in them, youth workers or peers who set an example.

But resilience is not only linked to childhood experience: it continues to be shaped throughout life. A chance to escape a life of misfortune can present itself at key transition points, Werner (1995: 83) noting that 'Among the most potent second chances for such youths were adult education programs in community colleges, voluntary military service, active participation in a church community, and a supportive friend or marital partner'.

Breaking the chain later: Turning points

As shown earlier, conduct disorder in childhood is more likely to persist than is an emotional problem. One of the earliest studies to demonstrate this was the follow-up by Robins (1966) of 475 children seen in a child guidance clinic in St Louis, between 1924 and 1929, along with 100 children from neighbouring schools. She found that boys seen due to 'antisocial behaviour' had a 70% risk of later arrest, girls a 70% chance of divorce, and a considerably raised rate of sociopathic personality, sometimes alcoholism, or schizophrenia. Children who were fearful, withdrawn, shy, had tics, speech defects, insomnia, nightmares or temper tantrums were no more likely to have adult mental ill-health than those lacking such traits in childhood. She argues that children with conduct disorder in school should be identified before they reached the age of 10, and provided with close supervision to ensure completion of assignments and regular attendance, and their use of leisure time should be controlled.

Malmgren and Meisel (2004) would make the date for trying to turn around the child's difficulties somewhat earlier. They found high rates of abuse and neglect, and current emotional or behavioural disorder (EBD) in juvenile correctional facilities. Average age of entry to special education was 10 years, but 90% had already been considered to have EBD before this and over half were known to at least one of the three agencies (young offenders' service, special school system or child welfare services) before the age of eight. They suggest that children under 10 considered to have special educational needs due to EBD should be a priority for preventive support, starting with attempts to break their early cycle of failure, finding opportunities for them to achieve.

A long-term follow-up through to age 70 of men who attended reform school at age 14 by Laub and Sampson (2003) suggests that the most important 'turning points' away from a life of crime in adult life were establishing a close relationship, getting a job, moving to a new neighbourhood or doing military service. These factors combine social controls, routines, and purpose; critically, they provide 'connective structures'. But it is more than this. Laub and Sampson argue that it is the event – the gaining of a job or romantic partner – that is the turning point, that the individual does at this time exercise a conscious choice to stay out of trouble. But where the marriage, work or military service went badly, the experience of rejection, alienation, and injustice puts men at greater risk of offending than if they had not had a wife or job.

Conclusions

The main threats to the child's wellbeing in the longer term are parental mental ill-health, child maltreatment and family discord. Later evidence of vulnerability to adult ill-health often becomes apparent in a consideration of special educational needs due to emotional or behavioural disorder or learning difficulty. Social disadvantage plays a role in terms of its effects on family harmony, and in turn, maternal mental health.

The child needs, above all else, to feel secure: that at least one person cares about him enough to stand between him and danger, and is capable of keeping him safe, as Luthar also concludes (2006). Reviewers (e.g. Hackett, 2003) summarize work suggesting that this is best fostered by parenting that is 'authoritative' (i.e. warm and loving, not too critical (responsive) and firm about well-defined boundaries for behaviour, but permissive within those boundaries (demanding)). This is better than permissive parenting (responsive but undemanding), neglectful parenting (unresponsive and undemanding) or authoritarian parenting (unresponsive and demanding). Parenting is shaped not only by social disadvantage, the support available to the parent, and parenting skills, but also by inheritied qualities of both parent and child, and intervention to strengthen parenting is likely to be most effective during the child's sensitive early years.

The potential for reducing rates of parental mental ill-health, child maltreatment and family discord were considered. These included reducing teenage pregnancy, supporting depressed mothers (more assertively if domestic violence or drug misuse is also suspected), ensuring that mental heath workers address child care responsibilities of adults they support, education programmes for separating couples, improving detection of ongoing child maltreatment. Secondary prevention opportunities exist as child emotional and behavioural problems emerge among children from troubled homes. Intensive fostering to reduce repeated placement breakdown and to reverse epigenetic effects is likely to be particularly important. Later strategies should include help with school work and setting firm boundaries for behaviour together with close supervision of troubled children well before the child is eight years old, along with extra efforts to find them some positive experiences in their school life to compensate for the lack of them at home.

Mentoring or support for children with early adversity might include helping to strengthen a relationship with another member of the family, or even another adult figure in a position to provide ongoing support, such as the parent of a good friend. It may also help if it creates a 'second chance' situation – a move to college, a lead involvement in a community football team. This applies throughout adulthood: chances will come from what goes right, often after a change that brings a real opportunity for happiness – a relationship with a stable partner, a good job, a 'fresh start'.

Note

1 Legislation is now developing rapidly in many countries and by 2010 most European countries (though not the UK) had prohibited corporal punishment in the home. Corporal punishment of children is prohibited in all settings, including the family home, in 25 countries as at March 2010 (Children are Unbeatable! 2010). Governments in a further 24 have made a public commitment to full prohibition and/or are actively considering draft legislation which would achieve this.

10 Strengthening support for children

Effective interventions

A clear story emerges that intervention as early in life as possible stands the best chance of influencing long-term vulnerability. We know much more now about those children most likely to have enduring problems, and can in theory target help where it should make most difference. This chapter aims to evaluate the evidence that we can do those two things: identify and recruit to preventive programmes children or young people known to be most vulnerable to mental ill-health in adult life; and provide an intervention focused on changing a salient factor known to be part of the explanation for their vulnerability that works.

Logically, help needs to start before conception, aiming to improve the proportion of babies born to parents who planned and wanted them, who are not still children themselves, and have sufficient material resources and social support to facilitate good parent–child relationships. During pregnancy, young mothers whose circumstances indicate they are likely to face some difficulty in parenting are an obvious target group for additional help – those with a learning disability, poor mental health, a home characterized by angry, conflictual relationships, drug misuse or violence, or lacking good support from another adult with the expected child. Taking the stages of childhood in order, earlier chapters suggest that the raised probability of emotional and conduct disorder in a child born to a parent with any of these difficulties can be reduced through help for the parents: to cope with difficult behaviour, providing firm boundaries without resort to violence, or too much shouting; to ensure children in step-families are treated equally; to equip parents to support a child with special needs, ill-health or a disability; in each case with the aim being to increase the child's security – his sense that his parents care for him and will support and protect him.

As noted in the previous chapter, a high-risk group are those children whose family difficulties have led the state to take parental responsibility for them. Their wellbeing is best protected if the new caring arrangements bring stability and good relationships. At the transition to independent living, support is again crucial to reduce their raised risk of homelessness, unintended pregnancy, mental ill-health and social difficulty (Stein, 2006).

Schools play a key role in helping young children with emerging special educational needs, and can help those with little support at home to find some positive experiences in their school life. Help to avoid any further abusive relationships, and instead to find reliable support and friendship and to learn to become an authoritative parent to their own children, is the type of support indicated by earlier discussion, and takes us full circle.

Does it work?

Preventing teenage pregnancy

According to the UK's review of its Teenage Pregnancy Strategy (DH, 2010), about three quarters of teenage pregnancies are unplanned, and about half end in abortion. The first 10 years of the strategy reduced births to those under 18 by 25%, but conceptions fell by less than this, and the target for reducing births had been 50%. Their review concluded that the two most important factors in reducing teenage births are comprehensive advice, information and support from family, school and other professionals; and young people friendly contraceptive and sexual health services; and the strategy has focused resources primarily in these two areas. They describe numerous innovative examples, which include: an outreach nurse to visit young people who recently had a live birth, miscarriage or abortion to help them choose effective contraception to prevent repeat unplanned pregnancies; a GP practice based weekly 'youth space' providing contraceptive and STI advice in a young person friendly style, open to all whether patients at the practice or not; a similar service based in a high school. They also note that a low-income background, low educational attainment, poor attendance in school, no post-16 education or low aspirations are underlying factors that increase risk, and should inform the targeting of support (DH, 2010). One example given is a collaborative project between housing, health and education services to support 16- and 17-year-old mothers in supported housing to interest them in developing vocational skills and to complete or continue their education. This was expected to delay, or reduce the number of, additional pregnancies.

Reviewing school-based preventive programmes from randomized controlled trials published in the 1980s and 1990s, Moore and colleagues (2002) conclude that they can and do improve self-efficacy beliefs about practising safe sex, and they reduce the number of partners, decrease the frequency of unprotected sex, and increase use of condoms. They can also delay the start of sexual activity among inexperienced young people. All effective programmes included communication skills rehearsal (assertiveness, negotiation skills), and most also included behavioural skills (avoiding sexually risky situations, escape; acquiring, carrying and using a condom). They were on the whole relatively brief interventions – an hour a week for 3 to 18 weeks – and effect sizes on knowledge were sometimes quite strong; on attitudes and communication skills they were sometimes moderate (0.4 or 0.5), while for behavioural change outcomes, using a condom for instance, effect size was usually small (0.2). The systematic review by DiCenso and colleagues (2002) involving 26 RCT evaluations of primary prevention educational programmes was, however, less positive about effects on behavioural change – delaying start of sexual intercourse, use of contraception, or pregnancy.

On some outcomes they found some positive results, but in the overall review these were counterbalanced by an equal number finding no benefit, or superior outcomes for those in the comparison group.

Some programmes place greater emphasis on overall youth development, on the assumption that it is the social determinants of teenage pregnancy that should be addressed, such as poor material circumstances, an unhappy childhood, dislike of school and low expectations for the future (Harden et al., 2009). Again the evidence of effectiveness of this strategy is mixed. It worked well in the Carrera Program in the United States, when first implemented by its charismatic leader in New York, where the prospective RCT evaluation showed a 50% reduction in pregnancies over the three study years (ages 13–16) among the high-risk target youth (a large proportion being children of lone parents, African American, living in unemployed households) (Kirby, 2009). The programme was expensive and time consuming, with up to three-hour after-school sessions totalling at least 16 hours a month, for up to three years, in job clubs, homework assistance, sex education sessions, arts and sports workshops, medical checks and counselling. It had no significant effect on the sexual behaviour of boys.

Unfortunately, attempts to replicate the very positive effects on the girls in three further sites by other practitioners failed to show any benefit in terms of reduced pregnancies or behaviour of the boys. But this may be in part related to their problems in maintaining an appropriate control group, and problems recruiting and retaining teens or good staff (Kirby, 2007). In fact the British study based on the Carrera approach found the opposite of a benefit in this strategy – a significant benefit for the comparison group girls (receiving standard youth provision, not in targeted groups), 6% of whom became pregnant compared to 16% of the intervention group (Wiggins et al., 2009). These authors speculate on their negative findings, and consider the likely explanation to be the effect of bringing similarly disadvantaged young people together (those considered at risk of teenage pregnancy, substance misuse and school exclusion), and the labelling inherent in the recruitment process that identifies them as at risk and therefore problem children.

On the other hand, a Teen Outreach Program (TOP) focused on volunteer activities and community service in which the teenagers (ages 14 to 18 years) were *providers*, not recipients of this support (e.g. as aides in care homes or hospital, or peer tutors, a minimum of 20 hours in total) found significant effects on rates of unplanned teenage pregnancy, school failure and drop-out (Allen et al., 1997), though the latter two outcomes changed more than the former. It consisted of three components: supervised community volunteer activities, classroom-based discussions of those experiences, and of key social and developmental stages of adolescence. There was a deliberate decision not to focus on the behaviours they aimed to change: sexual activity and school failure. Unfortunately their account suggests they were not fully convinced that schools adhered to their randomization, as small group differences in favour of the experimental group were already evident within a week or two of the start of the study.

However, a later evaluation by Allen and Philliber (2001) provides additional data confirming its effectiveness, and that it works particularly well with the highest risk young people in the sample – those who have already had or caused a pregnancy, been suspended or failed courses previously. Comparing 1673 young people receiving the intervention with a part randomly selected, part matched pairs group of 1604 young people, on questionnaires completed at the beginning and end of the school year in which the intervention occurred, showed that 8–9% of these high-risk young people dropped out of both groups, but that those very high-risk young people who stayed in the study, compared to similarly high-risk students who stayed in the comparison group (i.e. completed all questionnaires), had substantially fewer pregnancies. Numbers were not supplied, but they cite an odds ratio of 0.18, i.e. the ratio of the odds of an additional pregnancy by TOP participants in relation to the odds of pregnancy in the comparison group. Similarly, academic failure was reduced most among those who had previously been suspended. But again, these results are open to criticism as it is not an 'intention to treat' analysis.

Some of the reasons for disappointing results in other studies relate to their focus, which might encourage abstinence, or offer discussion or activities that are not well informed by the interests, beliefs and values of the adolescents themselves. A programme fully involving and largely delivered by other young people might be expected to be particularly effective, and this was explored by Stephenson and colleagues (2004) in a randomized intervention of a pupil peer-led sex education programme (RIPPLE) involving over 9000 children from 27 secondary schools in England.

A randomly selected half of the schools provided the usual teacher-led sex education, while in the other half, 16- and 17-year-old pupils were trained to provide three one-hour classroom sessions with 13–14-year-old pupils from the same schools, using participatory learning methods designed to improve skills in sexual communication, condom use, knowledge about pregnancy, sexually transmitted infections, contraception, and local sexual health services (Stephenson et al., 2004). Effects on outcomes were modest, but significantly fewer girls in the peer-led sessions reported having heterosexual intercourse by age 16 (35% versus 41%), though it did not reduce the proportion of girls or boys who had unprotected sex. Girls in the intervention group were slightly less likely to have an unplanned pregnancy (2.3% compared to 3.3%), were more confident about using a condom, and both boys and girls were more satisfied with peer-led sex education. Many reported that they would have preferred to have the peer-led sex education in single-sex groups, and many also felt it was not the right time for them. Peer educators volunteered for the role, rather than being selected by teachers, and tended to be more academically able than the average pupil. A further tracking of the young women through standard record systems to obtain data on abortions and live births by age 20 showed that 5% of both intervention and control groups had had an abortion, and 7.5% compared to 10.6% had had a live birth – a difference in the right direction, though not statistically significant (Stephenson et al., 2008).

Hence it might be concluded that effective programmes include skills as well as knowledge, and that much of this is best delivered by suitably prepared and supported peers; that programmes aimed at youth development need to give the young people some responsibility and the chance to help others, not just being passive recipients of information or skills; that single-sex programmes have advantages over mixed groups, and that adolescent development programmes should not reinforce high-risk norms by bringing together many others with a similar perspective, but ensure that they spend time with peers with a more aspirational, self-confident and sexually cautious outlook.

Supporting young disadvantaged mothers

One of the most important aspects of a secure family home for the child is that parents are supportive of one another, assuming there are two; and if only one, that the one gains some respite and support from another adult. One of the disadvantages of teenage parenthood is that they frequently lack either of these. The study described in the previous chapter of the mothers of twins (Moffit et al., 2002), 562 of whom had their first child in their teens and 554 who had their first child after the age of 20, showed that the young mothers had more often spent the first five years of their twins' lives as a single parent (6.4% compared to 1.8%), and their twins had contact with their biological father less frequently (less than weekly – 27.7% compared to 10.3%). Those with a partner were less likely to have reliable support, having more quarrels and more physical abuse. Parenting was also shaped by the presence of step-children (in 41.6% compared to 8.7% of homes), perhaps partly explaining the much lower parent–child time engaged in activities together.

The new young parent with little or no emotional and/or financial support from a partner or other adult may also find that their new baby is not the source of unconditional love they might have been looking for either, and parenthood is in fact an altogether less rewarding, more challenging and more limiting role than expected. The most well-known programme of research on how the parenting of disadvantaged mothers might best be supported is the nurse-led home visitation scheme set up and evaluated by the team led by David Olds from Colorado, and now known as the Nurse–Family Partnership (NFP) programme. They used randomized controlled designs, a broad range of measures of effectiveness and have the longest follow-up data of all family support programmes (retaining at least 86% of the samples into six-year follow-ups, and 81% at 15 years). Their New York evaluation remains the strongest evidence that home visiting can prevent child abuse, hence some detail of this approach will be described, though it is only one of numerous similar programmes across the US.

Their early study (Olds et al., 1986a) compared outcomes for four randomly allocated groups of women – 90 who received standard services; 94 who were provided with free transport to existing prenatal and well-child clinics; 100 who received an average of nine prenatal home visits from a nurse, lasting about 1.25 hours; and 116 who received home visits from the nurse for a further two years, once a week, diminishing over time to once every six weeks. The women were pregnant with their first child, aged under 18, single and/or of low socio-economic status, living in a poor, semi-rural county in the Appalachian region of

New York State, well served by services. The area had the highest rates of reported and confirmed cases of child abuse and neglect in the state, and high rates of infant mortality. The ante-natal programme was intended to enhance the social support and health habits of the mother and the length of gestation and birth weight of the child; the post-natal programme to prevent child abuse and neglect. Home visits concentrated on foetal and infant development and health, but the nurse would also chat to the woman and her friends and relatives about how they could help each other, and about the services that existed to help. The strengths of the women and their families were a central focus.

Comparisons between groups showed considerable advantages gained by the women receiving home visits from the nurse – compared to those randomly assigned to the comparison groups, they attended more childbirth classes, made greater dietary improvements, more often had a person with them at the birth, had fewer kidney infections, and smokers and women under age 17 had longer pregnancies and heavier babies (Olds et al., 1986b). Only 4% of women receiving continuing home visits were involved in verified cases of child abuse or neglect, compared to 19% of comparison groups over the two years of study, and observational data suggested that they were less likely to punish and restrict their child, and they had a wider range of play materials (Olds et al., 1986a).

These exciting results led to further follow-ups of this sample, and the initiation of two further experimental programmes – one in Memphis, Tennessee in 1988 focused on low-income black women; another in Denver, Colorado in 1994 (Olds et al., 2007). The Colorado study specifically investigated whether suitably trained paraprofessionals, recruited for their strong 'people skills', could achieve the same outcomes as nurses, and found that paraprofessionals had a more marked effect on mothers than did nurses, but did not significantly improve child outcomes (Olds et al., 2004). The follow-up when children were aged two showed benefits from paraprofessionals that were half as great as those in nurse-visited families, mostly non-significant, but by the follow-up at age four more effects of paraprofessional visiting became apparent.

Women visited by paraprofessionals were at this stage more likely than control group mothers to be in work, reporting a better sense of competence and mental health. They were less likely to be married, or living with the father of the child. But outcomes for the children were still not significantly different to control group children, whereas children in nurse-visited families showed stronger effects – in language, behaviour and executive function performance – leading the team to conclude that public money could be justified for nurse visitation programmes, but not for paraprofessional schemes (Olds et al., 2004). A further important improvement in the environment of nurse-visited families but not paraprofessional visited families was a reduction in domestic violence. Early follow-up of the New York State samples appeared to show strongest effects for women who were most disadvantaged (poor, unmarried and teenage) – particularly those judged as low in 'psychological resources' (intelligence, mental health and sense of mastery; Olds, 2002), hence the Memphis and Denver studies concentrated on those women who were on a low income and unmarried.

The Memphis programme involved 1139 women who were under 29 weeks pregnant with their first child, attending one large obstetric clinic between 1990 and 1991, and black (92%), unmarried (98%), age 18 or younger at registration (64%), at or below federal poverty level (85%) (Olds et al., 2007). As in New York State, the women were randomly allocated to four groups, and the nurse visits followed a detailed guide. Significant benefits were found to derive from the two-year nurse visitation programme at each follow-up (one, two, four and six years) compared to the group who were taxied to standard screening appointments and referral checks at 6, 12 and 24 months but received no home visits by the nurses. By the child's ninth birthday, two-year nurse-visited women showed continuing gains – a longer gap between pregnancies, greater stability in partner relationships. The children of mothers rated as low in psychological resources also showed significant benefits in academic achievement in their first three years of school, and higher receptive vocabulary, as well as fewer behaviour problems at age six (Olds et al., 2007). In terms of abuse, state-verified cases were too low in the sample to be used as the main measure, but in the first two years nurse-visited children overall had 23% fewer health-care encounters than control group children involving injuries and ingestions (Olds et al., 2007).

Gomby (2005) reminds us how much has been invested in the assumption that home visiting prevents abuse and neglect, improves parenting, promotes child health and development, and enhances the lives of mothers, with 37 states in the US having state-run programmes reaching as many as 400,000 families a year and costing between 0.75 and 1.0 billion dollars a year. Early Head Start has run in 708 sites nationally, Healthy Families America (HFA) in 430, Parents as Teachers (PAT) in 3000, compared to 166 for Old's NFP, and 137 for the Parent–Child Home Programme. Many use paraprofessional visitors, and they vary in intensity and duration. Their success hinges of course on the relationship between visitor and parent. Drawing from 13 meta-analyses and 11 literature reviews of the effectiveness of home visiting published between 1999 and 2005, and more than 100 other papers either evaluating programmes or commenting on aspects of them, including the disappointingly small number of studies (13) that had followed up participants of randomized or quasi-experimental trials until children reach at least age six, Gomby concludes that if asked, 'do these programmes work?' her brief answer is 'they can but they do not always do so', and many of the benefits found have been small.[1] However, the cost–benefit analyses to date, which are at best a rough indication given the difficulty of attaching a monetary value to all components or knowing all benefits over time and among siblings, suggest that the NFP is cost-effective in terms of taxes and welfare benefits alone, though for many other programmes this is not the case. Olds (2008) notes that as their New York study showed that their middle class participants did well without nurse visits, cost-effectiveness derives primarily from the support to low-income unmarried mothers.

Some additional evidence on who benefits most is provided by another intensive programme by a university group at UCLA, which had a particularly strong focus on strengthening family relationships. They provided weekly home visits for a year from late pregnancy, bi-weekly in year two, telephone calls and periodic follow-up tailing off over a further two years, weekly parent–child group meetings, and engagement of partner and relatives whenever possible (Heinicke et al., 1998). Children of intervention group mothers showed better ability to cope with brief separations at 12 months, and the mothers more responsiveness to their child's needs, in an RCT involving 70 vulnerable women pregnant with their first child. The expectation that these benefits were mediated by the relationship with the child's birth father, which was also improved, was not fully confirmed, however. Mothers who benefited most were those with a good level of security and autonomy in their ability to make and maintain relationships before the birth, who showed greater engagement with the home visitor and the intervention, and as a consequence had other improved social relationships. Motivation appeared to be increased by their own unresolved traumatic childhood experience (Heinicke et al., 2006).

Hence, although Olds suggests that the most high-risk women with a low sense of control benefit most, Heinecke suggests that they must have sufficient security and autonomy to engage well with the home visitor.

As Gomby (2005) notes, most of these studies find that effects on child outcomes were not as clear as they hoped. The best evidence for reduction in recorded incidents of abuse or hospitalization for injury is demonstrated by the NFP study in New York State, which showed a 50% reduction for the intervention group over the 15-year follow-up. The effectiveness even here was low among the one in five families where there was a good deal of domestic violence (Eckenrode et al., 2000). Many studies found decreases to injuries and some improvement in the method of child control used by mothers, but data on reductions in state-verified abuse was usually lacking (Gomby, 2005). Together with the numerous important gains in child care skills and child outcomes reported in the majority, most authors are convinced of the value of the overall approach, and new insights are being gained from targeted programmes for adolescents, and for mothers who misuse drugs (Olds et al., 2007).

Support for children with emerging behavioural problems

While the home visiting programmes are primary prevention approaches to assist young mothers from before the birth of their first child in order to try to avoid the types of difficulty that may lead to problems in the parent–child relationship, other interventions aim to help the parent as child behaviour problems emerge. These more commonly take a group approach. For instance, Scott and colleagues (2001b) evaluated the Incredible Years parenting programme as delivered to parents of three- to eight-year-olds referred to one of four south London child mental health services due to behaviour problems (uncomplicated by major developmental delay or an additional condition requiring specialist treatment).

An English version of the training videos (Webster-Stratton and Hancock, 1998) was shown to groups of six to eight parents in two-hour sessions lasting 13–16 weeks, in which 'right' and 'wrong' responses to children were shown, which they then practised at home with telephone support from the research team.

The group sessions emphasized that behaviour problems are normal, ensured the sessions were fun, with good-quality refreshments and crèche, and empathy for difficulties experienced, in a collaborative style of teaching. The training and supervision of facilitators ensured a close adherence to the programme content and methods. The parents and the behaviour problems of their children changed significantly on all outcome variables assessed over the five to seven month follow-up, which was all that could be assessed as the control group were a waiting list control hence received the programme themselves after this. An intention to treat analysis on the full 141 parents reduced the size of the differences but they remained moderate to large and statistically significant. Of course many assessments must be based on interviews with or ratings by parents, where it is not unreasonable to suspect a little bias. But an independent blind rating of a video recording of an 18 minute parent–child play task confirmed that praise rather than inappropriate comments increased threefold among intervention parents, but declined by a third in the comparison group (Scott et al., 2001b).

There are several other well-evidenced parenting skills development programmes – the one used across Switzerland and developed in Australia is known as Triple P (positive parenting programme). It has a range of levels of intensity (from information sheets for all parents, to videos, through to conflict resolution training), of which 'level 4' is intended for parents whose children have marked behaviour problems. However, in Switzerland, level 4 is offered in group form to all parents as a universal primary prevention strategy (Bodenmann et al., 2008). One randomized evaluation there compared 50 couples allocated to receive the four workshops (two to three hours each, 8 to 10 parents per group) and four telephone sessions, using the programme parenting manual, with 50 couples randomly allocated to each of two other groups – a no treatment control, and those following an equivalent number of hours of workshops in a marital distress prevention programme designed to enhance coping skills (CCET).

Triple P led to significantly greater improvements at one-year follow-up compared to either of the other groups in self-esteem and parenting skills of mothers (particularly their tendency to over-react to child misdemeanours), and their perception of child misbehaviour. Changes in fathers and in CCET participants were non-significant (Bodenmann et al., 2008). The ratings were by parents and there was no independent verification of these. But these broadly positive findings are supported by qualitative data from Swiss parents who rate the programme highly, from evaluation by its originators in Australia (Sanders, 1999) and from meta-analyses (e.g. Thomas and Zimmer-Gembeck, 2007).

The value of improving parenting as soon as problem behaviours emerge has been discussed in the previous chapter, in terms of preventing the accumulation of difficulties over time that tend to be associated. This argument has been expressed in influential papers by Gerald Patterson (Patterson, 1982; Reid and Patterson, 1989), who argues that intervention is important while the behaviours are still malleable, before they become an entrenched part of family life and self-reinforcing. His ideas, and the programmes developed from them, draw on social learning theory (Bandura, 1977). This emphasizes how much we learn from observing behaviour modelled by others that receives positive reinforcement, particularly when the observer believes that it is possible they can emulate that behaviour and receive similar rewards. Parent Management Training (Oregon model) (PMTO) is one of several similar types of programme developed to use these insights (including The Incredible Years and Triple P).

The theory suggests that when anger or aggression in a child, or non-compliance, results in the parent dropping their request, the oppositional behaviour has been rewarded. The parent may then avoid asking for action that might result in another angry response, thus further reductions in control by the parent are reinforced. Or they may get really angry to force compliance, both modelling aggression and demonstrating that it works. As interactions become more hostile, prosocial behaviour can pass unremarked and unrewarded, and warmth and encouragement from the parent is in short supply. A coercive cycle can develop that maintains itself, and may continue into school life. If there is poor regulation of homework or behaviour, problems mount, and peer relationships are also affected (Reid and Patterson, 1989). If the main parent is also depressed, the poor monitoring, inconsistent responses, antisocial behaviour and depression continue to reinforce one another.

Hence Patterson and colleagues (2004) have since argued that where intervention improves parenting, and starts to bring improved behaviour in the child, there can be other benefits, in particular to the parent's self-perception as competent and in turn to her level of depression. These will link – a reduction in depression leading to greater improvements to parenting – effectively, a virtuous circle replacing the coercive one.

They were able to test these ideas on a sample of 238 recently separated single mothers from Oregon and their sons (average age eight years, 85% white) randomly allocated to parenting intervention or control group. Three quarters of the mothers were receiving public assistance. The intervention consisted of 15 weekly early evening group meetings (an average of 10 mothers per group) supported through use of a parenting manual, a video and step-by-step sessions on effective parenting practices, decreasing coercive exchanges through responding early and effectively to misbehaviour, and positive reinforcement of prosocial behaviour. The sample was followed up at 6, 12, 18 and 30 months, assessments including judgements of mother–son interactions through eight videotaped tasks totalling 45 minutes. Their expectation that a reduction in maternal depression would be associated with continuing gains in child behaviour was strongly supported. Depression reduced in the treated group and was unstable in controls over 30 months, a significant difference in an intention to treat analysis. Reductions in child antisocial behaviour covaried with maternal depression (Patterson et al., 2004). However, the findings did not allow certainty over the direction of effects – whether the first change was to depression or to parenting – though it was considered more likely to be the start of the parenting programme that brought the early improvements in depression.

These group teaching models are seen to have advantages over home-based approaches in terms of cost-effectiveness, hence are recommended by the UK

National Institute for Health and Clinical Excellence (NICE) (2006). The decision on how widely to offer such programmes also needs to be informed by effectiveness. Olds' own review of well-evaluated home visiting schemes includes some that target particular groups, such as mothers of low birthweight babies, or drug misusing families. The former have some powerful data showing benefits up to 18 years later in educational achievements of the children, but these were significant only for the marginally underweight group (2000–2500 g), not the markedly underweight group, and the cost of the service (including a day-care enrichment programme) was considered to be prohibitive, given that no findings of special education cost avoided could be set against these (see Olds et al., 2007).

Established family problems

Norway has recently implemented the Oregon model (PMTO) throughout the country for parents of children with serious behaviour problems aged 5 to 12 (Ogden et al., 2005). The government invested in recruiting highly qualified teams to lead the programmes, providing them with comprehensive training for 18 months to ensure high fidelity to the model, with a view to considering these as a potential alternative to out-of-home placements. Their work is entirely with parents, and the parenting challenges faced by step-families are a particular focus. Evaluations since implementation are showing considerable benefit. Ogden and Hagen (2008) demonstrated that participation in PMTO in their RCT involving 121 parents across Norway (therefore a real-world effectiveness rather than researcher-controlled efficacy trial) improved their disciplinary skills (effect size 0.3), and this in turn had a significant effect on child compliance, from pre- to post-treatment. The control group received standard care, which could include family therapy, cognitive therapy or behaviour therapy, also using highly trained practitioners. PMTO did not result in improved academic competence or internalizing disorder, however, although the researchers expect that these may emerge in longer follow-ups. Effects were stronger on younger children, those under eight years on whom the change to behaviour problems represented two thirds of a standard deviation, a difference likely to be visible and have real impact. Significant direct effects on teacher ratings of social competence of the children were also demonstrated.

Two Norwegian districts (using the Incredible Years programme rather than PMTO) examined some of the factors associated with benefit (Drugli et al., 2010). They found some evidence to suggest that female children of single mothers benefited less, as did children of depressed mothers, two factors they suspected might be linked. However, the main parental predictor of poor response at this stage was contact with child protection services, suggesting that families with multiple problems needed more than a parent training programme in order to cope with the many other difficulties they were facing (Drugli et al., 2010: 564).

A similar conclusion was reached by authors of a Canadian RCT evaluation of a nurse home visiting scheme involving 163 parents of children under 13 years (average age five) who had been referred to child protection services for a reported episode of abuse or neglect in the previous three months. They found it to be ineffective in preventing a recurrence during the following three years (MacMillan et al., 2005). They tailored their 1.5 hour visits to the needs of the family, with a focus on family support, parent education and linkage to services. Both intervention and control groups also received standard child protection services. Only a subgroup of families known to the child protection service for under three months showed any benefit. Overall, more than one in three children experienced further physical abuse; nearly half, further neglect, confirming the difficulty of changing established problems, and suggesting that 'Successful remediation with families in which child maltreatment has already occurred might need very different services from those offered in early prevention programmes' (MacMillan et al., 2005: 1792).

However, although this study used public health nurses with experience in working with disadvantaged families or in child protection work, who visited families weekly for six months, bi-weekly for a further six months, then monthly for 12 months, they did not adhere to a model programme with existing evidence of efficacy.

When problems have reached a point where a custodial or other out-of-home placement is a consideration, one option that has been explored is a short 'intensive fostering' placement. In this, highly trained and supported foster carers offer mentoring, structure, encouragement, specified boundaries and consequences for behaviour, close supervision of the young person's whereabouts and activities at all times, promotion of relationships with more positive peers, earning points for positive behaviour that will enable them after six to nine months to move on, or back to their family. There is also work with both the young person in other settings to develop their problem solving and social skills and to find positive recreational activities, and with the family to encourage their reinforcement of what has been learned. Biehal and colleagues (2011) have completed one of the first independent evaluations in a prospective, quasi-experimental study involving 48 15-year-old repeat offenders in England. They demonstrated marked benefits in the first year following completion of the placement, though once the young person left a closely supervised foster care home, the benefits 'washed out'.

Rushton and colleagues (2010) argue that some elements of this kind of support should be offered routinely to families adopting young children from care, children known to have serious behaviour problems, to prevent disruption to the arrangement, and they describe some tentative evidence of the benefits of doing so. Currently almost one in four disrupt, slightly more than this continue despite ongoing problems with which they receive little support, while only about half seem relatively trouble-free (Rushton et al., 2010).

There is some evidence that greater financial investment in foster care might improve outcomes for children, with Kessler and colleagues (2008) tracing 479 alumni from Casey homes, and finding they fared significantly better than an equivalent group of alumni from publicly funded foster care (young people who met the eligibility criteria but for whom a Casey place did not become available). The former cost 60% more than the public care system, as they pay staff higher wages, seek higher staff qualifications, provide more financial resources for foster carers to use with children, more caseworker support, and have much lower turnover of staff and foster carers than the public system. For the young person, they also pay costs of job training and college attendance, providing the young person maintains an acceptable grade point average. This investment meant the Casey group spent up to two years longer in foster care than those in the public care service, had significantly better placement stability, and lower risk of foster carer neglect or abuse. Mental health and physical health outcomes at follow-up (up to 13 years later) were significantly different – roughly half as many having depression, anxiety or substance misuse disorders, or ulcers or cardiometabolic conditions. Further research into the cost-effectiveness of foster care enhancements and which components are the most important should help inform policy development.

Once a child reaches their early teens, and problems remain in the home and in school life, there is the possibility of helping them directly through the support of a 'mentor'. Evidence for this now popular strategy is discussed below.

Support for vulnerable adolescents through mentoring

Most of the studies on mentoring of school-age children come from the US. Jekeliek and colleagues (2002) provide an overview of five large-scale US programmes that have been evaluated through experimental research, quasi-experimental studies and non-experimental methods. The majority offer unstructured social and emotional support; many also help with academic work (homework), and meet their 'mentees' once, twice or three times a month. They select 'at risk' youth using differing definitions of risk, including: low income, from a single-parent household, living in an impoverished neighbourhood, a young offender or teenage mother ('Linking Lifetimes'). Most draw on volunteers from the community, provide mentor training and support; over half offer support lasting a year or more, several for many years. As Jekeliek and colleagues describe the differing arrangements:

> The *Big Brothers/Big Sisters* program takes applications from volunteers in the community, and subjects each application to an intensive screening process. The *Buddy System* program also recruits (and pays a small stipend to) mentors from the community. In the *Hospital Youth Mentoring Program*, mentors are employees at the hospitals sponsoring the program. *Across Ages* and *Linking Lifetimes* make a special effort to recruit older members of the community (ages 55+) to mentor youth. The *Campus Partners in Learning* program and *Project Belong* recruit college students to be mentors, with the goals of benefiting both the youth and the college student mentor. Most programs also screen mentors, both for safety and to assure successful matching to children.
>
> (Jekeliek et al., 2002: 6–7)

The BB/BS and Linking Lifetimes programmes offered one-to-one mentoring only, the Buddy programme group mentoring only, while others combined mentoring with other project components providing differing forms of academic tutoring. Drawing on the results of those studies that had used a randomized controlled trial, sample sizes providing comparison groups of at least 25 mentees, and at least 60% successful in retaining their engagement, Jekeliek and colleagues listed their benefits. These most commonly included improved attitudes to school, school attendance, sense of academic competence, and behaviour at school. Two also reported reduced take-up of drugs or alcohol. BB/BS reported some additional benefits, suggesting recipients felt they were less likely to hit someone, had more support from friends, and communicated better with their parents, and if this was the case they also had improved self-esteem. Positive effects in all programmes were affected by the quality of the mentor/mentee relationship and/or their frequency of contact and/or the length of the relationship. Where mentoring relationships did not last (finished in under three months), Jekeliek and colleagues (2002) found that these might in fact be harmful to the young person, contributing another failure and loss experience.

One of the larger of the evaluations reported above was of the BB/BS scheme (1138 youth randomized to the two groups – intervention and waiting list (18 months) control). Meetings lasting about four hours with their 'little brothers and sisters' who are aged between 10 and 14 years take place roughly three times per month. Both the children and the volunteers are asked about the qualities they look for in the brother or sister, and the activities they would wish to be involved in, and this is used for matching pairs. The screening of volunteers is extensive, and the screening, training and matching were costed at $1000 per volunteer (Tierney et al., 2000). The parent or guardian must approve the volunteer, and a supervisor or 'case manager' keeps in telephone contact with parent, young person and mentor monthly in the first year, quarterly thereafter. The BB or BS is unpaid – the sample in the study were on average aged 28 (women) or 30 (men), mostly well-educated young professionals. The little brothers and sisters are from disadvantaged home circumstances, with only one parent actively involved in their life; 40% of the sample also had a family history of drug use, 28% of domestic violence, 27% had experienced one or more forms of abuse. Roughly one in five of the sample were not matched with a BB/BS or changed their mind about involvement.

However, as other evaluations of one-to-one support have also indicated (e.g. Heinicke et al., 2006), successful befriending or mentoring relationships tend to be with those children or adults who are the more sociable. The funders themselves have expressed this concern. Several evaluations have been funded by Public/ Private Ventures, Philadelphia, and its president, Gary Walker (2007), notes the popularity of mentoring as a strategy for alleviating social problems in youth – because it has an intuitive appeal, fits well with dominant American cultural values (not 'big government', but emphasizing volunteerism, the personal touch, and the belief that with a little outside help, major problems can be overcome), and has evidence that it works – even if only so far for 18 months. But he sees disadvantages in its success – that it will reinforce the view that just a little help from some caring unpaid people is both sufficient and an easy solution – neither of which is true; at least as importantly, he draws attention to those not served by this, those who need it the most.

> No, mentoring's limit on the youth is not that the youth it usually gets can't benefit from mentoring; it's that the youth it usually doesn't get have the bigger problems. Mentoring's strengths, based on experience and data, are generally in the 8- through 13-year age range and concentrated in 9- to 11-year-olds. They are youth with responsible parents or teachers who want to connect them with mentors.

He continues:

> Youth who are older; who don't have a parent caring, knowledgeable, or insightful enough, or a teacher who finds them sympathetic; who are on the streets or in homeless shelters; who are in foster care or a juvenile institution—these youth do not often get volunteer mentors in the course of ordinary mentoring programs. Yet their "at riskness" is clearly magnitudes higher than the 10-year-olds who now make up the majority of mentees.
>
> (Walker, 2007: 12)

In addition, there is concern that a focus on this kind of intervention works against an argument for fundamental social change. However, Walker does not believe these projects will hinder change, hence he rejects the 'change not charity' arguments. He suggests that while it remains unclear exactly what needs to change and how, and until communities and politicians can be convinced to fund whatever 'it' is, voluntary mentoring programmes should continue.

Where mentoring might also be expected to play a preventive role is at the transition to independence – as young people from troubled homes, and children from foster homes and institutional care prepare (or probably fail to prepare) to leave school and home. The early and rapid transition to independent living that is so common among young people 'looked after' by the state is markedly different from the staged and protracted path through leaving school, leaving home, becoming financially independent, and finding independent accommodation before becoming a parent themselves, which is the more likely experience of the average young person (Biehal et al., 1995). For instance, Wade and Dixon (2006) followed up 106 care leavers from seven English local authorities, assessing the support available from family, friends and services, and the young people's success in finding work, stable accommodation, further education and reasonable mental health in their transition from care to independence. Three out of four of the sample moved to 'independent living' before the age of 18. Those with mental health problems, persistent offending, drug misuse, or emotional or behavioural difficulties before they left care fared worst in terms of engaging in further education, training or employment, and achieving stability of accommodation. Far too many were trying to live independently before most parents would consider that they were ready, and were not succeeding.

This discussion comes full circle, as these young people are leaving school and home with markedly lower educational attainment to the average young person, at a significantly younger age, with more than double the rate of unemployment of their peers (ages 16–19), and with a significantly raised rate of early parenthood – between one quarter and one half bearing a child before age 19, compared to 5% of 16–19 year-olds in the general population (Stein and Wade, 2000).

A qualitative evaluation of volunteer one-to-one mentoring schemes for care leavers in 13 parts of the UK aged 15–23 years, by Clayden and Stein (2005), described the initial goals the young people set themselves – tasks related to finding employment, accommodation, training or practical skills, or expressive goals linked to confidence and self-esteem. Almost all of them reported some benefits, three quarters of the 181 pairings felt they achieved their goals, and 39% had future plans in place, more of these occurring among those whose mentoring relationship lasted at least 12 months. Mentors too gained a good deal, feeling more skilled and more interested in working with young people as a result. However, nearly half the arrangements lasted under six months, and over one third had unplanned endings – a few of these due to the mentor withdrawing, which did not have a good impact on the mentee.

Unfortunately there is very little systematic evaluation of mentoring older teen-agers in relation to measureable outcomes such as employment, education, preg-nancy or depression. Some detailed consideration of the process and its effects is provided by Dubois and colleagues (2002), but these derive from their analysis of the many evaluations of BB/BS programmes, and hence relate to younger teen-agers. In this analysis, they conclude that the arrangements bring benefit only when the mentor achieves 'trusted adult' status in the eyes of his or her mentee. But only 40% of mentees spontaneously named their BB or BS as a significant adult when asked, even after 6 or 12 months of involvement. In fact, an important confounding factor to the evaluation of mentoring projects is that both interven-tion and control group subjects often have a pre-existing relationship with a 'natural mentor' – a family friend, school teacher, uncle, friend's parent. Dubois and colleagues suggest that the presence of such a person needs to be assessed at referral, and given the long waiting list for mentoring, priority could be given to those without such a natural mentor.

The challenge of delivering preventive support

In all these evaluations, the benefits are derived through a good-quality relation-ship between the person offering support and the intended recipient. Good engage-ment, however, is far from routine. For instance, the review by Gomby (2005) shows the wide variation between and within parent support programmes, with some evaluations finding as many as 40% of parents declining to participate, and up to 50% of those who initially participate dropping out before completion of the programme. In addition, these programmes typically assign some 'homework' to be completed between visits, such as reading to the child, and many parents fail to complete the recommended tasks (Gomby, 2005). Hence these are the first and most obvious requirements of a successful programme – effective recruitment and retention, effective engagement in the intervention.

One of the problems noted earlier occurs where the person wishing to help feels overwhelmed or powerless, such as when meeting problems in the family home of violence, drug or alcohol misuse. These will not be uncommon – the British Crime survey 2009–10 claims that one in four women in the UK will experience domestic abuse at some time in their lives. Figures cited in the review of violence in the UK by Hosking and Walsh (2005) are somewhat higher – one in three, with one in 10 women experiencing physical violence from a male partner every year. The evaluation of Healthy Families Florida (HFF) found that four of the six 'successful' or 'immediately bonded' parents who then did not complete the programme had become involved in alcohol or drugs. The home visitors 'felt they were powerless to influence the families at this point.' (Williams, Stern & Associates, 2005: 36).

Often the reluctance will come from the family, particularly if they have a combination of such problems and a visitor who perhaps expects too much of them. Shinman (1981) describes 'alienated' families who also have difficulties in relationships with family members and friends. Eyken (1982) suggested that what is often needed first is friendship, an opportunity to extend social contacts, before statutory services can hope to engage with them. A later European exploration of the views of excluded families in Greece, Hungary, Ireland and the UK quoted a UK father who put this succinctly:

> I didn't need social services, or the health visitor, never mind how nice she was. It needs other people, like you and me, to say 'I had that problem' – I found that was easier – and not to judge you, just be there for you.
>
> (French and Shinman, 2005: 56)

They sum up along the same lines:

> Towards the disengaged end of the continuum offers of child care, training and job opportunities tend to fall on deaf ears. The obstacles that preoccupy these parents have to be identified and addressed before formal information, established social groups, medicine or employment can help. Time-limited support can also increase mistrust rather than provide a kick-start. Depressed, worn out isolated parents are more likely to respond to low profile, undemanding and sustained social support from one and the same person who will listen without strings, than professional advice and assessments, or enthusiastic invitations to join groups. That is not to imply that they never will respond to them, it is to signal the necessity for informal groundwork that can be challenging and not immediately rewarding. The small early changes take time and patience and are not easy to measure. They are about the parents at rock bottom gaining a sense of self confidence and self esteem. These are the first and absolutely necessary steps out of social exclusion.
>
> (French and Shinman, 2005: 67)

Details provided in the Appendix to the HFF evaluation also illustrate how the befriender can succeed well if they engage first with the priorities of the individual. One 16-year-old mother of a three-month-old baby who already had two children and was living in a trailer with her own mother and eight siblings considered the most beneficial outcome was that she gained paid employment. Another teenage mother benefited from help to return to college. The first home visitor to the 16-year-old made little progress when focusing on birth control, whereas her replacement prioritized the housing situation and had much greater success in engaging her. The case studies leave the reader with less surprise about the difficulty these women experienced in parenting and the risk of child maltreatment.

Not all mentors are well suited or effective in their role, as Joseph Tierney and colleagues (2000) found in their evaluation of BB/BS. Some took the aim of changing their 'little brother or sister' very seriously and formed 'prescriptive relationships' where they set the goals, the pace, the ground rules, and did not adjust well if they met any resistance to change, leading to some frustration on the part of both parties. Others were better able to form 'developmental relationships' through which they increased their range of activities only as the trust and friendship strengthened. A great deal is demanded of a mentor, a role that in the BB/BS version and a majority of the US schemes is unpaid, and can be demanding as well as satisfying, sometimes frustrating more than fun, and takes a large proportion of the person's leisure time – Walker (2007) calculates it as at least 100 hours a year. There is therefore a natural limit on how many even the best organized programme could recruit.

The motivation of the mentor, befriender or home visitor is also central to their perseverance. The role is likely to be easier when they share an interest with their 'mentee' and key relatives are not opposed to their involvement, and more rewarding when working with those with fewer social and emotional difficulties. This latter point was emphasized in early evaluations of community mental health centres. When not compelled to prioritize the most resistant, often least grateful referrals – people who very often experienced the most severe and enduring mental disorder – workers gradually spent more and more time with those who at the time were described as the 'worried well' (Boardman et al., 1987; Levine, 1981). Yet policy in the US and elsewhere is viewing mentoring as an ideal social policy response to help a wide variety of very troubled citizens – young offenders, those released from juvenile detention, children of prisoners, and foster care youth.

Recruiting and retaining sufficient numbers of volunteer mentors and befrienders can be challenging, as Walker (2007) noted. However, payment of a low wage may in fact deter many of those currently offering support, who do so for reasons other than financial reward, and therefore include young middle class managers and professionals. Lessons from a comparison of the blood donor service in the US and UK suggest that financial incentives change the population willing to supply the service: they reduce the numbers of those who are not motivated by the money, increasing the numbers who are. In relation to blood supply, they increased the proportion of blood samples carrying hepatitis (Titmuss, 1970). The ideal might be to use volunteers for those with fewer problems, and well-paid staff to support those with complex needs.

The process of offering support, as argued in Chapter 7, must avoid reinforcing any negative self-perception on the part of the recipient, which poorly judged and inadequately skilled intervention can do. Scott and Dadds (2009) recognized that early drop-out, and problems in gaining the sense of collaboration needed between practitioner and parent, are often the result of the parent feeling blamed, or their strong views about their child associated with their resistance and pessimism being inadequately addressed.

The challenge of supporting families with multiple problems suggests that multiple types of support might be required. Combining home- and school-based support can double the effect size; longer interventions achieve effects that last longer (see Gomby, 2005). Biehal (2008) noted that supporting troubled adolscents needed also to work with parents, followed by a renegotiation sometimes of the terms of their relationship. The BB/BS evaluations too suggested that self-esteem of young people was improved most if the intervention also improved family relationships, not just through a good relationship between child and the BB/BS.

Should change to problem behaviour of young children be achieved through these programmes, a powerful cost-efficiency case for investment can be made. Scott and colleagues (2001a) followed up 142 young people in 1988 at the age of 28, from a sample first assessed as 10-year-olds in 1970, and drawn from a sample of all 2281 10-year-olds attending state primary schools in one London borough. They had originally been designated as falling into one of three groups – no problems, conduct problems, or conduct disorder – and those in the third group had each required services and support costing on average 10 times the amount incurred by the average 'no problem' child. The largest costs incurred were those in response to criminal behaviour, special educational need, foster care, residential care, and state benefits.

Karoly (2010) has undertaken a careful analysis of the differing ways benefit–cost ratios have been calculated by the six centre-based and home-based early childhood interventions with the most data in the US, and provides a set of recommendations to improve standardization. Many of the benefits are impossible to assess reliably in monetary terms, though become clearer with time, including cost savings deriving from reductions in child abuse and neglect, gains in child IQ, or even reduced teenage pregnancies. For outcomes that can more readily be valued, she finds that the returns vary from $2 to $16 for every $1 invested. While the studies show that early intervention brings financial benefits to society, the lack of comparability in costing method means that a higher estimated benefit–cost ratio is not necessarily the best guide to the most effective programme; for example, one citing minimal benefit–cost ratio had not attributed a financial benefit to improved IQ, home environment or mother–child interactions.

In other words, it is difficult and costly to intervene effectively, but it's worth it.

Conclusion

There are some general pointers emerging here for what works, for whom, and when. One of these relates to the expectations of people who matter. The effectiveness of teaching adolescents about contraception will be limited where the expectation of those teaching them and their peers is that they will be sexually active from a young age, they will take risks in search of pleasure, and this is normal behaviour. Targeted programmes that bring many 'high-risk' people together are more likely to backfire if participants then identify with undesirable group norms, shared expectations for low achievement. Similarly, if those offered support know this is because they are expected to have some difficulty in parenting, managing relationships, or because they are identified as having any other negative aspects of family behaviour, the result may be counterproductive. Whose expectations matter is worth noting – in the case of child care issues, the views of nurses matter more than those of paraprofessionals, particularly with parents with the lowest psychological resources; in the case of issues relating to employment and romantic partners, peer opinions may be more important than those of a professional. For young children, the most important expectations come from the parent, particularly the mother, an importance that is gradually matched or passed by the influence of peers. Some of the conclusions from earlier chapters spring to mind here – the importance of the placebo effect, the negative effects of labelling, the value of optimism.

As an earlier chapter made clear, getting help and advice when one asks for it is altogether different from being offered help because you are thought to need it. Also seeing others that we respect behave in ways that achieve desirable goals that we might also be able to achieve is central to how we learn. The achievements must come from our own efforts in order to improve confidence and competence.

Befrienders, mentors and paraprofessionals can be effective in enabling young people and struggling parents to achieve some of their goals, if their relationship achieves 'trusted adult' or 'trusted friend' status. That is, they become someone whose expectations matter. Older peers working hard at school, with aspirations in which parenthood is neither wanted nor expected as part of their immediate future, may be most effective in reducing unwanted pregnancies. Advice on specialist issues is taken more seriously when it comes from specialists.

But success in achieving a change for the better needs to come early. It is easier to help those with fewer and less severe difficulties. Entrenched problems appear to need more than family support. Changes do not always come from intervention targeting the change required, but may come from unrelated activity that brings a sense that one is valued by others. It is notable that mentors and befrienders often gain more than their mentee (see the accounts of Homestart by Eyken, 1982, and Newpin by Newton, 1992).

It is not just those on low incomes with multiple social problems that face parenting difficulty, although many argue that the raised rate of childhood emotional and behavioural problems in disadvantaged families is mediated by effects on parenting (e.g. Reid and Patterson, 1989). It is the overall family environment and the relationships between all those in the home that matters, and their expectations for their future. In this sense, whole population changes might be more important, and possibilities for these will be considered in the following chapter.

Note

1 Experimental studies typically assess whether, compared to a group that are as similar as possible to the intervention group, the difference in outcomes between them is more than might be explained as chance – that is, a probability of less than 1 in 20, or 0.05 – and is therefore considered 'statistically significant'. With large samples very small differences found can be statistically significant. Hence to convey the importance as well as significance of the difference, researchers may also cite the 'effect size', as a proportion of a standard variation. To simplify, an effect size of 0.2 is considered small, 0.5 moderate, while anything above 0.8 is large (McCartney and Rosenthal, 2000, cited by Gomby, 2005).

11 Society, status and participation

man's needs for "being held in esteem, having honor, dignity, wealth, fame, which though they may be factitious, always distressing and rarely fully satisfied, often give way to the overturning of reason"

(Pinel 1801; cited by Gerard, 1997: 388)

This review has repeatedly returned to the issue of social disadvantage and its link with mental ill-health. There is an equally clear link with physical ill-health, of course. Within any society, those low in social status and material resources live shorter, less healthy lives than those further up the hierarchy (Marmot, 2004). Not surprisingly, many assume that this is about the psychological effects of social status and income inequality; the effects of wealth on life opportunities; the physical quality of the home and neighbourhood; the control over one's life that money can bring, to make choices, take holidays, eat good food, feel free of financial worries and related stressful events. Undoubtedly these are a major part of the story, but much of this review suggests that the effects on mental health are often in fact through what low social status and low incomes do to close relationships and to parent–child relationships, and through the ways in which they raise the probability of humiliating and entrapping events and difficulties.

It is also observed that the wealth–health correlation is reflected in geographic differences in health, as discussed in Chapter 3, between cities and rural areas, between rich areas and poor, between rich countries and poor. Among rich countries, some differences are not as would be expected. Wilkinson (1996) has argued that countries with the largest gap between those at the top and those at the bottom of the income hierarchy are bad for everyone, as inequality affects the social fabric of communities, its 'social cohesion' and 'social capital', the extent to which it supports individuals and families within.

This chapter will explore these two factors – status and social capital – and their link with the mental health of individuals and of families. Can we learn from studying social factors associated with social status how to improve the mental health of those low in status? Might there be changes that could be made to housing or neighbourhoods or 'social capital' that might make a difference?

High socio-economic status is associated with good mental health

The understanding that status and mental ill-health are linked goes back a long way. Dohrenwend (1975) explains how Jarvis reported in 1855 in his report to the Commission of Lunacy in Massachusetts that 'the pauper class furnishes, in ratio of its numbers, sixty-four times as many cases of insanity as the independent class' (Dohrenwend 1975: 270). Numerous studies since confirm this relationship, as Dohrenwend shows, particularly when urban areas are studied. Jarvis explained this association as mental ill-health causing the lack of occupational success, a process of *social selection*, whereas most investigators since explain the association as the other way around; that is, that social disadvantage and associated more stressful lives lead to higher rates of ill-health – the *social causation* thesis. Of course, Jarvis would have been considering the more severe disorders and psychoses, whereas 100 years later there was more concern with the broader range of ill-health, and this helps explain their differing conclusions. Particularly influential texts among the latter group were *Social Class and Mental Illness* (Hollingshead and Redlich, 1958), and *Social Status and Psychological Disorder: A Causal Enquiry* (Dohrenwend and Dohrenwend, 1969), both demonstrating the strong inverse relationship with social class of both severity and prevalence of mental disorder.

In the early years of the twentieth century, medical statisticians collating mortality data in the UK defined five hierarchical groupings of social class according to occupation. According to David Rose (1995, and joint author with David Pevalin of the recently revised UK census tool), T.H.C Stevenson was the principal author of what has become known as the 'British' scheme, or the Registrar General's Social Class Scheme, as explained in Stevenson's lecture to the Royal Statistical Society in 1928 entitled 'The Vital Statistics of Wealth and Poverty'. The measure was not simply reflective of the income associated with the occupational group, but also of the associated 'culture' (knowledge and education), which he deemed more important than material factors in determining mortality. Hence his allocation of occupations to classes I to V was to some extent dependent on individual judgement, based on the 'standing within the community' of particular job roles, placing professionals (class I) always above managers (class II), no matter how senior the manager. Managers were in turn above administrators (IIIa) and skilled manual workers (IIIb), these above semi-skilled (IV) and unskilled (V) manual workers. Typically the rating was applied to the 'head of household', and the status of the family linked to this, whether or not other members of the household were in work. A revised version more restricted in focus – income security, job security and opportunities for advancement – has been used since 2001 by the Office for National Statistics in the UK.

As Cooper (2005) has noted, early studies have shown rates of schizophrenia of those in social class V up to four times those in social class I, the former having a worse clinical prognosis, and more likely to have been compulsorily admitted for treatment. The UK National Psychiatric Morbidity Survey (NPMS) also showed that the small proportion of people with probable psychosis and in work were much more likely to be in manual occupations than non-manual (Singleton et al., 2001). The difference has been most marked in cities, and not always significant in rural areas (Warner, 2004). The differences are not believed to come from living in disadvantaged family homes, as parental social class does not follow the same pattern, and the drift towards lower social class status often starts in adolescence with poor scholastic or work achievement, possibly due to early problems associated with the condition (84% not gaining exam passes higher than GCSE level compared to 63% of those with no signs of psychosis; Singleton et al., 2001). However, this does not fully account for class differences found, which are now thought to be compounded by periods of unemployment and difficulty gaining or retaining work leading to a drift toward low status jobs and poor accommodation in disadvantaged inner city communities after people become ill (social selection), where the person's lack of work, poor neighbourhood and housing can increase a sense of exclusion and impede recovery (social causation) (Cooper, 2005).

Social class differences are also marked in the prevalence of many physical disorders, and in mortality, though less marked in *incidence* rates of common mental disorder. A well-known and well-used data set demonstrating the links between physical health, mortality and current social status in London is the 'Whitehall study' involving 18,000 40–64-year-old men working in the British civil service from 1967, and a second cohort from the same source (the 10,000 British civil servants employed in 1985, interviewed for the fifth wave of data in 1997). The British civil service is a strongly hierarchical bureaucracy where all have reasonable job security and are in non-industrial, office-based jobs, of which 'administrative' roles are perversely the label for the highest grade, professional and executive roles next most senior, followed by clerical workers, with 'other' roles such as messengers and unskilled manual workers the most junior. From the beginning, marked average differences between men in each grade were noted, in blood pressure, lifestyle factors (smoking and exercise) and even height (20% of administrators but less than 10% of 'other' men were over six feet tall; Marmot et al., 1978). Deaths from coronary heart disease (CHD) in the 7.5-year follow-up showed a clear gradient between the four hierarchical groupings, with fewer deaths as status rose, the lowest grade having a mortality rate from CHD 3.6 times as high as the highest grade. In fact they noted that 'a man's grade of employment was a stronger predictor of his subsequent risk of CHD death than any of the other major coronary risk factors' (Marmot et al., 1978: 247).

But the NPMS showed that the class differences were not so marked in rates of common mental disorders, other than the low prevalence among those in class I. Rates were 10%, 14.5%, 18.2% in the three non-manual classes, and 15.8%, 18.2%, 18.5% in the three manual classes (Jenkins et al., 2003). As the great majority of the Whitehall sample fall into the first three groups (non-manual employment), socio-economic status (SES) differences in depression might be expected to be more marked in this study than in a population survey. However, Stansfeld and colleagues (2003) found grade differences in depression in women in Whitehall jobs only in those who also had symptoms of physical ill-health, and grade differences increased during the years of follow-up, suggesting that as the cohort aged and their symptoms of physical ill-health increased, so depressive symptoms also became more common, leading to a significant degree of comorbidity in women in the lowest occupational grades. For men, the features of their job (control, work demands, work support, effort–reward balance) held the clearest relationship to the gradient in depressive symptoms. The well-known health behaviours – smoking, alcohol and exercise – explained a good deal of the variation in physical health; that is, people in lower status jobs are more likely to smoke, take less exercise and drink more alcohol than those further up the occupational tree.

Earlier research has shown that for women, a distinction needs to be made between new onsets and chronic depression, as chronic depression shows a clear relationship with class, which is absent for new onsets, unless the woman has children at home (Brown and Harris, 1978). In Brown and Harris's research, the greater number of stressful life events experienced by depressed women and by those in the lower social class did not explain class differences in rates of depression. Instead these appeared to be explained by the greater *vulnerability* of working class women in the face of such events – their own childhood lack of care, current absence of a close confiding relationship, and perhaps a lack of a job outside the home. This means that those with long-term depressive ill-health would have a lower probability of being in the labour force at all.

Hence, although threatening life events and major difficulties are more common among people with low socio-economic status, and many assume this is the main reason behind class differences in mental ill-health, much common mental disorder appears to be linked to class differences in vulnerability to mental ill-health, and to raised rates of physical disorder. By contrast, class differences in serious mental ill-health are to a greater extent a consequence of their ill-health for their occupational success.

Child maltreatment and adolescent depression can limit adult achievement

The most important vulnerability factor for a wide range of adult mental ill-health is of course child maltreatment. The evidence for marked effects on academic achievement of a young person has already been discussed in Chapter 9, and is reflected in the profile of young people in the care of local authorities, who gain markedly fewer exam passes compared to their age group average (DCSF, 2009), and show lower college participation and higher rates of unemployment (Stein, 2006). Further supporting evidence can be cited from data from the longitudinal National Comorbidity Survey on 5004 people in the US. Controlling for several indicators of childhood socio-economic status, and age, race and sex, Zeilinski and David (2009) found those who had experienced child maltreatment or whose adolescence was characterized by behavioural difficulty were more likely to be in low-paid work or unemployed, and users of Medicaid. Similarly, using the British 1946 birth cohort of 3652 people, Colman and colleagues (2009) showed that children rated by their teachers as having conduct problems at age 13 and 15 were much more likely than better behaved school children to experience a range of negative socio-economic outcomes in adult life. Twice as many of the 10% with 'severe externalizing behaviour' at age 13, compared to those without problems, left school with no formal qualifications, and at ages 36, 43 and 53 they were more likely to have experienced unemployment (though not as often as might be supposed), to be in manual work, and to experience financial difficulty.

Colman and colleagues argue that it is the continuing interpersonal difficulty that is more damaging to the person's life chances than educational under-achievement, as after controlling for sex, father's social class, cognitive ability, educational achievement and depression in teenage years these results remain. However, as one correspondent noted (McClusky, 2009), the findings should not lead to dire predictions for these troubled teenagers, given that well over half of even the severe group had one marriage that lasted, and over 88% were in work.

Employment: Higher status jobs offer better security

Although being in work is beneficial to mental health, this does not apply to all jobs. One of the many studies that demonstrate this is a cross-sectional survey of 2497 mid-aged Australians by Broom and colleagues (2006). They found that people whose jobs combined insecurity and job strain (high demands, low control), and whose chances were slim of finding a comparable job if they lost this one, were more likely than unemployed people to be depressed (measured by GHQ score). Artazcoz and colleagues (2005) avoided the problems associated with asking people their own view of the security of their employment by asking instead about their job contract. They drew on data on 2472 salaried adults in Catalonia, Spain (a region with a particularly high level of casual labour), a sub-sample of those interviewed as part of the national health survey, which included GHQ scores. They found that those in temporary jobs with a fixed-term contract were no more likely to have poor mental health (high GHQ scores) than those in permanent work. But both these groups had significantly lower levels of mental ill-health than those with temporary contracts with no fixed term or with no contract at all. This was most clear among women, and among men in manual work (Figure 11.1). (There were too few non-manual workers with no contract to report data.)

Control for social selection was achieved through excluding all those with longstanding limiting health conditions. Artazcoz and colleagues speculate that some of the mental ill-health linked with this poor employment protection is linked also with other poor features of these jobs, such as the requirement to work long hours and the pressure not to take sick leave. Spain is a country with a strong 'male breadwinner' culture, and long-term full-time work is widely seen as a prerequisite for the transition to married life and having children, hence they were not surprised to find also that men in all types of temporary work (fixed term included) were about half as likely to have ever married or have children. In other words, the inability to plan for the future due to temporary or precarious

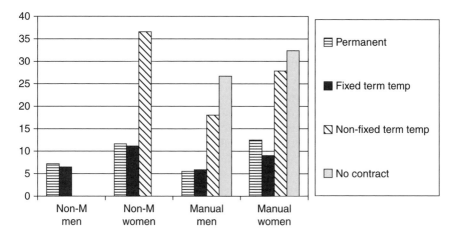

Figure 11.1 Percentage of poor mental health among workers in Spain by type of contract (drawn from table in Artazcoz et al. (2005), with permission).

employment is linked to decisions relating to marriage and parenthood, but the greater lack of control in not being able to predict when a job and income will end has the stronger link with mental health (Artazcoz et al., 2005).

Siegrist and Theorell (2006) argue that an evaluation of stress associated with work needs to take account of the 'effort–reward balance', and particularly the unfairness felt by those who believe they have no choice but to accept poor pay and conditions, due to the lack of alternatives, perhaps their low skill or a disability, and their low value to their employer due to the high numbers of others who would quickly fill the vacancy – a situation ever more common with globalization of labour. 'Job strain', defined as high job demands – the psychological demands of the work, alongside low control – the lack of freedom to decide how best to undertake the work, has also been described by Karasek and Theorell (1990). The review of research by Siegrist and Theorell (2006) provides persuasive evidence that high job strain and low effort–reward balance each produce at least a twofold increase in coronary heart disease compared to those in jobs with low strain or high effort–reward balance, and that having little freedom to make decisions makes long spells of sick leave more likely. Both features of employment appear also to be linked to mental ill-health. As noted above, Stansfeld and colleagues (2003), using Whitehall study data, show both job strain and low effort–reward balance to be associated with raised rates of depression in men.

Unemployment is associated with raised rates of mental ill-health

A review by Waddell and Burton (2006) finds numerous sources of evidence confirming the negative effects of unemployment on mental health, which they argue are partly mediated by effects on financial anxiety and relative status. Being unemployed in the West carries a stigma, and can be a humiliating and shameful experience (Smith, 1985). Furaker and Blomsterberg (2003) showed that this was still the case: drawing on telephone survey data in Sweden with a random sample of 1824 adults, they found that one in three believed that those without work could get work if they tried harder. It was also common to find attitudes suggesting that people must have some shortcomings if out of work, and that the state should expect more from them in return for the benefits paid. Those who have come closest to redundancy, or experienced it themselves or through a family member, were found to be more understanding, while young people were more likely to hold stigmatizing attitudes than older groups. These attitudes may of course have changed with the recent rise in rates of unemployment in young people.

Many researchers have provided insights into how being unemployed for a lengthy period of time affects people. Perhaps the best-known and most succinct summary is that from Marie Jahoda (1979), drawing on research in the 1970s, but also her classic study of the Austrian town Marienthal in the 1930s, devastated by mass unemployment, which led her to conclude that there are five main reasons why employment is important, beyond the financial returns.

> First among them is the fact that employment imposes a time structure on the waking day. Secondly, employment implies regularly shared experiences and contacts with people outside the family. Thirdly, employment links an individual to goals and purposes which transcend his own. Fourthly, employment defines aspects of status and identity. Finally, employment enforces activity.

The only positive aspect of unemployment that one might note here is that its effects have been shown to be less marked when that experience is shared widely because unemployment is high (Platt and Kreitman, 1984; Clarke, 2009). But health effects of unemployment often increase as time goes by (Bartley and Plewis, 2002), and contact with friends can diminish as a short period of unemployment stretches towards 12 months (Economic Intelligence Unit, 1982).

While Jahoda's account clearly links unemployment with a poor sense of wellbeing, this is not the same as causing mental ill-health. However, there is no shortage of evidence for this too, as well as a clear link with suicide. Admissions to psychiatric hospitals have been shown to follow the economic cycle of recession and growth, and the well-known studies by Harvey Brenner (1973) that illustrated this have been supported by other research since (see Warner, 1994; Catalano and Hartig, 2004). Although suicide is rare, it remains more common in those without work. Blakely and colleagues (2003) tracked the records of two million people aged 18–64 completing the 1991 census in New Zealand, matching them to mortality records three years later, and showing that suicides were between two and three times as common among the unemployed compared to those in work, after controlling for the raised rate of mental ill-health among the unemployed. Those not working, but not seeking work either, had a similarly raised rate of suicide. Being married reduced the risk of suicide by about half.

Employment, unemployment and mental health:
Some implications

Improve working lives: Control, rewards, support, security

Some methods to reduce the stressfulness of certain jobs are self-evident. The provision of an employment contract with terms and conditions that offer some security is one (Artazcoz et al., 2005). Management development programmes to help assess how job strain and the 'effort–reward balance' can be improved might be another (see Siegrist and Theorell, 2006). The many textbooks on management theory describe how successful businesses are those that place an appropriate value on their staff, providing stability, staff development schemes, fewer levels in the hierarchy, transparent information sharing, and devolved decision making (Peters and Waterman, 1982; Pfeffer, 1998).

Wilkinson (1996) has suggested that the work environment in Japan reflects a greater application of such practices, and helps to explain workers' superior health there. He claims that as well as a lesser gap in pay between those at the top and those at the bottom as compared to many Western countries, the culture of the workplace is one where concern is shown for both the worker and their families, and there is a greater emphasis on loyalty, cooperation and group performance. He also describes how Japanese directors are more likely to have worked their way up from within the company, and workers at all levels take an equal share of pay restraint when the company is less successful, so that job security of low-status workers is not the first target for savings.

Employees who have some control over their working hours (start and finish times, control over days off, taking unpaid leave, choice of dates for holidays) take fewer days of sick leave, particularly for women in stressful jobs, as Ala-Mursula and colleagues (2004) demonstrated in a prospective study of 16,139 public sector workers in Finland. Numerous other examples of good employment practice have been collated by the European Agency for Safety and Health at Work (2002). One drawn from nursing home providers in Spain illustrated how staff can often provide the most useful suggestions on how to improve the workplace. Their proposals included improved staffing at peak times to reduce workload, the reorganization of shifts to improve holiday and staff cover and flexibility; improved staff training; and designating specific responsibilities to auxiliaries both to improve role clarity and to provide greater autonomy. Prior to the research, sickness absence rates had been 18%. Within a year of implementing the proposed changes they had reduced to 2%, and they did not rise significantly above this level over the next three years.

Seymour and Grove (2005) found 31 of these sorts of programme that had strong evaluative data, mostly RCTs, including many that aimed to help employees with existing mental ill-health that had an individual rather than organization-wide focus. The review considered common disorders, not the more severe conditions, and job retention and return after sick leave. There was some evidence for benefits from greater employee involvement in decision making and problem

solving, management training in these areas, and the provision of stress management training for staff in preventing sickness absence. However, they found much
stronger evidence in relation to supporting those with exisiting mental ill-health,
and through individual programmes that offered a combination of coping skills
training and support. After two weeks of stress-related sick leave, they show that
providing four or five sessions of CBT can improve job retention.

The strategies needed to minimize work stress are now widely understood and
are reflected in relevant policy in many countries. For instance, the Health and
Safety Executive in the UK has produced a set of 'management standards' that
employers are required to adhere to which relate to workplace stress in the same
way organizations have had to do in relation to physical safety (e.g. HSE, 2007).

Help those recovering from mental ill-health to gain work

In the middle of a marked economic downturn, unemployment is affecting all
sections of society. But some groups are always disproportionately affected. For
lone parents, ethnic minority groups and people without formal qualifications, the
rate of unemployment is roughly double the rate for the total working population
in the UK (HM Treasury and Department for Work & Pensions, 2003). For school
leavers of 16 and 17 it is four times as high, with about one third of them unemployed and seeking work in 2009 in the UK (Marmot Review, 2010).

People with disabilities and ill-health vary by condition as to how far their
employment is affected. Citing UK Labour Force data for 2008, the Marmot
Review (2010) shows that of 17 different chronic health problems and disabilities,
those with a serious mental health condition have the lowest rate of employment
(about 12%), and those with depression and bad nerves were only slightly more
likely to be in work – well under 30% of this group. This compares to the average
employment rate of those in the workforce in 2008 of over 90%.

A substantial proportion of people who are out of work due to mental ill-health
would much prefer to be working, and want mental health services to help them
do so (Secker et al., 2001). One reason so few succeed in many Western societies
is the disincentives created by the welfare benefit system that is provided to
support those unable to work. People are reluctant to lose safe financial benefits
from the state when they are unsure whether paid work will endure or whether
they will be able to cope with it long-term (Warner, 2004). The pay they may
initially gain may also be so low that their situation is no better financially, and
much less secure.

A second problem relates to the low expectations that can come with a diagnosis of a mental illness. Often work is not seen to be a realistic option, nor
employers expected to find them valuable employees. Where these expectations
can be changed, and the financial disincentives avoided, the employment rate can
also change, as Warner (2000) illustrates, quoting the employment rate in south
Verona in Italy in 1994 when as many as 60% of a randomly selected sample of
people being treated for schizophrenia were found to be in work (although most
not employed full-time). His own area in Boulder, Colorado now has double the

expected US rate of employment for those with a diagnosis of schizophrenia. Warner suggests several policy changes that would help, including increases to the weekly 'earnings disregard' (the amount someone is entitled to earn before their benefits are reduced), or providing wage subsidies to increase the net reward of working.

Crowther and colleagues (2001) reviewed 18 randomized controlled trials comparing schemes that aim to prepare people recovering from serious mental ill-health to go back to work (sometimes referred to as 'train and place') with those that aim to support people through the process of finding suitable vacancies, applying, and starting work (the 'place and train' approach). They provide convincing evidence of the advantages of the latter over the former approach in terms of hours per week worked in open employment in the year following.

Currently, a model known as 'individual placement and support' (IPS), developed by Drake and Becker and refined over time (e.g. Becker et al., 2001; Bond, 1998, 2004), has the strongest evidence of efficacy. It is based on the assumption that given careful matching of job and candidate, and the right support, all those who express a desire to work should be able to do so (Rinaldi et al., 2008). Diagnosis is not important, and people are not judged by others as 'not ready' to work, with either too many symptoms or symptoms that are too challenging. The support is crucial, and it needs to be clear it is there for a considerable time after the person finds work, should the person need it. If the individual has chosen to disclose their mental health diagnosis to the employer, the worker may be able to help resolve any early workplace difficulty. The vocational support worker should be based with the mental health team as this also helps to overcome the assumptions by so many mental health workers that the employment of the service user is an unrealistic aspiration, and possibly harmful to their health. For young people, supported education is an equally important option (Rinaldi et al., 2008).

The IPS model has been subject to numerous RCT evaluations, and almost all those based in the US have demonstrated marked benefits in terms of getting people into work, achieving employment rates of 30–40% compared to other methods that report 10–12% (Crowther et al., 2001). Several randomized controlled trials of the method across Europe and in the UK have also shown its effectiveness; only one recent study in south London did not. However, even this study found that slightly more gained work (11% compared to 8% of the control group – a dismally low figure either way), but it also showed marked savings for the health service as on average the intervention group spent fewer days in hospital over the following year, so even after the cost of the IPS scheme was deducted, NHS savings were significant (Howard et al., 2010).

In reflecting on the low success of the programme, the authors recommended that individuals should be screened for motivation so only those who are 'active' job seekers are offered the help, and that benefits counselling should be provided. (This was already part of the approach as implemented in other areas, and is particularly important in the UK with its harsh welfare benefit regime.) However, it is important too that further work explores how the greater benefits reported in the US might be achieved in the UK and the rest of Europe, and at the same time, not to oversell this as a certain way to ensure mental health service users gain work. At its best it can help about 40% of those recovering from serious mental ill-health to gain work, 30% more than would have worked otherwise – a considerable achievement, but not a magic wand. In Warner's (2000) more cautious overview, he recommends that provision should still include the full range of vocational support, from the most sheltered to the most independent (sheltered work, social enterprises and supported employment), aiming for as satisfying, normalizing, and integrated arrangements as possible in all.

Warner and Mandiberg (2003) describe how small work enterprises can be created to provide work to those recovering from a psychosis in a mixed workforce, citing good examples of these in many European countries, but relatively few in the US or UK. The high rate of employment achieved by northern Italy is largely through these schemes. The firms are non-profit-making, with a large proportion of the workforce with a history of serious mental ill-health, and may for instance produce health foods or provide domestic services, office services, printing, or painting and repairs (Warner and Mandiberg, 2003). However, they are not often viable without some subsidy from mental health services. Their viability can also be assisted by mental health service providers seeking to contract their services with agencies or companies that employ those with a history of mental ill-health. This approach could be strengthened by finance departments making this a mandatory part of the contracting process; that is, to first consider such agencies. By contrast, the development of sheltered work is no longer considered a good method of rehabilitation, as it can simply confirm to the worker that they are not capable of open employment, which rarely follows (Rinaldi et al., 2008).

Increase employment opportunities for school leavers

While the poorly qualified young person leaving school may have faced relatively little difficulty in finding some paid employment 30 or 40 years ago, their opportunities are declining. The average young person is entering the labour market later, after gaining more qualifications, and becoming a parent later, while those who leave school at 16 with few or no qualifications also move to parenthood at a much younger age (see Bynner et al., 2002). The gap is growing between early and late school leavers, as shown by a comparison of the transition to adulthood of young people from two longitudinal studies of British birth cohorts – those born in 1958 and those born in 1970 (Bynner et al., 2002). There were fewer 17-year-olds not in employment, educaton or training (NEETs) in the 1970 cohort, but four years later many more of this cohort were unemployed. Many more of the 1970 cohort of young women who were not in education or work at 21 declared their occupation as 'housework', reflecting their earlier exit from the labour market to have children.

Those who had periods of unemployment showed raised rates of non-clinical depression (measured on a malaise inventory of self-esteem and depression), and rates of both unemployment and depression increased substantially in the later cohort. Bynner and colleagues (2002) noted how the traditional school leaver 'entry' jobs – craft apprenticeships and secretarial work – were declining and being replaced with sales, catering and caring jobs, often low paid and part-time.

In the current recession, the disturbingly high level of unemployment in young people in all OECD countries has raised great concern about long-term effects – the likelihood of 'scarring' – leaving these young people at a significant employment and earnings disadvantage for many years into the future. Scarpetta and colleagues (2010) describe two groups for whom we should be most worried: first, those 'left-behind youth' who have left school without qualifications, come from an immigrant or minority ethnic background, and/or live in disadvantaged, remote or rural neighbourhoods – estimated (from data on NEETs) as 11% of 15–25-year-olds across OECD countries in 2007. They found that two thirds of this group had already become disenfranchised, and were not actively seeking work or had been unemployed for over a year. The second group are 'poorly integrated' new entrants, not necessarily unqualified, but who move in and out of temporary jobs, unemployment and inactivity. The two groups together mean that 30–40% of school leavers face great problems in finding secure employment.

Policy directions

No-one wants to be unemployed. It is demoralizing and often demeaning, and one of the greatest policy challenges is how more of those who wish to work can be enabled to do so. Perhaps more job sharing may be needed if there are too few jobs – half a job may be better than none. Some types of 'welfare to work' strategies or compulsory training schemes can increase stigma, according to Bambra (2010), while providing limited help in gaining employment. Rinaldi and colleagues (2008) suggest the same is true for sheltered work for those with existing mental ill-health or disability.

One of the most important features of any job is its security, yet many options for reducing unemployment might reduce the security of those in work. For instance, Saint-Paul (2008) discusses the relative merits of the tough stance in the UK where there is little employment protection (i.e. it is easy to fire people in a downturn, but also therefore not risky to hire more in a recovery) and little unemployment benefit (lasting only six months) with the stronger employment protection in France (hard to fire, so risky to hire) and higher unemployment benefit (about three times as much, lasting 30 months). One might prefer to live in France – except that this system is not conducive to getting young people into the labour market. The French unemployment rate was double the UK rate (see Saint-Paul, 2008). Countries with a low level of regulation in the labour market such as the UK and US have fewer (two thirds as many) poorly integrated youth, and under half as many left-behind youth (6% in the US, 15% the European average; Scarpetta et al., 2010).

Many would like to return to the times when large numbers of training roles were available in the form of apprenticeships, which were real jobs, perhaps now subsidized by the state (e.g. Scarpetta et al., 2010). They describe a range of differing initiatives by governments across the OECD, but little clear evidence yet on which work best and why. The solution is unclear, but the need to find one is urgent. The age group for whom poverty is rising fastest across the OECD is the 18–25-year-olds (OECD, 2008). Also of concern are single parents, who are three times as likely to be poor as the average person. The raised risk of parenting problems among these two groups has been revisited throughout this review.

As Bambra (2010) notes, the employment that is available is also changing, as a 24-hour society needs more shift workers and work during unsocial hours, and this affects 'work–life balance'. More employment is temporary, with short-term contracts (or no contracts), and as traditional permanent positions decline this affects job security. Those in low-paid, unprotected posts will be easiest to make redundant, and so also least likely to have a redundancy payment to soften the fall. Bambra argues that these factors make ill-health a higher risk in the current recession than in those of the 1980s and 1990s. Economic recovery may see poor employment security continue, however, as it would seem that the labour market changes are unlikely to be reversed, and many more people will be learning to live with financial insecurity.

Status: Housing and neighbourhood disadvantage

Low-paid workers and unemployed people inevitably have restricted choice in where they can afford to live. As government policy during the twentieth century sought to provide housing for all, including those with the lowest financial resources, many cities across northern European countries moved increasingly toward segregated areas of the poorest people, often into large purpose-built estates of social housing. Anne Power (1999) describes how social, income and housing problems combined with poor estate management and planning produced unpopular places to live, and a downward spiral during the 1970s, with real concerns of chaos and danger. Property that became 'difficult to let' left empty apartments, attracting drug misuse and vandalism. Some of the largest estates across Europe had rates of unemployment of more than 80%, over half the families with children were lone-parent families, crime rose to four times the average, and most young people left school with no qualifications (Power, 1996).

Power documented the proportion of children in poverty in the UK (defined as households earning less than half of national average income after allowing for housing cost) as rising from 10% to over 30% between 1979 and 1991. This was reflected in social housing: a drop by one third of households in employment over the same period; and a doubling of households headed by a single parent. She notes also the markedly lower educational achievements of children attending schools linked to these large estates, and how once their reputation becomes tarnished, living there carries a stigma.

Good examples of the 'rescue' of some social housing schemes were also described (Power, 1999). These experimental projects across Europe in the 1980s devolved decisions and resources to the local level, ensuring that residents participated fully in planning improvements. They were backed by higher level commitment to support change, with offices based on the estates, and a person engaged to fulfil the role of community facilitator. One example is described where the gradual shift to local control enabled them to create local services and jobs, strengthen management, tackle the backlog of repairs, and resist the 'dumping' of troublesome and criminal families to poor estates. The policing of drug trafficking was improved; self-help groups were established. However, the poverty remained, and Power (1996) argued that the viability of these estates depends on improved employment opportunities and better transport.

Stable communities can provide support to families

Early responses to areas of poor housing had involved large-scale demolition, moving residents into better accommodation, but dispersed, and much was written about the loss of social networks in this process. Young and Willmott (1962) was one of the first – a now classic account of the dispersal of families from a close-knit working class area in Bethnall Green, London, to new housing estates in a suburb in Essex, where families were often cut off from relatives and lonely. While this may have romanticized the life of those formerly in the inner city terraced housing, it had a substantial impact on regeneration processes thereafter. It is now better understood that renewal processes must also attend to economic regeneration and community life, and, if possible, avoid destroying existing networks.

The support that was often central in these early accounts was that between mother and daughter, and the daughter's new family. The importance of such family support has not diminished, even if its availability may have done. Power and Willmot (2007) describe the lives of parents in two urban low-income areas in the north of England – including two large social housing estates. Detailed interviews with the main carer illustrate the importance of support from relatives and to a lesser extent from neighbours. One in five saw their mother every day, and over half saw their mother at least once a week. The most common type of support provided was help with child care, sometimes enabling the mother to go out to work. Between half and two thirds of the samples could name at least a few people locally they could trust, and trust was judged by them as important in terms of feeling safe in their homes, able to go out without being robbed, in 'looking out for each other', in crime prevention. A majority (about two thirds) could also give an example of an exchange of favours such as providing access to a phone, passing on unwanted baby clothes, leaving a spare key with them. Power and Willmot (2007: 24) comment that 'A dominant theme in the respondents' narratives on friends and family was the importance not so much of the actual support received from them, as *knowing it is there to draw on when ever it is needed*' (emphasis in original).

These networks are strongest among stable communities of course, as Power and Willmot (2007) illustrate. So too do Sampson and colleagues (1999) in their study of the 342 neighbourhoods of Chicago, which demonstrated that residential stability was more important to adult–child relationships and to the frequency of exchanges of favours and information among parents than was the ethnic mix or poverty of the area.

Arguably these stable social networks explain some of the better mental health often found in rural areas compared to cities. For instance, Glendinning and West (2007) studied over 600 young people in Siberia, one of the most materially deprived regions of the OECD, finding that although village children were poorer than city children and more often lived with a lone parent, rating their own physical health as considerably worse, their mental health was significantly better. The authors' analyses led them to argue that young people in villages drew on support from family, peers, kin-based networks, and tradition, and shared the values of their parents for hard work and cooperation. There was greater respect for the advice and guidance of parents and teachers, they were better engaged with school than city children, and had traditional views relating to gender roles. In the city, the mental health of children related more to good peer support, doing well at school and seeing good prospects for work in the local area. Those who did not engage well in school and dropped out early had worse mental health, which Glendinning and West (2007) suggest may be linked to the implications for their social position in terms of their opportunities in the city. That is, kin are key to future security in small communities, while personal academic achievement and your parents' education matter more to you in the city.

Individual, more than neighbourhood, 'social capital' links to mental health

The term increasingly used to describe the trust between neighbours and the social networks linking people within communities is 'social capital', particularly since Robert Putnam's book *Bowling Alone: The collapse and revival of American community'* (2000). His use of the term is to describe the 'connections among individuals – social networks and the norms of reciprocity and trustworthiness that arise from them' (p. 19). He argues that we need face–to-face contacts with people in order to develop trust and that both trust and social contacts are declining, lamenting the changes to our way of life, our changing values.

Social capital is a very different concept to the terms *social integration* and *social isolation* as they were used by researchers in earlier years, though they might sometimes have been confused since. The latter were usually simply the descriptive terms used for those who were or were not married and in work (e.g. Myers et al., 1975). Myers and colleagues followed up a random sample of 720 adults over two years in Newhaven, Connecticut, studying their health, life difficulties and community support, and finding that life events and crises played the greatest role in health, but that people with few events yet many symptoms were more likely to be 'poorly socially integrated'. By this they meant never married, lower occupational status, unemployed, dissatisfied with role, and/or recently treated for physical ill-health. Conversely, those with many events and few symptoms were better educated, in higher status jobs, more satisfied with their role, and had less physical ill-health. Social integration, particularly through marriage and satisfactory employment, were the factors they argued to be important to mental health.

Putnam's ideas relating to social capital, although linked with research findings on inner city mental ill-health, were not in fact focused on family life. His interest was less on the inner-city housing estate, or the rise in divorce, single parenthood, or unemployment, and more on the average family and their lifestyle. These are changes that have come with technology and higher average incomes: we can communicate without leaving the home, and link status more to increasing individual material wealth rather than to our role in our communities. He argues that 'Television, two-career families, suburban sprawl' along with 'generational changes in values' lie behind a reduced interest in active involvement in voluntary groups or clubs, or even outings to the park with friends. 'Our growing social-capital deficit threatens educational performance, safe neighbourhoods, equitable tax collection, democratic responsiveness, everyday honesty, and even our health and happiness' (Putnam, 2000: 367).

Putnam suggests that participation in local organizations and groups not only provides useful social contacts but also acts to sustain rules of conduct. They often involve a sense of mutual obligation – an exchange of favours, fostering strong 'norms of reciprocity' that can produce a culture of, or generalized expectation, of reciprocity. Social networks come in many forms – from the extended family, our colleagues at work, and parents of the classmates of our youngest children. Those with whom we are strongly bonded are good for maintaining us, while those in more distant or diffuse networks might be more important to creating new opportunities; the two are described by Putnam as 'bonding' and 'bridging' networks. (Szreter and Woolcock (2004) proposed a third type of social capital, 'linking' people vertically through formal institutions such as community or local government structures, though Putnam (2004) feels that this addition tends to confuse the effects of social capital with those of state intervention.) He characterizes it thus: 'Strong ties with intimate friends may ensure chicken soup when you're sick, but weak ties with distant acquaintances are more likely to produce leads for a new job' (Putnam, 2000: 363). He documents persuasively the changes in these over time, the increasing and strengthening community life in the decades before the 1960s, and the marked decline in the United States in the decades to follow.

Putnam's scale uses 14 indicators from lifestyle and social trend surveys routinely carried out across the US. It includes: served on committee for local organization in last year; civic and social organizations per 100,000 population; did voluntary work: frequency last year; entertained at home: frequency last year. It also includes items relating to feeling safe: most people can be trusted versus can't be too careful; agree: most people are honest. Hence the term 'social capital' brings together many differing aspects of community life into a single index, and different researchers since have included differing components in their own measures, making evidence difficult to compare and conclusions hard to draw (De Silva et al., 2005).

Reviewing 21 studies of social capital and mental illness, De Silva and colleagues find seven that define small and large communities in terms of aggregated responses to such statements (ecological social capital), from which few if any effects on mental health are apparent. But the 14 that report people's *individual* responses to the questions (individual social capital) found good evidence of a link with mental health, but only in relation to questions about 'cognitive social capital' (e.g. trust of neighbours), rather than behaviour (e.g. attending groups).

Measures of social capital correlate with child wellbeing and achievement

Putnam shows that his measure of social capital calculated for each state in America has a close to linear relationship with the 'Kids Count' index of child wellbeing data also collected across the US. The latter measure collates scores from 10 indicators including child deaths, low birth weight, teen births, school drop-outs and children living in unemployed or lone-parent households. As both Kids Count profiles and social capital correlate with education, income and employment, firm conclusions about causal links cannot be drawn with confidence. However, Putnam's analysis after multiple regressions suggests that while poverty is more important, social capital does play an important role – 'in keeping children from being born unhealthily small and in keeping teenagers from dropping out of school, hanging out on the streets, and having babies out of wedlock' (Putnam 2000: 297–8).

Similarly, he supplies considerable evidence of the correlation between his measure of social capital and the performance of schools. He reminds us that the early use of the term 'social capital' was to describe the importance of community involvement in successful schools as long ago as 1916. L.J. Hanifan described it in terms of the good will, fellowship, sympathy and social exchanges of the school community as a resource sustaining the whole. This seems intuitively important – when a young child starts at a school that is in a dilapidated condition, and seemingly poorly run, parents can decide to get involved in the parent–teacher association and mobilize other parents and neighbours to help improve it, or they can opt out, and buy a place at a private school, or move house to be in reach of a smarter school. 'Sink schools' can quickly be created, and perpetuated in this way, suggesting that social capital – or, at least, parent involvement – matters.

Strong social capital can mitigate material disadvantage for children

The most important components of social capital, according to the review by De Silva and colleagues (2005), were the cognitive elements – knowing the neighbours, feeling a sense of belonging, liking the neighbourhood, a sense of trust. One possibility for beneficial effects is the way these may also shape expectations and exert a controlling influence on behaviour, through low crime, improved aspirations, challenges to extreme views. Statistics for violent and non-violent law-breaking vary dramatically between districts, and have been shown to influence young people to behave in ways their peers with identical social and educational circumstances in a low-crime neighbourhood do not. This tends to provide some support to the argument that the the neighbourhood matters as well as the individual's feelings about it. Certainly Putnam (2000: 312) argues that 'My fate depends not only on whether I study, stay off drugs, go to church, but also on whether my neighbors do these things'.

Parents who try to persuade their 15-year-old son to return home before midnight have a much greater challenge if other parents among his social group do not set these boundaries. But in any locality, only contact with the parents of his friends will tell you whether they are trying to hold the same boundaries and that their son is also telling them, as yours tells you, that other parents allow it. Putnam argues that seeing good behaviour, and seeing adults challenge antisocial behaviour when it occurs (rather than 'turn a blind eye'), is also needed to help steer young people away from temptation towards crime, hence there needs to be a good proportion of the families in a neighbourhood willing to do so.

This is a large part of how schools can exert their influence on pupils, through the involvement of pupils and their parents in decision making, in creating an ethos, or culture of expectations for good behaviour and academic work. This was the claim made by Michael Rutter and colleagues (1979) in their landmark study of secondary schools that remains relevant today, which recommended that in order to create this ethos, schools needed a good cross-section of children from the local community. In particular, they need to have a representative proportion of intellectually able students. These students, and those with disabilities, disadvantage, from ethnic minorities and with behavioural problems, are not distributed equally between schools, placing some schools very much at a disadvantage. A preponderance of low-ability children, or of disadvantaged children, was associated with low expectations and with raised delinquency rates.

A 'good' school was characterized by its 'ethos' rather than individually talented teachers or excellent facilities, and this ethos had the most powerful effect on pupil behaviour and achievement. A 'good' school has a balanced intake of ability levels, widespread opportunity for pupil participation and individual responsibility, good classroom management and discipline, often an academic emphasis, and a wide use of rewards and incentives (Rutter et al., 1979). Studies on the reduction of bullying in schools since this time have also placed an emphasis on the school 'climate' or 'culture'.

For instance, the study in 20 Canadian high schools, set up to evaluate a violence reduction intervention (and described in Chapter 7), also reported substantial variation between schools in rates of delinquency independent of the intervention. The three with the lowest rates averaged 5% of grade 11 pupils engaging in violent delinquent acts, while three schools at the other end of the range averaged 16%, with one school having 32% of pupils showing such behaviour (Crooks et al., 2011). Controlling for differences in intake, they demonstrate a major effect of school:

> Given the same individual profiles or risk, students were more likely to engage in violent delinquency if they were attending a school perceived by the entire student body as an "unsafe" climate than if they were attending a school perceived as a "safe" climate.
>
> (Crooks et al., 2011: 398)

Together these studies suggest that achievement and behaviour will be improved more through changes to the social fabric of school institutions than by interventions focused on traditional educational goals – skills of teachers, books, class size. That is, through ensuring a balanced intake of ability and socially disadvantaged pupils; developing sports teams to play outside designated lesson time; after-school clubs; perhaps a school play where parents also assist; where the ethos is one of mutual respect, consideration; where misbehaviour is well controlled, and pupils feel safe. Putnam cites studies showing that private religious schools have some of the most frequent parent–teacher contacts outside the classroom, and seem to produce particularly well-adjusted children, connected, he believes, to what he defines as their strong social capital.

Policy directions

Unemployment or insecure low-paid work means people are also more likely to be in social housing, and to live in poor neighbourhoods. There appears to be increasing polarization of rich and poor people in richer and poorer areas. Hills (2007) suggests that policy designed to improve such problems is not working.

> Nearly half of all social housing is now located in the most deprived fifth of neighbourhoods, and this concentration appears to have increased since 1991. If ensuring that social tenants can live in mixed-income areas is a key potential advantage of social housing, we do not seem to be achieving it.
>
> (Hills, 2007: 11)

He describes the areas originally built as flatted council estates as having marked problems with drug users or dealers, and a general fear of crime (both reported by one in five tenants); and '18% . . . feel unsafe alone even at home or outside in daylight. One in seven social tenants in these areas says they are *very* dissatisfied with their neighbourhood' (emphasis in original).

It was not always so, and need not be so. It is not long since social housing was a desirable option for low-income working families (Hills, 2007).

Housing policy also needs to support and if possible strengthen family connections, by enabling relatives to stay close to one another, or move closer. Arguably, the support the family provide to each other is the most important component after feeling safe that is reflected in measures of social capital – knowing help is there if you need it. Some examples of active intervention to do this exist – Singapore is an exceptional example, with assertive policy to shape living arrangements. Numerous financial incentives and preferential housing options are offered to married children wishing to move to live close to their parents (Teng, 2007). Bambra and colleagues (2010), in a wide-ranging examination of eight policy areas that aim to reduce inequality, drawing on 30 systematic reviews since 2000 in developed countries, show that housing and employment are the policy areas with best evidence of benefit. For instance, programmes in the US to offer assistance with rent so that people had more choice about where they lived, leading to more mixed neighbourhoods and reducing segregation, were found to have benefits to perceived safety, and to reductions in distress, anxiety, alcohol and substance misuse. Changes to work environments that increased individual control at work, and increased control over shift work patterns, have also shown benefit to self-reported mental health, and those that decreased control or decreased job security increased self-reported mental ill-health.

Conclusions

No surprises. People need to feel safe – in their homes, in their schools and in their jobs. There needs to be a route to security for everyone, particularly those aged 16–24, not just one that requires more and more qualifications. The correlation between status and mental ill-health is partly shaped by early childhood adversity and emotional and behavioural problems in adolescence, limiting adult achievement and raising risk of unemployment. In employment, status is related to better job security, less job strain, better effort–reward balance, greater flexibility in working hours to accommodate individual needs, and this explains at least in part the link with mental health in men.

Those living in existing poor neighbourhoods low in social trust, or working in high-strain, insecure, unrewarding jobs, are best placed to lead improvements to them, if they can be given the power and resources to do so. As well as safety, people's jobs, schools and neighbourhoods will be associated with lower levels of mental ill-health if they succeed in creating a climate of expectation that workers, school pupils and residents will achieve, behave well, be treated fairly, help one another out, and show respect for others. Neighbourhoods that have a good level of residential stability, particularly with family members close by, are important in supporting families with young children. Vulnerability to mental ill-health is higher and socio-economic status is lower among those with low levels of safety and of positive expectations at home, at school and at work.

As more of the world's population move to the cities (from 40% in the mid-1970s to perhaps 60% by 2025, according to the World Bank (2000)), and work shifts from agriculture to industry to trade and services with profound changes to working lives, the need to address the challenges of inner-city life becomes more urgent.

12 Ready to change

This review has ranged far and wide. Probably too far. But this reflects the shift over the past 20 years in thinking about mental health, and the extent of the research accumulating on every aspect. The aim here has been to be even-handed and to consider the merits and usefulness of progress in each area – from biology and genetics to psychology, sociology and epidemiology, to the insights of those who have personal experience. What it shows is that all of these provide part of the story, and need to be incorporated into any explanation of mental ill-health, or into attempts to prevent it. Genetics, biology and life experience shape who we are. What matters to the individual can be described in terms of their lives from before conception through to adult life, and those who play the most important role are the person themselves, their parents, their wider family, close friends and sexual partners. Those in health or social services or in community support organizations can play a role in helping to strengthen the resilience of individuals, and the support available to them. But vulnerability, coping and support, not just that available through public services, are shaped, perhaps more than we realize, by decisions made – or not made – by government.

In this final chapter, there is some reflection on the insights gained about what matters, and what works, and why it might be that in each area reviewed there have been numerous examples of well-planned programmes that did not work. These have often been for people who were considered most in need of the help offered.

These discussions are intended to be helpful to practitioners and policy makers, hence are framed in terms of 'mental ill-health'. However, earlier chapters have for illustrative purposes placed emphasis on schizophrenia and depression, particularly what we know about why the problems so labelled may relapse or follow a chronic course. Intervention with troubled children and adolescents has also been a core focus, given the links between early maltreatment and anxiety and depression, particularly chronic depression. The use of labels – not necessarily the broad diagnostic groupings, but labels of the core symptom types – continues to be central to the growing research on vulnerability, and a strong case has been made for the continued use by researchers of the more subtle distinctions (e.g. Tremblay, 2010). But detailed categories are not necessarily useful to practitioners. For service users they can carry all the disadvantages of any label conveying a 'problem status', as discussed below. This has been a tricky balance to achieve in reviewing evidence from research and distilling more general messages for practice. Hence a cautionary note about these generalizations should be added, that the conclusions drawn here are heavily influenced by research on the case study areas, and it is unlikely that the general statements will apply to all types of mental ill-health. On the other hand, depression is associated with many other conditions, and a key causal factor is child maltreatment which clearly does have wide relevance to a wide range of disorder, and there are many general issues discussed here that can be defended and should prove useful.

What matters?

There are at least four recurring themes in the research discussed.

(i) Feeling loved as a child – avoiding neglect, rejection or maltreatment

Adverse child experience is top of the list. Neglect, abuse and rejection increase risk of conduct disorder and emotional disorder in children. Each also contributes substantially to risk of depression in adult life, through increasing the numbers of stressful life events likely to be experienced; increasing the person's vulnerability to those events; lowering self-esteem; affecting the likelihood of finding and staying with a supportive partner, and possibly the quality of those relationships (perhaps through decreased trust); and through decreasing the likelihood that any depression will clear up quickly. While the evidence has been studied here in relation to depression, people with a wide range of other types of mental ill-health in adult life are also found more frequently than those without ill-health to have experienced abuse, neglect or rejection in childhood.

Much of this we have known for very many years. What is new is a greater understanding of the interplay between personality, social, psychological and genetic factors that mediate the link between early adversity and adult mental ill-health, with implications that may assist in planning preventive programmes.

(ii) Feeling safe

A second theme relates to feeling safe from current threat, and feeling protected from future threat. A secure source of income, living in a low-crime neighbourhood, feeling safe at school are some of the wider sources of security. Social support from important relationships is essentially about feeling protected: knowing your military peers and seniors are competent and will do their best to keep you safe, that they have placed you in a position for which you are adequately prepared; that in the face of life difficulties, a lover, relative or close friend will be there for you, neighbours will respond if you scream for help, and will contribute to, rather than damage the safety of your immediate environment for yourself and your family. And being loved as a child is not enough, if one is not also confident of protection from harm.

(iii) Feeling valued

A third theme links to the concept of shame, or humiliation, seen for example in a sense of inferiority, extreme shyness, or loneliness as a child, the experience of humiliating events in adulthood, the shame of unemployment or demeaning work, the discrimination and rejection that is associated with psychiatric diagnoses, the stigma associated with psychotic symptoms, and the humiliation of regular personal criticism by those close. Humiliation is a powerful emotion capable of marked effect on mental health, and a key factor in aggression and violence. There are implications for how people are treated in a range of settings, in terms of ensuring dignity and respect, a sense that one is a full participating citizen with a valued role to play in the family, community or workplace.

(iv) A sense of control, able to shape one's future

A fourth theme links to the importance of a sense of control, or at least a sense of optimism about the future. It may be particularly important when a person does not feel safe, loved or valued. Having a sense that we have the autonomy and resources – intellectual, social, financial – to influence our future, to get out of difficulties, is important; when it has been lacking, an event or change that conveys hope of a 'fresh start' – an opportunity to change things for the better – can aid recovery from a depressive episode. For others, a belief in a God who will ensure things turn out well can sometimes compensate for a lack of individual control. People with a history of antisocial behaviour who find a good relationship, or a secure job, appear less likely to reoffend, probably in part due to seeing the value of exerting control now they have more to lose. Doing a job well, giving to others and being appreciated for this, using one's strengths, first and foremost provides a sense of value, but also increases the sense that one has some control over one's future, a possibility of maintaining love, safety and value. Hope and optimism can play an important role in recovery from both physical and mental ill-health, and in coping with adversity, having a sense that a positive future is not only a possibility, but can be brought through one's own determination and effort.

It seems likely that love, safety, value and control make some contribution to the onset and course of most types of mental ill-health, although current evidence is clearest for depressive episodes. It is also possible that threats to one more than another will interact with differing types of genetic profile or personality characteristic to increase the likelihood of one type of disorder over another. Such speculation has some support from research in terms of the course of disorder.

A strong constitution/resilience: Developed through life

Vulnerability or resilience develops from the earliest stage in life. The first three years may be most important. This is also true for much physical ill-health. David Barker has influenced many in public health with his analysis of life-course effects, concluding that models of degenerative disease, for instance, have for too long been based on an assumption that their causes lie in the interaction of genetic susceptibility with *current* adverse life circumstances and lifestyle, when in fact the individual's susceptibility will also to a considerable degree be shaped by their foetal and infant life. His paper in 1991 showed that deaths from chronic obstructive lung disease correlated strongly with lower respiratory tract infection before the age of two years, that weight at one year correlated strongly with death from ischaemic heart disease 60 years later, that prenatal growth was even more important, with low birth weight in relation to placenta weight a better predictor of blood pressure 50 years later than any other factor in the person's current circumstances. He suggests therefore that we are to some extent already 'programmed' for the health problems we experience in later life during pregnancy and early childhood, and the early health factors described are in turn associated with material and social disadvantage at the time. With a theme that is echoed over and again in contemporary analyses of the determinants of public health, he concludes that 'The seeds of inequalities in health in the next century are being sown today – in inner cities and other communities where adverse influences impair the growth, nutrition and health of mothers and their infants' (Barker, 1991: 67). It would appear that a similar argument is likely to hold for a good deal of mental ill-health.

Three main types of explanation have been proposed to account for the role of experiences through the life course on current vulnerability: latent, pathway and cumulative effects (Graham, 2002). Latent effects suggest a critical period in infancy when a specific vulnerability can be created in the way Barker suggested (meaning parental biography will be the key focus); a pathway model indicates that disadvantage at one point creates increased risk of further disadvantage (suggesting that childhood experience and child-to-adult transition should be the key focus); and the accumulation model indicates a focus on chronic disadvantage at all life stages.

Research reviewed earlier, particularly the cohort studies, confirms the complexity of the life course effects on mental health – all three apply. For instance, regression analyses of data on the UK 1946 birth cohort found that parental divorce and adolescent physical and mental ill-health had pathway effects (e.g. on adult support, social class, marital breakdown), but that there was also a latent effect remaining after these were controlled, linked with affective disorder at age 53 (Kuh et al., 2002).

More light has been shed on all these pathways through the life-course and how they increase adult risk of clinically relevant depression in a series of analyses by Brown, Craig and Harris and their colleagues, revisiting the role of childhood maltreatment. In five papers, culminating with Brown et al. (2008b), they draw on data from three of their earlier studies, and confirm the crucial role of child maltreatment in adult depression and both its indirect and direct effects (see Chapter 5), or as Graham (2002) phrases these – pathway and latent effects. The indirect effects, deriving from maternal indifference and rejection but also from physical abuse by either parent, increase depression through a pathway including increased childhood behaviour problems, early risky sexual behaviour and leaving home with inadequate support. These factors in turn increased risk of later threatening adult life events, ongoing social difficulties and poor emotional support. Together these factors markedly increase risk of an onset of depression when a severe life event or marked difficulty occurs and will also contribute to it taking a chronic course (Brown et al., 2008b). However, when all such pathway effects were controlled, a direct effect on chronic depression remained – primarily of childhood experience of maternal indifference (neglect) and maternal rejection (emotional abuse). An early interplay of childhood maltreatment with genetic vulnerability appears largely to explain this (Brown and Harris, 2008).

The mediating links are by no means always one way. For example, the role of conduct problems can in turn sometimes increase the parenting problems, as suggested by the fact that low affection from a mother appeared to move to rejection more often for a rebellious child than for a compliant one

Tracing these factors back further in the life-course, parental discord showed a marked association with child maltreatment. It was related to the likelihood of rejection or physical abuse by the mother, and poor control over her child or children, both of which were linked with the child's behavioural problems. Depression in the mother also reduced her control over her children, and in turn led to more conduct problems. One step further back, financial hardship made family discord more likely (Brown et al., 2007).

It is these sorts of complexities that lead researchers such as Biehal (2008) to note their concern about efforts to help multiply disadvantaged adolescents lacking family support that only address current problems. The latent vulnerability of these young people will affect their ability to benefit from some of the support offered and is likely to mean that a more extensive intervention is needed to take account of this, in order to achieve lasting benefit.

Effective intervention to build resilience: Does it work?

Love, protection, value, and control – is it so surprising that short-term experimental programmes struggle to show lasting change to these? It has been a disappointing finding in this review that a well-designed randomized blinded trial has rarely demonstrated large effects of an intervention that there is good reason to expect will bring measurable benefit. To take one example – parents struggling with their parenting role can be offered weekly support by a home visitor, and some of these programmes are highly effective in doing so (mainly the nurse–family partnership; Olds, 2002). But hundreds of evaluations of home visiting programmes have been undertaken over the years, and an examination of just the most rigorous RCTs shows that for every outcome studied, half of the evaluations found minimal or no effect (Gomby, 2005). As Gomby notes, programmes deliver 20–40 hours of intervention over the course of a few years, and

> that is not much time in which to address issues as complex as child abuse and neglect, school readiness, and deferral of second pregnancies. But, that is the task that has been set for home visiting programs. It is therefore important

for policymakers and practitioners to keep their expectations modest about what can be accomplished through any single intervention.

(Gomby, 2005: 44)

A second example is the negative effect of criticism and over-involvement of family members, and the positive effect of warmth and understanding on the rate of relapse in psychosis, which is well supported (see Chapter 6). Despite numerous replications of the association, and of the beneficial effect of reducing high 'EE' (expressed emotion in critical comments), an effectiveness study by Garety and colleagues (2008) testing the implementation of family psycho-education and CBT in general clinical practice produced disappointing results. Despite taking particular care to ensure excellent adherence to demonstrated techniques of CBT and family intervention, with well-qualified therapists, fully supervised and trained by those with long experience in the methods, they failed to show an effect on either relapse or hospital admission in a careful randomized controlled study with 301 patients.

At first glance, the reasons for disappointing results seem quite different to those affecting efforts to help families dealing with multiple social disadvantage. In the Garety study poor results for family intervention were due to the unexpected finding of a low number of relapses in either intervention or control group among service users living with relatives, so that any potential benefits could not be adequately assessed. But exploring participation and benefit shows overlap with issues arising in other studies (see below). Participants living with families tended to be white families, in the more suburban areas, already low in EE, and whose presence seems to have helped the service user respond to treatment of all three types as compared to the less favourable outcomes of the larger group of service users not living with relatives. The absence of benefits of CBT appeared to be due to the severity of the problems of the sample who were at an acute stage of a relapse, often having ceased taking medication, rather than a group who had stabilized.

In discussing this kind of efficacy–effectiveness gap (the gap between trials of an intervention in a targeted sample led by researchers, demonstrating the potential of the intervention to bring significant benefit, and the reduced effectiveness when transferred to real-world implementation in a larger scale study), Scott (2008) discussed some of the problems. These include the drop-out rates from the intervention group (often more than one in four), the less than optimal attendance in sessions among many of those not 'dropping out', the large proportion of potential participants who decline to participate at the sampling stage, but particularly the greater reluctance of those most likely to benefit. Many other implementation problems are discussed by Glasgow and colleagues (2003), who have developed an 'implementation science' website (RE-AIM) to help researchers address these issues.

The complex multifactorial nature of mental ill-health, and the narrow focus of most intervention research, particularly the RCT, presents major difficulties for their use in real-world settings. Not least among the problems is the apparent lack of motivation of some potential participants, perhaps unconvinced the service offered will change their lives for the better, not convinced they have a problem, and/or who don't want to be helped. It will be argued that in fact the whole approach to how we currently go about trying to help high-risk individuals and families might need to be rethought, if intervention is to bring improvements to their sense of control over their lives, and their expectation that they can be valued and safe.

Problems with methodology

The recommended method for building evidence for effective health intervention is to test changes to factors that are thought to play a causal role, or interventions thought to be therapeutic, in an RCT, preferably double blinded. Subjects have often volunteered, so are well motivated and self selected, and are then randomly allocated to one of two or more conditions. They may also have been invited to participate because they have no comorbid conditions, and few other complications. The protocol for the often intensive and complex intervention must be rigidly followed by skilled practitioners fully trained in the approach. If significant results are found, replications are ideally obtained, preferably from studies by different research groups in different settings, before the effectiveness of the intervention is tested in a real-life situation with the whole of the population it is intended to help, including those with additional problems. If all is well, the intervention might then become part of recommended health policy.

The approach derives from clinical medicine and drug trials, responding to concerns about the extent of waste on treatments of no proven value (Cochrane, 1972). It is also the 'prevention science' approach recommended for evaluating mental health interventions in the US (Mrazek and Haggerty, 1994, and described in Chapter 4). In the UK, the National Institute for Health and Clinical Excellence (NICE) was formed in 1999 to produce reviews of best evidence, the ranking of which places the double blinded RCT close to the top. Reviews of multiple RCTs, and merging data from multiple RCTs in meta-analyses, are considered even better. Benefits are sometimes measured in QALYs – quality-adjusted life years bought by the treatment.

Public health was added to the remit of NICE in 2005, leading to some reflection on the appropriateness of this approach (Kelly et al., 2010). The complex forms of public health evidence mean there is a paucity of good RCT data: it becomes expensive and unwieldy with the length of causal chains to be examined, and with the time delays needed to evaluate a preventive programme. In mental health there are additional issues about the random allocation of vulnerable people, the reluctance of professional staff to adhere to what is agreed, and the costs of doing this well. And how do you test the effects of improving social capital? And can you randomly allocate a supportive partner?

Problem 1: Random allocation of subjects

The difficulty of recruitment and data collection is invariably underestimated, as Simkiss and colleagues (2010) show in their fascinating account of the progress of their RCT evaluation of a parenting programme in Wales. They wished to test the effectiveness of the 10-week Family Links Nurturing Programme that aims to strengthen family relationships and the parents' ability to manage difficult behaviour in a young child. Sound evidence of benefit from before and after studies, and from qualitative research, suggested that the proposed intervention was likely to work well. It was initially welcomed enthusiastically by practitioners, but it took a full 12 months longer than anticipated to recruit the sample families. Both practitioners and families often conveyed fear about being judged, did not want to wait for the intervention in the control condition (six months after the completion of the programme by the intervention group), and expressed numerous anxieties, all threatening the viability of the programme. More funds than budgeted had to be expended to keep the staff on side as well as the sample.

Problem 2: Sticking to the protocol but adapting it sufficiently to fit wider needs

Glasgow and colleagues (2003) argue that an *effective* method must appeal to a broad group of potential recipients and providers, be easily implemented by a range of practitioners, and able to work if they adapt it to the constraints of the setting or the particular needs of participants. This is quite different to the requirements of an assessment of *efficacy*, as discussed above. Glasgow and colleagues suggested a number of additions to the CONSORT guidance criteria for the RCT to ensure the efficacy trial produces better information to inform those who may apply the method in routine practice. These include more detail about who participated and who benefited and why, what features should not be varied, clarifying too if and why some people were excluded. They also suggest that many implementation problems could be avoided with greater participation of the intended target group in the initial design of both efficacy and effectiveness trials.

Problem 3: The additional time and cost of gaining biographical detail on participants

The kind of qualitative data needed to judge the effectiveness of a mentoring programme for young people living in a family home where domestic violence and drug misuse are known problems might include the existence of a close relationship with a participant's grandfather who lives next door and provides all that any mentor can offer and more. The young person's school success might also counteract a lack of support from the parent. A common technique is to use complex statistical modelling to estimate the relative impact of each of the important factors, but inevitably some of the important detail of context is lacking unless a qualitative analysis is embedded within the RCT.

At best, mental health interventions work for some of the recipients. Not surprisingly, limited help tends to work best for those with limited problems. Jessop and Stein (1991) found that monthly or more frequent visits or phone calls from a specialist multidisciplinary health care team for at least six months to low-income urban parents of children with a long-term health condition (e.g. congenital disorders, epilepsy, asthma, sickle cell anaemia) benefited those with low resources (sources of help and support, social, financial, educational) when their child's needs were at the lower end of the range. The help was insufficient for improvement in the children's adjustment or the mother's symptoms of mental ill-health when the child's needs were high, and was not important if the family already had good coping resources. It is perhaps unsurprising that the meta-analysis of 177 prevention programmes for children by Durlak and Wells (1997) showed low effect sizes for parent training programmes for disadvantaged families, but greater impact achieved by those interventions focused on children who were not necessarily socially disadvantaged, but were going through stressful transitions – parental divorce, change of school, frightening medical procedures. It means that targeting people at the more vulnerable end of the spectrum needs intervention that addresses more complex components of their risk status, and to assess effectiveness accordingly.

Those with more serious problems may sometimes be less open to offers of help, and the work might be less rewarding for practitioners.

Problem 4: Participants are not ready to change

Many difficulties underpinning someone's risk of mental ill-health represent patterns of negative behaviour and thinking that have become entrenched, self-perpetuating, resistant to change. It can be hard to engage them in preventive programmes (see French and Shinman, 2005; Gomby 2005; and Chapter 10). In the field of addictions, and in health promotion practice aiming to help people change patterns of eating, alcohol use and smoking, two theories developed in the 1980s have been particularly influential: the 'stages of change model' (Prochaska and DiClemente, 1984) and 'motivational interviewing'. The latter method is to help the person explore and resolve their ambivalence, and build their commitment to change (Miller and Rollnick, 1991).

Despite heavy criticism of the stages of change model, for instance in an editorial by West (2005) and discussion papers that follow, its popularity with clinicians has been barely dented. Its value to practitioners has been its simplicity, showing stages from 'pre-contemplation' to 'maintenance', and proposing that intervention should be tailored to the 'stage' of readiness to change of the individual. It suggests that service users will not all be equally ready to change, and that it does not always make sense to offer the same type of help as if they were; that relapse is a normal part of the process before new patterns can be maintained; and maintaining change will sometimes need as much support as making change.

Recognizing that some of the target group are less ready to change while others are already motivated to do so should both inform the approach and help predict likely attendance problems and drop-out. When time and resources are limited it may assist choices relating to target group (Prochaska and colleagues, 1992). There will be some whose behaviour may be seen as a problem by others, but who have no intention of changing in the immediate future, may fail to see anything wrong with their behaviour, or fail to see it as something that is possible to change. If seeking therapy, they may be doing so under pressure from others. Similarly, those who wish to change may not yet be ready to do anything about it, or may see the obstacles to change as too great, including competing social pressures. This is not a reason not to offer intervention to those less easy to engage, but a way to assist a realistic appraisal of the investment that might be required.

Motivating people to change behaviour

Probably all practitioners find that some of those they aim to help are more receptive than others, and that differing approaches will be required accordingly. Some commitment to change is required. For instance, Biehal (2008) discusses the challenges of shifting the behaviour of troubled adolescents and their families through family support. She compared those receiving (but not randomly allocated to) a specialist intensive and less intensive standard support service. She explored why in both groups, some families benefited while others did not, as well as why the more intensive help brought so little additional benefit. The families had multiple problems reflected in violence, special educational needs, poor health, relationship difficulties and material disadvantage, and marked concern about neglect or abuse. But those whose difficulties reduced the most, in both groups, were those where the commitment to the children by their parents, despite all difficulties, was strongest.

Caplan as early as 1964 concluded that a crisis situation increases receptivity to offers to help, where desire for change has not been strong. As noted earlier, home visiting brought most benefit to parents of a child born with special needs, pre-term or low birth weight where there was a perception of a need for help (Gomby, 2005; Olds et al., 2007). Biehal (2008) also found that those families whose difficulties had endured less than three years, and who were currently facing a crisis situation, were more likely to benefit. It may not be a difficult matter to assess readiness to change – for instance, the Newpin mother-to-mother befriending project in London simply asks the question. A written statement about what it is the parent wishes to change about her life and her child's life is a prerequisite for acceptance of the referral (see Newton, 1992).

'Motivational interviewing' can be taught to practitioners to help them engage with service users, whatever their level of interest. It starts by clarifying degree of committment in order to shape the discussions and help appropriately (Miller and Rollnick, 1991). First developed for contacts with problem drinkers in the 1980s, it has been applied more broadly, including during the past 20 years in family support and in partner abuse programmes (e.g. Murphy and Maiuro, 2009). There is no manual; it is a method centred on a set of principles: empathy, respect, developing autonomy, exploring pros and cons of changing, and building intrinsic motivation. It develops skills in the practitioner in building a 'therapeutic alliance' and avoiding a directive, judgemental or moralistic stance.

Such motivational skills can be as essential to managers as to practitioners, as they need to gain the wholehearted support for the method of those charged with delivering it. Any reservations can easily be transmitted to the service recipient (Simkiss et al., 2010), or lead to other blocks being found to the successful implementation of the programme (Glasgow et al., 2003).

People may not want 'help'

The disadvantages of a focus on a person's 'problems' or deficits are commonly discussed. Chapter 7 noted the potential cost to self-esteem of being identified as needing help. The value of an alternative focus on opportunity, aspirations and strengths lies behind the proposals of service users who argue for a recovery model of care (Anthony, 1993), of proponents of positive psychology (Seligman et al., 2005), of the 'strengths model' of rehabilitation (Rapp, 1998) and the theory of motivational interviewing. It appears, for example, to have been more successful with teenagers identified as at high risk of unplanned pregnancy to provide an opportunity to gain work experience rather than classes on the avoidance of risky sexual behaviour (see Chapter 10). Arranging for some to offer befriending to others will often bring greater benefits to them than being befriended (see Newton, 1992). People value help when they seek it, but not necessarily when offered, or when the help offered is for problems that are not those they perceive to be most important. Although at one level this is self-evident, there often remains a mismatch between intervention objectives and service user priorities.

Help can stigmatize

Avoiding the potential stigma of being identified as needing 'help' is one of the advantages a universal programme has over the targeted one. It is not unknown for the identification of the problem status of the target group to lead to adverse effects. It can convey that others believe they have a problem, and one that needs special help for them to be able to surmount it. Second, the behaviour is common to a problem group, to which they now belong – an ineffective parent, a difficult teenager, a naughty child, an unsupportive relative, a psychiatric patient. Third, spending time with others in this problem group will strengthen their relationships and identification with them, possibly reinforcing their sense of social exclusion.

The purpose of an efficacy trial as defined by Flay (1986: 451) is to test whether a programme 'does more good than harm when delivered under optimum conditions'; an effectiveness trial is one that does the same under real-world conditions. An illustration of the problems that can be inadvertently created is supplied by Hallfors and colleagues (2006). Teenage substance misuse is a serious concern in many countries, enough to justify a substantial state budget, for which efficacy of proposed intervention is a prerequisite for funding allocation. One intervention achieving the approved US list for funding, known as Reconnecting Youth, was evaluated in a trial that was as faithful as could be managed to the original intervention, with five times as many students as the original efficacy study (Hallfors et al., 2006). It consisted of classes delivered to 15-year-olds in nine schools across two large urban districts in different parts of the US. Half the 1360 'high-risk' (poor school attendance, poor achievement) students were assigned to receive it in classes of 10–12 students, half not, for half the school year, as a credit-bearing option with 55 core lessons focused on self-esteem, decision making, personal control and interpersonal communication. Using the measures developed by the original research team, they assessed school attendance and achievement, and self-rated assessments of substance use, mood, weekend activities and peer relationships.

The study had the problems of participation shown by so many interventions – only half the students attended regularly, and despite supposedly random allocation, there were some baseline group differences. After the intervention, the experimental group were significantly more angry than controls. After six months, they had significantly increased their high-risk peer bonding, reduced conventional peer bonding and reduced their prosocial weekend activities (homework, club or church attendance, family activities). In addition, the programme often competed with attendance of remedial classes for missed core academic assignments.

The answer to 'building resilience in childhood – does it work?' is that efficacy trials demonstrate that a change to known risk factors to mental health using a number of carefully developed preventive programmes, with a strong theoretical base, frequently achieves intended benefits. In translating these to everyday practice the results have not infrequently been disappointing, particularly in relation to the group who appear most in need of change.

Implications for policy and practice: Targeted or universal strategies?

The long list of problems associated with targeted strategies discussed above suggest that a far better way forward might be a universal measure – offering support to all parents of young children. Programmes such as Head Start and Early Head Start in the US and Sure Start in the UK have taken this approach, but in areas likely to recruit many disadvantaged families. However, like health education, these programmes do not tackle individual exposure to risk, in place of changing individual response to risk, in the way Rose (1985) proposed. They also have some of the other disadvantages that Becker (1993) described for health education (see Chapter 4), including the tendency for the benefits to be gained by those whose need is less. This is sometimes described as the 'middle class capture' in universally offered services (OECD Family Database, 2009a), perhaps at the same time also stigmatizing and alienating those whose need for change is most obvious (very overweight, heavy drinkers or smokers, or with particularly unruly children).

Sure Start centres in the UK offered family support to all families within defined geographic areas, these areas selected on many standard indicators of deprivation, so that in theory, disadvantaged families could receive support in a non-stigmatizing way. The centres were not required to follow defined protocols, but were free to set their own priorities, in partnership with local parents. They were charged with offering home visiting, family support, play and learning, family and child health care and support for children and families with special needs. However, the evaluations of this programme have so far found disappointingly small gains for the least disadvantaged families, and some evidence that the most disadvantaged families may have been affected adversely. That is, although there were a range of benefits to mothers over the age of 20, there were some adverse effects on the social functioning of children of teenage mothers and single parents, and on the verbal ability of children whose parents did not work (Belsky et al., 2006). Rutter (2006) argues that such universal strategies will do nothing to reduce inequality, as for this you need targeted programmes, like those offered by Olds' nurse–family partnership.

In the US, there have been comparable initiatives: the Head Start (HS) programme (mainly a pre-school education service, from 1965) for children from four years, and an Early Head Start (EHS) (from 1994, home visiting and centre based support) for up to three–year-olds. EHS was the model for the UK Sure Start, but had an evaluation strategy with some advantages, including some standardization of programmes, measures of programme fidelity and randomized controls. However, the divergence of benefits to those with high and low needs was again clear. Their many positive effects (best for those enrolled during pregnancy, and for African American mothers, and experienced over a large range of parenting and child performance and adjustment outcomes) were not shared by the most disadvantaged mothers, i.e. those with four or five risk factors: teenage, single parent, NEET, no high school diploma, on benefits. On these mothers the programme appeared to have an unfavourable impact, and they became, for instance, more harsh towards the child during the research interview of the parent (Love et al., 2004). However, these high-risk mothers did reduce the number of subsequent pregnancies, and their involvement helped them to access more state benefits.

Mothers with one or two risk factors also gained little, except to reduce the likelihood of using physical chastisement, slightly fewer reporting smacking their child in the previous week. Benefits to mother and child were concentrated among those with three risk factors. Of the high-risk participants (four or five factors), evaluators of EHS concluded that the programme did not provide sufficient support to meet their high needs, programme staff found them difficult to work with (particularly depressed mothers), and the scheme was not the right approach to help this group, who appeared to be overwhelmed by yet another demand on their unstable, unsupported lives. It is not that those with a particular *type* of disadvantage were more difficult to help than others facing different types of challenge. For instance, where the local programme focused intensive work on teenage mothers – their education and employment aspirations as well as the needs of their child or children – they brought positive effects to this group as a whole. Similarly, depressed mothers benefited when they participated, although it was suggested they needed more help for their own mental health needs (Love et al., 2004). The challenge was the combination of numerous problems. Those who were, for instance, depressed, single mothers, teenage, unqualified *and* unemployed tended not to be among those who benefited.

Some might speculate here about latent vulnerability adding to pathway and cumulative life-course effects, including gene–environment interactions. Research in molecular genetics is reinvigorating the debate from decades previously of 'cycles of disadvantage', and reviews of the potential implications for overturning possible adverse epigenetic effects centres on intensive early support, possibly starting pre-birth (Tremblay, 2010). Such research is at an early stage, but is clearly an area to be watched.

Some solutions: Start earlier?

There is a substantial biological literature on critical and sensitive periods early in life, and the greater difficulty in bringing benefits from later intervention in relation to skills normally developed at those points. (Those of us learning to speak a second language in adult life know this.) Reviewing the bio-psycho-social development of disruptive behaviour in children, Tremblay (2010) concludes that intervention needs to start as early in pregnancy as possible. The importance of the emotional health as well as physical health and nutrition of the pregnant woman and the stressfulness of her environment may have been underestimated.

Heckman (2007) comes to the same conclusion. Examining evidence on the development of health, cognitive skills and non-cognitive skills, he explores implications for investment. His wide-ranging focus indicates not only that intervention is most cost-effective when at the earliest stage, but also that there will be 'dynamic complementarity' – a cross-fertilization of investment in one to benefits of later investment in another. Cognitive ability is of course a powerful predictor of success in education and employment, and associated with low crime and good health. Non-cognitive skills such as perseverance, motivation, risk aversion and self-control also have powerful effects on wages, schooling, criminal activity, teenage pregnancy and achievement (see Heckman, 2007). Good health and cognitive and non-cognitive skills, each affect the others. In fact in other work, Heckman shows that 'scores on achievement tests and grades, often used as measures of cognition, are determined in substantial part by personality' (Borghans et al., 2011: 316). This echoes the arguments of those conducting research on the value of optimism on health and achievement – that optimists don't give up easily (Segerstrom, 2006). It suggests not only that intervention should be early, but that it should address expectations, patience, motivation and self-control as much as reading or other cognitive skills and health.

Tremblay (2010: 361) further argues that 'the logic of the epigenetic process suggests that intensive prenatal interventions will have impacts on numerous aspects of physical and mental health as well as social adjustment, including the major modern health problems: low birth weight, obesity, cardiovascular problems, cancer, hyperactivity, mood disorders and substance abuse'. To realize the benefits of dynamic complementarity however, means following up early intervention with further intervention to improve cognitive or non-cognitive skills or health at a later stage in development: life course interventions to match a life-course perspective on vulnerability and resilience.

This could be done through targeting high risk, as childhood problems might be predicted from knowledge of the mother's mental health and family social circumstances, any adolescent behaviour problems, educational difficulty or depression. Along with known current vulnerability factors such as a dysfunctional relationship with her partner, young age and social difficulties, it might make sense to start here (Tremblay, 2010). However, the logic of the earlier parts of this chapter suggests that a universal approach is needed, which brings women with such risk factors into a programme with those with few problems, good mental health, good relationships with a partner. The key is to shift the norm: average beliefs, behaviour, expectations, without emphasizing the deficiencies of a minority. A first pregnancy is a potential turning point, certainly a transition, which usually brings a willingness to engage (Olds, 2008). The focus and label of the intervention should not be problem-focused, but a requirement for, say, all pregnant women aged under 20, to plan the best possible childhood experience for their children. To capitalize on other findings in this review, a pregnant woman might be asked to attend some sessions with a partner – the birth father if appropriate, another adult who will share the parenting and committment to the child if not, in order both to build support and to strengthen the expectation that this is a task that needs at least two people, and a safe 'nest'.

Earlier chapters have demonstrated the strong link between child mental health and maternal depression and that age under 20 at first pregnancy is an important marker for risk of mental ill-health in both parent and child. There is at least tentative evidence that intervention during pregnancy and the first weeks following childbirth from a health visitor trained in basic counselling skills and in how to assess the mental health of mothers can prevent and treat maternal depression (Brugha et al., 2011); and good evidence that nurse home visiting can improve the health of the pregnant mother and the newborn child and the mother's parenting, and reduce child maltreatment, particularly among disadvantaged teenage mothers (Olds, 2002). The focus is also an enabling one, including a focus on her own longer term goals, helping her to develop a vision for her future 'and then make smart choices about planning future pregnancies, completing their educations, and finding work. In the service of these goals, the nurses helped women build supportive relationships with family members and friends, and linked families with other services' (Olds, 2008: 7).

Some policy responses

The OECD (2009) report *Doing better for children* discusses numerous options, all of which require a substantial investment early in children's lives, concentrating on improving outcomes for vulnerable children. It argues for development of a comparable set of wellbeing outcomes across the life cycle, and clear targets, to facilitate cross-country comparisons. Its solution to the balancing of stigmatized targeted support and costly universal provision is to adopt a 'cascading service model' whereby everyone is offered a certain level of service (e.g. one home visit from a health visitor) and, based on judgements about need for support at this visit, a smaller number are offered further visits or invited to a parenting group.

The OECD report suggests using known risk factors, but also early signs of difficulty such as the child needing special educational support in the early years at school, as priorities for additional help. The strategy is similar to the 'disease modelling' approach described in Chapter 4 – that is, use risk indicators to reduce spending on some and increase it on others. Reduce the number of universal ante-natal or post-natal checks on low-risk families in order to provide more intensive support to those with higher risk. They also suggest increased conditional cash transfers for higher risk groups. That is, provide cash payments triggered by age milestones, which are dependent on completion of certain health programmes of prenatal care, post-natal checks and immunizations, and perhaps parenting educa-tion programmes (OECD, 2009). During school years, there could also be some financial prioritizing of disadvantage, such as providing pay incentives to attract good teachers to work with disadvantaged children.

Policy across countries varies in the extent to which it supports lone and couple parenting, or the parent who wishes to remain at home while the child is young. For instance, Lundberg and colleagues (2008) consider three prevalent models: dual earner, general family policy, and market-oriented family policy. Dual earner policy includes benefits that enable either parent to combine employ-ment and child care, and provides universal child benefits and child care support (Denmark; Finland; Norway; Sweden). General family policy supports a gendered division of labour, benefits accruing to the person with a dependent spouse with children (Austria; Belgium; France; Germany; Ireland; Italy; the Netherlands); while the third type is a combination of the two, but in much weaker form (Australia; Canada; Japan; New Zealand; Switzerland; UK; US). Using infant mortality data for each country as recorded each fifth year from 1970 to 2000, Lundberg and colleagues suggest that Nordic models are more protective, and that universal forms of family policy will have greater public health benefits, greater attraction to middle class voters and, by avoiding means testing, reduced stigma.

Some countries are also providing universal education to parents to help them manage common child care problems (see Chapter 10) – Switzerland uses Triple P, Norway uses PMTO or Incredible Years (but only with families with children with serious behaviour problems). Governments around the world are increasing the resources placed into improving parenting as the visibility of problems in children's behaviour draws ever more comment. Group-based parenting programmes have some of the best evidence of effectiveness but, as previous discussion conveys, must be implemented with fidelity to the model developed, by practitioners with skills and confidence to ensure it is an enjoyable and non-stigmatizing experience for parents.

A strong focus in public policy on family support and prevention is essential, but this must not detract from keeping an equally keen eye on the detection of existing abuse and neglect, and the need for assertive action to protect children. Davies and Duckett (2008) warn that when systems and training focus heavily on prevention there can be a danger that child protection becomes a secondary activity.

Society and government: Ready to change?

Introducing targeted measures to help a high-risk group is relatively easy for a government, so long as it does not affect the options, lifestyle and freedom of choice of the majority, in which case it may take decades (see Chapter 4). Commitment to change is evident in 2011–12 in the UK in new funding allocated to reducing unemployment in young people, helping families with multiple problems and facilitating early intervention with young people with psychotic symptoms, in part justified by potential economic benefit. A review of 15 types of preventive mental health programme – from parenting interventions, early intervention in psychosis, school bullying, to workplace programmes, suicide prevention, medically unexplained symptoms, to befriending older adults – estimated potential return on investment over the short, medium and longer terms (Knapp et al., 2011). Two areas of benefit stood out above others – preventing conduct disorder in children, and early detection and intervention in psychosis, both bringing estimated benefits to the NHS of nearly £10 for every £1 invested. Screening for alcohol misuse in general practice and safety barriers at suicide jumping points also bring substantial benefit to the NHS, workplace depression programmes benefit employers, suicide awareness training for GPs benefit families and the economy. The UK government published its policy *No Health without Mental Health* (DH, 2011) one year after a comprehensive review of health inequalities (the Marmot Review, 2010), both of which were wholeheartedly endorsed by the Royal College of Psychiatry (RCPsych, 2010).

However, some types of universal measure of the kind envisaged by Rose (1981) are likely to present greater challenges. How can a society change to improve love, safety, value and control of its citizens throughout life? Reducing the prevalence of child maltreatment can be traced back to social disadvantage and limited options available to young parents. Improving the safety and security of people in their homes, their work and their communities may require fundamental shifts in policy; as would reducing social exclusion, and the wider effect of wealth creation in a free market on the lives of those not well placed to compete.

Unpalatable problems can produce great efforts towards the less contentious solutions. In the years following the Poor Law in the early nineteenth century, William Farr's data on causes of death was showing that they were all too frequently associated with overwork and hunger. For Edwin Chadwick, entrusted as he was with promoting public health, such a claim looked like an accusation of his own criminal irresponsibility. He preferred the record to provide a diagnosis, such as 'fever'. He emphasized too other important factors in public health, such as filth and sewage, which did not bring medicine into politics or challenge the political economy. Starvation was too social and too political an issue (Hamlin, 1995).

Freud first brought to public attention the role of child sexual abuse in the 18 case histories published as *The Aetiology of Hysteria* in 1896, but quickly recognized that society was not ready to acknowledge that it existed, and nor did it seem was he, once he realized the implications for the prevalence of incest among all sections of society, including respectable bourgeois families of Vienna

(Herman, 1992). Within a year he repudiated these conclusions, and convinced himself and others that his patients were making them up, and in fact that these women longed for the sexual abuses of which they complained.

There is now at least a willingness to acknowledge both of these issues – the health effects of poverty and growing inequality in Western ecomomies, and the high prevalence of all kinds of child abuse and neglect. But solutions that restrict individual freedom or choice are those for which public support is difficult to achieve. Note how slow progress has been to gain signatories to the international commitment to prohibit corporal punishment in the home, or to enforce the law more rigorously against perpetrators of domestic violence.

Choice suggests a decision between options based on our judgement that one is inferior to the other; choices that work to the advantage of those most knowledge-able, articulate, or otherwise better placed to gain the best. Choice of school is one freedom that could be rethought, and school catchment areas redrawn to ensure all school intakes are as similar as possible, with no choice in which one attends. Choice did little to improve seatbelt use or smoking prevalence, as compared to compulsion through legislation. It is often social norms and societal wide expecta-tions that play the most powerful role in public health.

Conclusion

It may be 100 years since the start of the Mental Hygiene movement and the first child guidance centres, but the challenge remains – how best to help the many children whose risk of later mental ill-health is raised from early in life.

There are numerous strategies for preventing mental ill-health, but those who are most vulnerable to 'chronic' mental ill-health have complex vulnerability factors that make helping them a challenging process. It is hard to avoid the stig-matizing effect of offering support. Starting before birth has been proposed, with a focus on augmenting competence in the parents in areas that are important to them, working towards aspirations framed by them, strengthening their sense that they are valued by people who matter. Helping people cope with 'problems', particularly problems located in the person themselves, can be counterproductive. Most of us respond better to efforts to engage us in providing help to others, using our abilities and skills, for which we are valued. Perhaps more success will come from reframing the target.

There appear to be substantial overlaps in what makes us resilient to the chronic conditions affecting both physical and mental health. Vulnerability is key, and can also shape response to intervention, which can sometimes do more harm than good. There is some way to go before practice can be as effective as hoped. The business of providing support that works is far more complex, and far easier to get completely wrong, than some proponents acknowledge. But the pace of develop-ment in related areas of research and the commitment to change are grounds for optimism.

Bibliography

Abas, M.A. and Broadhead, J.C. (1997) 'Depression and anxiety amongst women in an urban setting in Zimbabwe' *Psychological Medicine*, 27: 59–71

Abel, K., Appleby, L., Cordingly, L., Friedman, T. and Salmon, M. (2003) 'Clinical and parenting skills outcomes following joint mother–baby psychiatric admission' *Australian and New Zealand Journal of Psychiatry*, 37, 5: 556–62

Abraido-Lanza, A.F. (2004) 'Social support and psychological adjustment among Latinas with arthritis: A test of a theoretical model' *Annals of Behavioral Medicine*, 27: 162–71

Abramson, L.Y., Seligman, M.E.P. and Teasdale, J.D. (1978) 'Learned helplessness in humans: Critique and reformulation' *Journal of Abnormal Psychology*, 87, 1: 49–74

Adams J.E. and Lindemann, E. (1974) 'Coping with long-term disability' in Coelho, G.V., Hamburg, D.A. and Adams, J.E. (eds) *Coping and Adaptation*, New York: Basic Books

Ader, R. and Cohen, N. (1993) 'Psychoneuroimmunology: Conditioning and stress' *Annual Review of Psychology*, 44: 53–85

Ahern, J., Jones, M.R., Bakshis, E. and Galea, S. (2008) 'Revisiting Rose: Comparing the benefits and costs of population-wide and targeted interventions' *Milbank Quarterly*, 86: 581–600

Ahrenfeldt, R.H. (1958) *Psychiatry in the British Army in the Second World War*, London: Routledge

Ala-Mursula, L., Vahtera, J., Linna, A., Pentti, J. and Kivimäki, M. (2005) Employee worktime control moderates the effects of job strain and effort–reward imbalance on sickness absence: The 10-town study. *Journal of Epidemiology & Community Health*, 59, 10: 851–7

Aldridge, J. and Becker, S. (2003) *Children Caring for Parents with Mental Illness*, Bristol, UK: Policy Press

Allen, J.P. and Philliber, S. (2001) 'Who benefits most from a broadly targeted prevention program? Differential efficacy across populations in the teen outreach program' *Journal of Community Psychology*, 29, 6: 637–55

Allen, J.P., Philliber, S., Herrling, S., and Kuperminc, G.P. (1997) 'Preventing teen pregnancy and academic failure: Experimental evaluation of a developmentally-based approach' *Child Development*, 64: 729–42

Alloy, L.B., Abramson, L.Y., Whitehouse, W.G., et al. (1999) 'Depressogenic cognitive styles: Predictive validity, information processing and personality characteristics, and developmental origins' *Behaviour Research and Therapy*, 37: 501–31

Allsop, J. and Freeman, R. (1993) 'Prevention in health policy in the UK and the NHS' in Mills, M. (ed) *Prevention, Health and British Politics*, Aldershot, UK: Ashgate

Amminger, G.P., Schäfer, M.R., Papageorgiou, K., et al. (2010) 'Long-chain Ω-3 fatty acids for indicated prevention of psychotic disorders: A randomized, placebo-controlled trial' *Archives of General Psychiatry*, 67, 2: 146–54

Anderson, J., Huppert, F. and Rose, G. (1993) 'Normality, deviance and minor psychiatric morbidity in the community: A population-based approach to General Health Questionnaire data in the Health and Lifestyle Survey' *Psychological Medicine*, 23: 475–85

Anisman, H., Merali, Z. and Hayley, S. (2008) 'Neurotransmitter, peptide and cytokine processes in relation to depressive disorder: Comorbidity between depression and neurodegenerative disorders' *Progress in Neurobiology*, 85: 1–74

Anthony, W. (1993) 'Recovery from mental illness: The guiding vision of the mental health service system in the 1990s' *Psycho-social Rehabilitation Journal*, 16, 4: 11–23

Antonovsky, A. (1979) *Health, Stress and Coping*, San Francisco: Jossey-Bass

Antonovsky, A. (1987) *Unraveling the Mystery of Health: How people manage stress and stay well*, San Francisco: Jossey-Bass

APA (American Psychiatric Association) (1994) *Diagnostic and Statistical Manual of Mental Disorders (4th edition)*, Washington, DC: APA

Appel, J.W. (1999) 'Fighting fear', *American Heritage*, 50, 6: 22

Arseneault, L., Cannon, M., Poulton, R., Murray, R., Caspi, A. and Moffitt, T.E. (2002) 'Cannabis use in adolescence and risk for adult psychosis: Longitudinal prospective study' *British Medical Journal*, 325: 1212–13

Artazcoz, L., Benach, J., Borrell, C. and Cortes, I. (2005) 'Social inequalities in the impact of flexible employment on different domains of psycho-social health' *Journal of Epidemiology & Community Health*, 59: 761–7

Associate Parliamentary Food and Health Forum (APFHF) (2007) *Minutes of the meeting of the FHF Inquiry into the links between diet and behaviour*. London: UK Parliament, www.fhf.org.uk/inquiry (accessed 16 August 2009)

Babcock, J.W. and Cutting, W.B. (1911) *Prevalence of Pellagra*, Washington, DC: US Government Printing Office

Baker, S. (2001) MIND exercise survey response, summarized in http://news.bbc.co.uk/2/hi/health/1338145.stm (accessed 23 August 2009)

Baker, S. and Read, J. (1996) *Not Just Sticks and Stones: A survey of the stigma taboos and discrimination experienced by people with mental health problems*, London: MIND

Bambra, C. (2010) 'Yesterday once more? Unemployment and health in the 21st century' *Journal of Epidemiology & Community Health*, 64: 213–15

Bambra, C., Gibson, M., Sowden, A., Wright, K., Whitehead, M. and Petticrew, M. (2010) 'Tackling the wider social determinants of health and health inequalities: Evidence from systematic reviews' *Journal of Epidemiology & Community Health*, 64: 284–91

Bandura, A. (1977) *Social Learning Theory*, Englewood Cliffs, NJ: Prentice Hall

Barberger-Gateau, P., Letenneur, L., Deschamps, V., Pérès, K., Dartigues, J-F. and Renaud, S. (2002) 'Fish, meat and risk of dementia: Cohort study' *British Medical Journal*, 325, 7370: 932–3

Barker, D.J.P. (1991) 'The foetal and infant origins of inequalities in health in Britain' *Journal of Public Health Medicine*, 13, 2: 64–8

Barter, C., McCarry, M., Berridge, D. and Evans, K. (2009) *Partner Exploitation and Violence in Teenage Intimate Relationships*, London: NSPCC

Bartley, M. and Plewis, I. (2002) 'Accumulated labour market disadvantage and limiting long-term illness: Data from the 1971–1991 Office for National Statistics Longitudinal Study' *International Journal of Epidemiology*, 31: 336–41

Bateson, G., Jackson, D.D., Haley, J. and Weakland, J.H. (1956) 'Toward a theory of schizophrenia' *Behavioural Science*, 1: 251–64

Bechdolf, A., Phillips, L.J., Francey, S.M. et al. (2006) 'Recent approaches to psychological interventions for people at risk of psychosis' *European Archives of Psychiatry and Clinical Neurosciences*, 256: 159–73

Beck, A.T. (1973) *The Diagnosis and Management of Depression*, Philadelphia: University of Pennsylvania Press

Beck, A.T., Rush, A.J., Shaw, B.F. and Emery, G. (1987) *Cognitive Therapy of Depression*, New York: Guilford Press

Becker, D.R., Smith, J., Tanzman, B., Drake, R.E. and Tremblay, T. (2001) 'Fidelity of supported employment programs and employment outcomes' *Psychiatric Services*, 52: 834–6

Becker, M.H. (1993) 'A medical sociologist looks at health promotion' *Journal of Health and Social Behavior*, 34, 1: 1–6

Beers, C.W. (1908) *A Mind That Found Itself*, New York: Longmans, Green

Belsky, J., Melhuish, E., Barnes, J., Leyland, A.H. and Romaniuk, H. (2006) 'Effects of Sure Start local programmes on children and families: Early findings from a quasi-experimental, cross-sectional study' *British Medical Journal* (International Edition), 332, 7556: 1476–8

Benedetti, F., Maggi, G., Lopiano, L., et al. (2003) 'Open versus hidden medical treatments: The patient's knowledge about a therapy affects the therapy outcome' *Prevention & Treatment*, 6, 1

Benjet, C., Borges, G., Medina-Mora, M.E., Zambrano, J. and Aguilar-Gaxiola, S. (2009) 'Youth mental health in a populous city of the developing world: Results from the Mexican Adolescent Mental Health Survey' *Journal of Child Psychology and Psychiatry*, 50, 4: 386–95

Benson, H. and McCallie, D.P. (1979) 'Angina pectoris and the placebo effect' *New England Journal of Medicine*, 300, 1424–9

Bentall, R. (2004) *Madness Explained: Psychosis and human nature*, London: Penguin

Berkowitz, R., Eberlein-Fries, R., Kuipers, L. and Leff, J. (1984) 'Educating relatives about schizophrenia' *Schizophrenia Bulletin*, 10: 418–29

Bertelsen, M., Jeppesen, P., Petersen, L., et al. (2009) 'Course of illness in a sample of 265 patients with first-episode psychosis—Five-year follow-up of the Danish OPUS trial' *Schizophrenia Research*, 107: 173–8

Biehal, N. (2008) 'Preventive services for adolescents: Exploring the process of change' *British Journal of Social Work*, 38: 444–61

Biehal, N., Clayden, J., Stein, M. and Wade, J. (1995) *Moving On: Young people and leaving care schemes*, London: HMSO

Biehal, N., Ellison, S. and Sinclair, I. (2011) 'Intensive fostering: An independent evaluation of MTFC in an English setting' *Children and Youth Services Review*, 33, 10: 2043–9

Bijl, R.V., Ravelli, A. and van Zessen, G. (1998) 'Prevalence of psychiatric disorder in the general population: Results of the Netherlands Mental Health Survey and Incidence Study (NEMESIS)' *Social Psychiatry and Psychiatric Epidemiology*, 33: 587–95

Bipolar UK (2011) *Self Management Training*, www.bipolaruk.org.uk/self-management-training (accessed 28 August 2011)

Birchwood, M., Jackson, C. and Todd, P. (1998) 'The critical period hypothesis' *International Clinical Psychopharmacology*, 12: 27–38

Birchwood, M., Trower, P., Brunet, K., Gilbert, P., Iqbal, Z. and Jackson, C. (2006) 'Social anxiety and the shame of psychosis: A study in first episode psychosis' *Behaviour Research and Therapy*, 45: 1025–37

Bird, V., Premkumar, P., Kendall, T., Whittington, C., Mitchell J. and Kuipers, E. (2010) 'Early intervention services, cognitive behavioural therapy and family intervention in early psychosis: Systematic review' *British Journal of Psychiatry*, 197: 350–6

Birley, J. (1999) 'Rehabilitation' in Freeman, H. (ed) *A Century of Psychiatry*, London: Mosby-Wolfe

Birley, J. and Hudson, B. (1983) 'The family, the social network and rehabilitation' in Watts, F.N and Bennett, D.H. (eds) *Theory and Practice of Psychiatric Rehabilitation*, Chichester, UK: Wiley

Black, C. (2008) *Working for a Healthier Tomorrow: Dame Carol Black's review of the health of Britain's working age population*, London: The Stationery Office

Blakely, T.A., Collings, S.C.D. and Atkinson, J. (2003) 'Unemployment and suicide: Evidence for a causal association?' *Journal of Epidemiology & Community Health*, 57: 594–600

Boardman, A.P., Bouras, N. and Cundy, J. (1987) *The Mental Health Advice Centre in Lewisham, Service Usage: Trends from 1989–84*, Research Report No. 3, London: Research and Development in Psychiatry

Bockting, C.L., Schene, A.H., Spinhoven, P., et al. (2005) 'Preventing relapse/recurrence in recurrent depression with cognitive therapy: A randomized controlled trial' *Journal of Consulting and Clinical Psychology*, 73: 647–57

Bodenmann, G., Cina, A., Ledermann, T. and Sanders, M.R. (2008) 'The efficacy of the Triple P-Positive Parenting Program in improving parenting and child behavior: A comparison with two other treatment conditions' *Behaviour Research and Therapy*, 46, 4: 411–27

Bolger, N., Zuckerman, A. and Kessler, R. C. (2000) 'Invisible support and adjustment to stress' *Journal of Personality and Social Psychology*, 79, 6: 953–61

Bond, G. R. (1998) 'Principles of individual placement and support' *Psychiatric Rehabilitation Journal*, 22: 11–23

Bond, G. R. (2004) 'Supported employment: Evidence for an evidence-based practice' *Psychiatric Rehabilitation Journal*, 27: 345–59

Borghans, L., Golsteyn, B., Heckman, J. and Humphries, J.E. (2011) 'Identification problems in personality psychology' *Personality and Individual Differences* 51: 315–20

Bowlby, J. (1969) *Attachment and Loss Vol. 1: Attachment*, London: Hogarth Press

Bowlby, J. (1973) *Attachment and Loss Vol. 2: Separation, anxiety and anger*, London: Hogarth Press

Bowlby, J. (1980) *Attachment and Loss Vol. 3: Loss, sadness and depression*, London: Hogarth Press

Bowlby, J. (1988) *A Secure Base: Clinical applications of attachment theory*, London: Routledge

Brandon, M., Belderson, P., Warren, C., et al. (2008) *Analysing Child Deaths and Serious Injury through Abuse and Neglect: What can we learn?* London: Department for Children, Schools and Families

Brenner, M.H. (1973) *Mental Illness and the Economy*, Cambridge, MA: Harvard University Press

Breslau, J., Aguilar-Gaxiola, S., Kendler, K.S. Su, M.,, Williams, D. and Kessler, R.C. (2006) 'Specifying race–ethnic differences in risk for psychiatric disorder in a USA national sample' *Psychological Medicine*, 36, 1: 57–68

Brevik, J.I., and Dalgard, O.S. (1996) *The Oslo Health Profile Inventory*, Oslo, Norway: University of Oslo

Brookmeyer, R., Johnson, E., Ziegler-Graham, K. and Arrighi, H.M. (2007) *Forecasting the Global Burden of Alzheimer's Disease*, Baltimore, MD: Johns Hopkins University, Department of Biostatistics Working Paper 130

Broom, D.H., D'Souza, R.M., Strazdins, L., Butterworth, P., Parslow, R. and Rodgers, B. (2006) 'The lesser evil: Bad jobs or unemployment? A survey of mid-aged Australians' *Social Science & Medicine*, 63, 3: 575–86

Brown, G.W. (1998) 'Genetic and population perspectives on life events and depression' *Social Psychiatry and Psychiatric Epidemiology*, 33, 363–72

Brown, G.W. (2002) 'Social roles, context and evolution in the origins of depression' *Journal of Health and Social Behavior*, 43, 3: 255–76

Brown, G.W., Adler, Z. and Bifulco, A. (1988) 'Life events, difficulties and recovery from chronic depression' *British Journal of Psychiatry*, 152: 487–98

Brown, G.W., Andrews, B., Harris, T., Adler, Z. and Bridge, L. (1986a) 'Social support, self-esteem and depression' *Psychological Medicine*, 16: 813–31

Brown, G.W., Bifulco, A. and Harris, T.O. (1987) 'Life events, vulnerability and onset of depression: some refinements' *British Journal of Psychiatry*, 150: 30–42

Brown G.W. and Birley, J.L.T. (1968) 'Crises and life changes and the onset of schizophrenia' *Journal of Health and Social Behaviour*, 9: 203–14

Brown, G.W., Birley, J.L.T. and Wing, J. K. (1972) 'Influence of family life on the course of schizophrenic disorders: A replication' *British Journal of Psychiatry*, 121: 241–58

Brown, G.W., Carstairs, G.M. and Topping, G. (1958) 'Post-hospital adjustment of chronic mental patients' *The Lancet*, 2: 685

Brown, G.W., Craig, T.J.K. and Harris, T.O. (2008a) 'Parental maltreatment and proximal risk factors using the Childhood Experience of Care & Abuse (CECA) instrument: A life-course study of adult chronic depression—5' *Journal of Affective Disorders*, 110: 222–33

Brown, G.W., Craig, T.K.J., Harris, T.O. and Handley, R.V. (2008b) 'Parental maltreatment and adulthood cohabiting partnerships: A life-course study of adult chronic depression—4' *Journal of Affective Disorders*, 110: 115–25

Brown, G.W., Craig, T.J.K., Harris, T.O., Handley, R.V. and Harvey, A.L. (2007a) 'Development of a retrospective interview measure of parental maltreatment using the Childhood Experience of Care and Abuse (CECA) instrument—A life-course study of adult chronic depression—1' *Journal of Affective Disorders*, 103: 205–15

Brown, G.W., Craig, T.J.K., Harris, T.O., Handley, R.V., Harvey, A.L. and Serido, J. (2007b) 'Child-specific and family-wide risk factors using the retrospective Childhood Experience of Care & Abuse (CECA) instrument: A life-course study of adult chronic depression—3' *Journal of Affective Disorders*, 103: 225–36

Brown, G.W. and Harris, T.O. (1978) *Social Origins of Depression*, London: Routledge

Brown, G.W. and Harris, T.O. (eds) (1989) *Life events and illness*, London: Unwin Hyman

Brown, G.W. and Harris, T.O. (2008) 'Depression and the serotonin transporter 5-HTTLPR polymorphism: A review and a hypothesis concerning gene–environment interaction' *Journal of Affective Disorders*, 111, 1: 1–12

Brown, G.W., Harris, T.O. and Bifulco, A. (1986b) 'Long-term effect of early loss of parent' in Rutter, M., Izard, C. and Read, P. (eds) *Depression in Childhood: Developmental perspectives*, New York: Guilford Press

Brown, G.W., Harris, T.O. and Hepworth, C. (1994) 'Life events and endogenous depression: A puzzle re-examined' *Archives of General Psychiatry*, 51: 525–34

Brown, G.W., Harris, T.O. and Hepworth, C. (1995) 'Loss, humiliation and entrapment among women developing depression: A patient and non-patient comparison' *Psychological Medicine*, 25, 7–21

Brown, G.W., Monck, E. M., Carstairs, G.M. and Wing, J. K. (1962) 'Influence of family life on the course of schizophrenic illness' *British Journal of Preventative Social Medicine*, 16: 55–68

Brown, G.W. and Moran, P. (1994) 'Clinical and psycho-social origins of chronic depressive episodes. 1: A community survey' *British Journal of Psychiatry*, 165: 447–56

Brown, S.L., Nesse, R.M., Vinokur, A.D. and Smith, D.M. (2003) 'Providing social support may be more beneficial than receiving it: Results from a prospective study of mortality' *Psychological Science*, 14, 4: 320–7

Brugha, T.S., Bebbington, P.E., Jenkins, R., et al. (1999) 'Cross validation of a general population survey diagnostic interview: A comparison of CIS-R with SCAN ICD-10 diagnostic categories' *Psychological Medicine*, 29, 5: 1029–42

Brugha, T.S., Jenkins, R., Taub, N., Meltzer, H. and Bebbington, P.E. (2001) 'A general population comparison of the Composite International Diagnostic Interview (CIDI) and the Schedules for Clinical Assessment in Neuropsychiatry (SCAN)' *Psychological Medicine*, 31, 6: 1001–13

Brugha, T.S., Weich, S., Singleton, N., et al. (2005) 'Primary group size, gender and future mental health status in a prospective study of people living in private households throughout Great Britain' *Psychological Medicine*, 35, 5: 705–14

Brugha, T.S., Morrell, C.J., Slade, P. and Walters, S.J. (2011) 'Universal prevention of depression in women postnatally: Cluster randomized trial evidence in primary care' *Psychological Medicine* 41: 739–48

Bunt, K., Shury, J. and Vivian, D. (2001) *Recruiting Benefit Claimants: A qualitative study of employers who recruited benefit claimants* (DWP Research Report No. 150), Leeds, UK: CDS

Burmeister, M., McInnis, M.G. and Zöllner, S. (2008) 'Psychiatric genetics: Progress amid controversy' *Nature Reviews: Genetics*, 9: 527–40

Butler, A.C., Chapman, J.E., Foreman, E.M. and Beck, A.T. (2006) 'The empirical status of cognitive behavioral therapy: A review of meta-analyses' *Clinical Psychology Review*, 26: 17–31

Butzlaff, R. and Hooley, J. (1998) 'Expressed emotion and psychiatric relapse: A meta-analysis' *Archives of General Psychiatry*, 55, 6: 547–52

Bynner, J., Elias, P., McKnight, A., Pan, H. and Pierre, G. (2002) *Young People's Changing Routes to Independence*, York, UK: Joseph Rowntree Foundation

Cahn, C.H. (1999) 'DSM classification', in Freeman, H. (ed) *A Century of Psychiatry*, London: Mosby Wolfe

Calnan, M. (1991) *Preventing Coronary Health Disease: Prospects, policies and politics*, London: Routledge

Cannon, M., Caspi, A., Moffitt, T.E., et al. (2002a) 'Evidence for early-childhood, pan-developmental impairment specific to schizophreniform disorder: results from a longitudinal birth cohort' *Archives of General Psychiatry*, 59: 449–56

Cannon, M., Jones, P.B. and Murray, R.M. (2002b) Obstetric complications and schizophrenia: Historical and meta-analytic review, *American Journal of Psychiatry*, 159: 1080–92

Caplan, G. (1964) *Principles of Preventive Psychiatry*, New York: Basic Books

Caplan-Moskovitch, R.B. (1982) 'Gerald Caplan: The man and his work' in Schulberg, H.C. and Killilea, M. (eds) *The Modern Practice of Community Mental Health*, San Francisco: Jossey Bass

Cardno, A.G., Marshall, J., Coid, B., et al. (1999) 'Heritability estimates for psychotic disorders: The Maudsley Twin Psychosis Series' *Archives of General Psychiatry*, 56: 162–8

Carrà, G., Montomoli, C., Clerici, M. and Cazzullo, C.L. (2007) 'Family interventions for schizophrenia in Italy: Randomized controlled trial' *European Archives of Psychiatry and Clinical Neuroscience*, 257: 23–30

Cartwright, A. (1974) *Exploratory studies of the services for maladjusted children*, Unpublished MPhil thesis, University of London

Caspi, A., Sugden, K., Moffitt, T.E., et al. (2003) 'Influence of life stress on depression: Moderation by a polymorphism in the 5-H-TT gene' *Science*, 301: 386–9

Caspi, A., Moffitt, T.E., Cannon, M., et al. (2005) 'Moderation of the effect of adolescent-onset cannabis use on adult psychosis by a functional polymorphism in the catechol-o-methyltransferase gene: Longitudinal evidence of a gene × environment interaction' *Biological Psychiatry*, 57, 10: 1117–27

Catalano, R. and Hartig, T. (2004) 'Economic predictors of admissions to inpatient psychiatric treatment in Sweden' *Social Psychiatry and Psychiatric Epidemiology*, 39, 4: 305–10

Cawson, P., Wattam, C., Brooker, S. and Kelly, G. (2000) *Child Maltreatment in the United Kingdom: A study of the prevalence of abuse and neglect*. London: NSPCC

CBI (2010) *On the Path to Recovery: Absence and workplace health survey 2010*, London: CBI/Pfizer

Chadwick, P.K. (1997) *Schizophrenia: The positive perspective*, London: Routledge

Children Are Unbeatable! (2010) Newsletter, Issue No. 2 – April 2010, www.childrenare-unbeatable.org.uk/pdfs/newsletters/CAU-Issue02.pdf (accessed 21 May 2012)

Clarke, A.E. (2009) 'Work, jobs and wellbeing across the Millenium' *OECD Social Employment and Migrations Working Papers No, 83*, Paris: OECD

Clayden, J. and Stein, M. (2005) *Mentoring Young People Leaving Care: Someone for me*, York, UK: Joseph Rowntree Foundation

Cleaver, H., Unell, I. and Aldgate, J. (1999) *Children's Needs – Parenting Capacity: The impact of parental mental illness, problem alcohol and drug use, and domestic violence on children's development*, London: Stationery Office

Cobb, S. (1976) 'Social support as a moderator of life stress' *Psychosomatic Medicine*, 38: 300–14

Cochrane, A. (1972) *Effectiveness and Efficiency: Random reflections on health services*, London: Nuffield Provincial Hospitals Trust

Cohen, A., Patel, V., Thara, R. and Gureje, O. (2008) 'Questioning an axiom: Better prognosis for schizophrenia in the developing world?' *Schizophrenia Bulletin*, 34, 2: 229–44

Cohen, S., Frank, E., Doyle, W.J., Skoner, D.P., Rabin, B.S. and Gwaltney, J.M. (1998) 'Types of stressors that increase susceptibility to the common cold in healthy adults' *Health Psychology*, 17: 214–223

Cohen, S., Doyle, W.J., Turner, R.B., Alper, C.M. and Skoner, D.P. (2003) 'Emotional style and susceptibility to the common cold' *Psychosomatic Medicine*, 65: 652–7

Colgrove, J. and Bayer, R. (2005) 'Manifold restraints: Liberty, public health, and the legacy of Jacobson v Massachusetts' *American Journal of Public Health*, 95: 571–6

Collishaw, S., Maughan, B., Goodman, R. and Pickles, A. (2004) 'Time trends in adolescent mental health' *Journal of Child Psychology and Psychiatry*, 45, 8: 1350–62

Collishaw, S., Pickles, A., Messer, J., Rutter, M., Shearer, C. and Maughan, B. (2007) 'Resilience to adult psychopathology following childhood maltreatment: Evidence from a community sample' *Child Abuse & Neglect*, 31: 211–29

Colman, I., Murray, J., Abbott, R.A., et al. (2009) 'Outcomes of conduct problems in adolescence: 40 year follow-up of national cohort' *British Medical Journal*, 338: a2981

Commission on Chronic Illness (1957) *Chronic Illness in the United States, vol. 1*, Published for the Commonwealth Fund, Cambridge, MA: Harvard University Press

Cooke, D., Newman, S., Sacker, A., DeVellis, B., Bebbington, P. and Meltzer, H. (2007) 'The impact of physical illnesses on non-psychotic psychiatric morbidity: Data from the household survey of psychiatric morbidity in Great Britain' *British Journal of Health Psychology*, 12: 463–71

Cooper, B. (2005) 'Immigration and schizophrenia: The social causation hypothesis revisited' *British Journal of Psychiatry*, 186: 361–3

Cooper, J. (1999) 'ICD-10: Mental disorders chapter of the international classification of diseases tenth revision' in Freeman, H. (ed) *A Century of Psychiatry*, London: Mosby-Wolfe

Cornah, D. (2006) *The Impact of Spirituality on Mental Health: A review of the literature*, London: Mental Health Foundation

Cornblatt, B., Obuchowski, M., Roberts, S., Pollack, S. and Erlenmeyer-Kimling, L. (1999) 'Cognitive and behavioral precursors of schizophrenia' *Development and Psychopathology*, 11, 3: 487–508

Crawford, M. (2007) *Presentation on 28.03.07 to the FHF Inquiry into the Links between Diet and Behaviour*, London: Associate Parliamentary Food and Health Forum, www.fhf.org.uk/inquiry (accessed 24 November 2011)

Crawford, M.A., Bazinet, R.P. and Sinclair, A.J. (2009) 'Fat Intake and CNS functioning: Ageing and disease' *Annals of Nutrition and Metabolism*, 55: 202–28

Creed, F. (2000) 'The study of life events has clarified the concept of psycho-somatic disorders' in Harris, T.O. (ed) *Where Inner and Outer Worlds Meet: Psycho-social research in the tradition of George W. Brown*, London: Routledge

Crisp, A.H., Gelder, M.G., Rix, S., Meltzer, H.I. and Rowlands, O.J. (2000) 'Stigmatisation of people with mental illness' *British Journal of Psychiatry*, 177: 4–7

Crooks, C.V., Scott, K., Ellis, W. and Wolfe, D.A. (2011) 'Impact of a universal school-based violence prevention program on violent delinquency: Distinctive benefits for youth with maltreatment histories' *Child Abuse & Neglect*, 35: 393–400

Crowther, R., Marshall, M., Bond, G. and Huxley, P. (2001) 'Vocational rehabilitation for people with severe mental illness' *Cochrane Database of Systematic Reviews*, issue 3

Crum, A.J. and Langer, E.J. (2007) 'Mind-set matters: Exercise and the placebo effect' *Psychological Science*, 18, 2: 165–71

Cutting, J. (1985) *The Psychology of Schizophrenia*, Edinburgh, UK: Churchill Livingstone

Davidson, R.J., Kabat-Zinn, J., Schumacher, J., et al. (2003) 'Alterations in brain and immune function produced by mindfulness meditation' *Psychosomatic Medicine*, 65: 564–70

Davies, L. and Duckett, N. (2008) *Proactive Child Protection – The social work task*. Exeter, UK: Learning Matters

Davis, C. G., Nolen-Hoeksema, S. and Larson, J. (1998) 'Making sense of loss and benefiting from the experience: Two construals of meaning' *Journal of Personality and Social Psychology*, 75, 2: 561–74

DCSF (2009) *Improving the Attainment of Looked After Young People in Secondary Schools*, London: DCSF

Deegan, P.E. (1988) 'Recovery: The lived experience of rehabilitation' *Psycho-social Rehabilitation Journal*, 11, 4: 11–19

De Silva, M.J., McKenzie, K., Harpham, T. and Huttly, S.R.A. (2005) 'Social capital and mental illness: A systematic review' *Journal of Epidemiology & Community Health*, 59: 619–27

DH (2004) *At Least Five a Week: Evidence on the impact of physical activity and its relationship to health. A report from the Chief Medical Officer*, London: Department of Health

DH (2008) *The Case for Change – Why England needs a new care and support system*, London: Department of Health

DH (2009a) *Work, Recovery and Inclusion*, London: Department of Health

DH (2009b) *Flourishing People, Connected Communities: A framework for developing wellbeing*, London: Department of Health

DH (2010) *Teenage Pregnancy Strategy: Beyond 2010*, Nottingham, UK: DCSF Publications

DH (2011) *No Health without Mental Health: A cross-government mental health outcomes strategy for people of all ages*, London: HM Government

DiCenso, A., Guyatt, G., Willan, A., and Griffith, L. (2002) 'Interventions to reduce unintended pregnancies among adolescents: Systematic review of randomised controlled trials' *British Medical Journal*, 324, 7351: 1426–30

Dixon, L., Hamilton-Giachritsis, C. and Browne, K. (2005) 'Attributions and behaviours of parents abused as children: A mediational analysis of the intergenerational continuity of child maltreatment (Part II)' *Journal of Child Psychology and Psychiatry*, 46, 1: 58–68

Doane, J.A., West, K.L., Goldstein, M.J., Rodnick, E.H. and Jones, J.E. (1981) 'Parental communication deviance and affective style' *Archives of General Psychiatry*, 38: 679–85

Dohrenwend, B.P. (1975) 'Socio-cultural and psycho-psychological factors in the genesis of mental disorders' *Journal of Health and Social Behavior*, 16, 4: 365–92

Dohrenwend, B.P. and Dohrenwend, B.S. (1969) *Social Status and Psychological Disorder: A causal enquiry*, New York: Wiley Interscience

Donaghy, M.E. (2007) 'Exercise can seriously improve your mental health: Fact or fiction?' *Advances in Physiotherapy*, 9: 76–88

Donelly, M. (1999) 'Franco Basaglia (1924–1980)' in Freeman, H. (ed) *A Century of Psychiatry*, London: Mosby Wolfe

Doyle, Y.G., Furey, A. and Flowers, J. (2006) 'Sick individuals and sick populations: 20 years later' *Journal of Epidemiology & Community Health*, 60: 396–8

Draper, B., Pfaff, J.J., Pirkis, J., et al. (2008) 'Long-term effects of childhood abuse on the quality of life and health of older people: Results from the Depression and Early Prevention of Suicide in General Practice Project' *Journal of the American Geriatrics Society*, 56, 2: 262–71

Drugli, M.B., Larsson, B., Fossum, S. and Mørch, W.T. (2010) 'Five- to six-year outcome and its prediction for children with ODD/CD treated with parent training' *Journal of Child Psychology and Psychiatry*, 51, 5: 559–566

DuBois, D.L., Neville, H.A., Parra, G.R. and Pugh-Lilly, A.O. (2002) 'Testing a new model of mentoring' *New Directions for Youth Development*, 93: 21–57

Dunn, A., Trivedi, M.H., Kampert, J., Clark, C.G. and Chambliss, H.O. (2005) 'Exercise treatment for depression: Efficacy and dose–response' *American Journal of Preventive Medicine*, 28: 1–8

Dunn, J. and Plomin, R. (1990) *Separate Lives: Why siblings are so different*, New York: Basic Books

Durlak, J.A. and Wells, A.M. (1997). 'Primary prevention mental health programs for children and adolescents: A meta-analytic review' *American Journal of Community Psychology*, 25: 115–52

DWP (2011) Employment rates of disabled people, by main impairment type, http://odi. dwp.gov.uk/docs/res/factsheets/b2-employment-rates-of-disabled-people.pdf (accessed 31 January 2012)

Easterlin, R.A. (1974) 'Does economic growth improve the human lot?' in David, P.A. and Reder, M.W. (eds.) *Nations and Households in Economic Growth: Essays in honor of Mozes Abramowitz*, New York: Academic Press

Easterlin, R.A., McVey, L.A., Switek, M., Sawangfa, O. and Zweig, J.S (2010) The happiness–income paradox revisited, www.pnas.org/cgi/doi/10.1073/pnas.1015962107 (accessed 28 January 2012)

Eckenrode, J., Ganzel, B., Henderson, C.R., et al. (2000) 'Preventing child abuse and neglect with a program of nurse home visitation: The limiting effects of domestic violence' *Journal of the American Medical Association*, 284, 11: 1385–91

Economic Intelligence Unit (1982) *Coping with Unemployment: The effects on the unemployed themselves*, London: EIU

Eisenberg, P. & Lazarsfeld, P. F. (1938) 'The psychological effects of unemployment' *Psychological Bulletin*, 35, 258–390

Emery, A.E.H., Watt, M.S. and Clack, E.R. (1973) 'Social effects of genetic counselling' *British Medical Journal*, 1: 724–6

Epstein, S. (1983) 'Natural healing processes of the mind' in Meichenbaum, D. and Jaremko, M.E. (eds) *Stress Reduction and Prevention*, New York: Plenum Press

Eriksson, M. and Lindström, B. (2006) 'Antonovsky's sense of coherence scale and the relation with health: A systematic review' *Journal of Epidemiology & Community Health*, 60: 376–81

ESEMeD/MHEDEA 2000 Investigators (2004) 'Prevalence of mental disorders in Europe: Results from the European Study of the Epidemiology of Mental Disorders (ESEMeD) project' *Acta Psychiatrica Scandinavica*, 109 (Suppl. 420): 21–27

European Agency for Safety and Health at Work (2002) *Prevention of Psycho-social Risks and Stress at Work in Practice*, Luxembourg: Office for Official Publications of the European Communities

Everson, S.A., Goldberg, D.E., Kaplan, G.A., et al. (1996) 'Hopelessness and risk of mortality and incidence of myocardial infarction and cancer' *Psychosomatic Medicine*, 58, 2: 113–21

Eyken, W. van der (1982) *Homestart: A four-year evaluation*, Leicester, UK: Homestart Consultancy

Falkov, A. (1995) *Study of Working Together Part 8 Reports: Fatal child abuse and parental psychiatric disorder: An analysis of 100 case reviews*, London: Department of Health

Falloon, I.R.H., Boyd, J.L., McGill, C., et al. (1985) 'Family management in the prevention of morbidity of schizophrenia: Clinical outcome of a two year longitudinal study' *Archives of General Psychiatry*, 42: 887–96

Fava, G.A., Rafanelli, C., Cazzaro, M., Conti, S., and Grandi, S. (1998) 'Wellbeing therapy: A novel psychotherapeutic approach for residual symptoms of affective disorders' *Psychological Medicine*, 28: 475–80

Fergusson, D.M., Boden, J.M. and Horwood, L.J. (2008) 'Exposure to childhood sexual and physical abuse and adjustment in early adulthood' *Child Abuse & Neglect*, 32, 6: 607–19

Festinger, L. (1957) *A Theory of Cognitive Dissonance*, Stanford, CA: Stanford University Press

Festinger, L. and Carlsmith, J.M. (1959) 'Cognitive consequences of forced compliance' *Journal of Abnormal and Social Psychology*, 58, 2: 203–10

Finlay-Jones, R. and Brown, G.W.B. (1981) 'Types of stressful life events and the onset of anxiety and depressive disorder' *Psychological Medicine* 11: 803–15

Fisher, H., Morgan, C., Dazzan, P. et al. (2009) 'Gender differences in the association between childhood abuse and psychosis' *British Journal of Psychiatry*, 194: 319–25

Fisher, P.A., Kim, H.K. and Pears, K.C. (2009) 'Effects of multidimensional treatment foster care for preschoolers (MTFC-P) on reducing permanent placement failures among children with placement instability' *Children and Youth Services Review*, 31: 541–6

Flay, B.R. (1986) 'Efficacy and effectiveness trials (and other phases of research) in the development of health promotion programs' *Preventive Medicine*, 15: 451–74

Foreman, D.M. (1998) 'Maternal mental illness and mother–child relations' *Advances in Psychiatric Treatment*, 4: 135–43

Foresight Mental Capital and Wellbeing Project (2008) *Mental Capital and Wellbeing: Making the most of ourselves in the 21st century*, London: Government Office for Science

Foshee, V.A., Bauman, K.E., Ennett, S.Y., Suchindran, C., Benefield, T. and Linder, G.F. (2005) 'Assessing the effects of the dating violence prevention program "Safe Dates" using random coefficient regression modeling' *Prevention Science*, 6, 3: 245–58

Fox, S.E., Levitt, P. and Nelson, C.A. (2010) 'How the timing and quality of early experiences influence the development of brain architecture', *Child Development*, 81, 1: 28–40

Freeman, M., Hibbeln, J.R., Wisner, K.L., et al. (2006) 'American Psychiatric Association's treatment recommendations for omega-3 fatty acids in psychiatric disorders' *Journal of Clinical Psychiatry*, 67: 1954–67

French, G. and Shinman, S. (2005) *Learning from Families – Transnational report: Policies and practices to combat social exclusion amongst families with young children in Europe*, London: Home-Start International

Friedman, S.H. and Resnick, P.J. (2007) 'Child murder by mothers: Patterns and prevention' *World Psychiatry*, 6, 3: 137–141

Furåker, B. and Blomsterberg, M. (2003) 'Attitudes towards the unemployed. An analysis of Swedish survey data' *International Journal of Social Welfare*, 12: 193–203

Gafoor, R., Craig, T., Garety, P., Power, P. and McGuire, P. (2009) 'Do the benefits of early intervention treatments for schizophrenia persist?' *European Psychiatry*, 24, S1: S113

Gaminde, I., Uria, M., Padro, D., Querejeta, I. and Ozamiz, A. (1993) 'Depression in three populations in the Basque Country: A comparison with Britain' *Social Psychiatry and Psychiatric Epidemiology*, 28: 243–51

Garber, J., Miller, W.R. and Seamen, S.F. (1979) 'Learned helplessness, stress, and the depressive disorders' in Depue, R.A. (ed) *The Psychobiology of the Depressive Disorders*, New York: Academic Press

Garety, P.A., Fowler, D.G., Freeman, D., Bebbington, P., Dunn, G. and Kuipers, E. (2008) 'Cognitive–behavioural therapy and family intervention for relapse prevention and symptom reduction in psychosis: Randomised controlled trial' *British Journal of Psychiatry*, 192: 412–23

Gerard, D.L. (1997) 'Chiarugi and Pinel considered: Soul's brain, person's mind' *Journal of the History of the Behavioral Sciences*, 33, 4: 381–403

Gesch, C.B., Hammond, S.M., Hampson, S.E., Eves, A. and Crowder, M.J. (2002) 'Influence of supplementary vitamins, minerals and essential fatty acids on the antisocial behaviour of young adult prisoners: Randomised, placebo-controlled trial' *British Journal of Psychiatry*, 181: 22–8

Gilbert, P. (1999) *Depression: The evolution of powerlessness*, London: Taylor & Francis

Gilbert, P. (2007) *Psychotherapy and Counselling for Depression*, (3rd edition), London: Sage

Glaser, R. and Kiecolt-Glaser, J.K. (2005) 'Stress-induced immune dysfunction: Implications for health' *Nature Reviews Immunology*, 5: 243–51

Glasgow R.E., Lichtenstein E. and Marcus A.C. (2003) 'Why don't we see more translation of health promotion research to practice? Rethinking the efficacy to effectiveness transition' *American Journal of Public Health*, 93, 8: 1261–7

Glendinning A. and West, P. (2007) 'Young people's mental health in context: Comparing life in the city and small communities in Siberia' *Social Science & Medicine*, 65: 1180–91

Goffman, E. (1963) *Stigma: Notes on the management of spoiled identity*, New York: Simon & Schuster

Goldberg, D. (1992) 'Early diagnosis and secondary prevention' in Jenkins, R., Newton, J. and Young, R. (eds) *The Prevention of Anxiety and Depression: The role of the primary care team*, London: HMSO

Goldberg, D. and Goodyear, I. (2005) *The Origins and Course of Common Mental Disorders*, London: Routledge

Goldberg, D. and Huxley, P. (1980) *Mental Illness in the Community: The pathway to psychiatric care*, London: Tavistock

Gomby, D.S. (2005) *Home visitation in 2005: Outcomes for children and parents*, Invest in Kids Working Paper No. 7, Washington, DC: Committee for Economic Development

Goodman, L.A., Rosenberg, S.D., Mueser, K.T. and Drake, R.E. (1997) 'Physical and sexual assault history in women with serious mental illness: Prevalence, correlates, treatment, and future research directions' *Schizophrenia Bulletin*, 23, 4: 685–96

Gordon, R. (1983) 'An operational classification of disease prevention' *Public Health Reports*, 98, 2: 107–9

Gottesman, I.I. (1991) *Schizophrenia Genesis: The origins of madness*, New York: W.H. Freeman

Gottesman, I.I. and Gould, T.D. (2003) 'The endophenotype concept in psychiatry: Etymology and strategic intentions' *American Journal of Psychiatry*, 160: 636–45

Gottlieb, B.H. (1983) *Social Support Strategies: Guidelines for mental health practice*, Beverly Hills, CA: Sage

Graham, H. (2002) 'Building an inter-disciplinary science of health inequalities: The example of lifecourse research' *Social Science & Medicine*, 55: 2005–16

Green, J.G., McLaughlin, K.A., Berglund, P.A., et al. (2010) 'Childhood adversities and adult psychiatric disorders in the national comorbidity survey replication I' *Archives of General Psychiatry*, 67, 2: 113–23

Gumley, A., Karatzias, A., Power, K., Reilly, J., McNay, L. and O'Grady, M. (2006) 'Early intervention for relapse in schizophrenia: Impact of cognitive behavioural therapy on negative beliefs about psychosis and self-esteem' *British Journal of Clinical Psychology*, 45: 247–260

Hackett, S. (2003) 'A framework for assessing parenting capacity' in Calder, M.C. and Hackett, S. (eds) *Assessment in Childcare: Using and developing frameworks for practice*. Lyme Regis, UK: Russell House

Hallahan, B. and Garland, M.R. (2005) 'Essential fatty acids and mental health' *British Journal of Psychiatry*, 186: 275–7

Hallfors, D., Hyunsan C., Sanchez, V., Khatapoush, S., Hyung M.K. and Bauer, D. (2006) 'Efficacy vs effectiveness trial results of an indicated "model" substance abuse program: Implications for public health' *American Journal of Public Health*, 96, 12: 2254–9

Hamer, M. and Chida, Y. (2009) 'Physical activity and risk of neurodegenerative disease: A systematic review of prospective evidence' *Psychological Medicine* 39: 3–11

Hamlin, C. (1995) 'Public health then and now: Could you starve to death in England in 1839? The Chadwick-Farr controversy and the loss of the "social" in public health' *American Journal of Public Health*, 85, 6: 856–66

Hammen, C. (1997) *Depression*, Hove, UK: Psychology Press

Hammen, C. (2010) 'Adolescent depression: Stressful interpersonal contexts and risk for recurrence' *Current Directions in Psychological Science*, 18, 4: 200–4

Hanifan, L.K. (1916) 'The rural school community center' *Annals of the American Academy of Political and Social Science*, 67: 130–8

Hann, A. (1993) 'The decision to screen' in Mills, M. (ed) *Prevention, Health and British Politics*, Aldershot, UK: Ashgate

Harbottle, L. and Schonfelder, N. (2008) 'Nutrition and depression: A review of the evidence' *Journal of Mental Health*, 17, 6: 576–87

Harden, A., Brunton, G., Fletcher, A. and Oakley, A. (2009) 'Teenage pregnancy and social disadvantage: Systematic review integrating controlled trials and qualitative studies' *British Medical Journal*, 339: b4254

Harris, T. (ed) (2000) *Where Inner and Outer Worlds Meet: Psychological research in the tradition of George W. Brown*, London: Routledge

Harris, T. (2008) 'Putting Newpin to the test: A randomised controlled trial of the antenatal and post-natal project' in Mondy, L. and Mondy, S. (eds) *Newpin: Courage to Change Together: Helping families achieve generational change*, Sydney, Australia: Uniting Care Burnside

Harris, T., Brown, G.W. and Bifulco, A. (1987) 'Loss of parent in childhood and adult psychiatric disorder: The role of social class position and premarital pregnancy' *Psychological Medicine*, 17: 163–83

Harris, T., Brown, G.W. and Bifulco, A. (1990) 'Loss of parent in childhood and adult psychiatric disorder: A tentative overall model' *Development and Psychopathology*, 2: 311–28

Harris, T., Brown, G.W., and Robinson, R. (1999a) 'Befriending as an intervention for chronic depression among women in an inner city. 1: Randomised control trial' *British Journal of Psychiatry*, 174: 219–24

Harris, T., Brown, G.W. and Robinson, R. (1999b) 'Befriending as an intervention for chronic depression among women in an inner city. 2: Role of fresh start experiences and baseline psycho-social factors in remission from depression' *British Journal of Psychiatry*, 174: 225–32

Harrison, G., Hopper, K., Craig, T., et al. (2001) 'Recovery from psychotic illness: A 15- and 25- year international follow-up study' *British Journal of Psychiatry*, 178: 506–17

Hawton, K., Simkin, S., Deeks, J., et al. (2004) 'UK legislation on analgesic packs: Before and after study of long term effects on poisonings' *British Medical Journal*, 329, 7474: 1076

Heckman, J.J. (2007) 'The economics, technology, and neuroscience of human capability formation' *Proceedings of the National Academy of Sciences of the United States of America*, 104, 33: 13250–5

Heinicke, C.M., Goorsky, M., Moscov, S., et al. (1998) 'Partner support as a mediator of intervention outcome' *American Journal of Orthopsychiatry*, 68, 4: 534–4

Heinicke, C.M., Goorsky, M., Levine, M., et al. (2006) 'Pre- and post-natal antecedents of a home-visiting intervention and family developmental outcome' *Infant Mental Health Journal*, 27, 1: 91–119

Helgeson, V.S. (2003) 'Cognitive adaptation, psychological adjustment, and disease progression among angioplasty patents: 4 years later' *Health Psychology*, 22, 1: 30–38

Heller, K. (1996) 'Coming of age of prevention science: Comments on the NIMH-IoM prevention reports' *American Psychologist*, 51, 11: 1123–7

Herman, J.L. (1992) *Trauma and Recovery: From domestic abuse to political terror*, London: Pandora

Hermanns, N. (2010) 'CS03-01 – Epidemiology of co-morbid diabetes and depression' *European Psychiatry*, Supplement 1, 25: 148

Hetherington, M.E. (2003) 'Social support and the adjustment of children in divorced and remarried families' *Childhood*, 10: 217–36

Hettema, J.M., Kuhn, J.W., Prescott, C.A. and Kendler, K.S. (2006) 'The impact of generalized anxiety disorder and stressful life events on risk for major depressive episodes' *Psychological Medicine*, 36: 789–95

Hibbeln, J.R., Nieminen, L.R.G., Blasbalg, T.L., Riggs, J.A. and Lands, W.E.M. (2006) 'Healthy intakes of n_3 and n_6 fatty acids: estimations considering worldwide diversity 1–5' *American Journal of Clinical Nutrition*, 83 (suppl): 1483S–93S

Hibbeln, J.R., Davis, J.M., Steer, C., et al. (2007) 'Maternal seafood consumption in pregnancy and neurodevelopmental outcomes in childhood (ALSPAC study): An observational cohort study' *The Lancet*, 369: 578–85

Hills, J. (2007) *Ends and Means: The future roles of social housing in England* (summary), London: LSE

Hirsch, S.R. and Leff, J.P. (1975) *Abnormalities in Parents of Schizophrenics*, Institute of Psychiatry Maudsley Monographs, London: Oxford University Press

HM Treasury and Department for Work & Pensions (2003) *Full Employment in Every Region*, London: The Stationery Office

Hoff, K. and Pandey, P. (2004) 'Belief systems and durable inequalities: An experimental investigation of Indian caste' *World Bank Policy Research Working Paper*, 3351

Hofmann, S.G., Sawyer, A.T., Witt, A.A., and Oh, D. (2010) 'The effect of mindfulness-based therapy on anxiety and depression: A meta-analytic review' *Journal of Consulting and Clinical Psychology*, 78, 2: 169–83

Hogarty, G.E., Anderson, C.M., Reiss, D.J., et al. (1991) 'Family psycho-education, social skills training and maintenance chemotherapy in the aftercare treatment of schizophrenia II: Two year effects of a controlled study on relapse and adjustment' *Archives of General Psychiatry*, 48: 340–1

Holahan, C.J., Pahl, S.A., Cronkite, R.C., Holahan, C.K., North, R.J. and Moos, R.H. (2010) 'Depression and vulnerability to incident physical illness across 10 years' *Journal of Affective Disorders*, 123, 1–3: 222–9

Hollingshead, A. and Redlich R.C. (1958) *Social Class and Mental Illness*, New York: John Wiley

Home Office (2010) *Crime in England and Wales: Quarterly update to June 2010*, London: National Statistics

Hopper, K., Harrison, G., Janca, A. and Sartorius, N. (2007) *Recovery from schizophrenia: An international perspective. A report from the WHO Collaborative Project, the international study of schizophrenia*, Oxford: Oxford University Press

Horn, M. (1984) 'The moral message of child guidance 1925–1945' *Journal of Social History*, 18, 1: 25–36

Horn, M. (1989) *Before It's Too Late: The Child Guidance Movement in the United States, 1922–1945*, Philadelphia: Temple University Press

Horwitz, A.V. and Wakefield, J.C. (2007) *The Loss of Sadness: How psychiatry transformed normal sadness into depressive disorder*, Oxford: Oxford University Press

Hosking, G. and Walsh, I. (2005) *The WAVE Report 2005: Violence and what to do about it*, Croydon, UK: Wave Trust

House, J.S. (1981) *Work Stress and Social Support*, Reading, MA: Addison-Wesley

Howard, L.M., Thornicroft, G., Salmon, M. and Appleby, L. (2004) 'Predictors of parenting outcome in women with psychotic disorders discharged from mother and baby units' *Acta Psychiatrica Scandinavica*, 110: 347–55

Howard, L.M., Heslin, M., Leese, M., et al. (2010) 'Supported employment: Randomised controlled trial' *British Journal of Psychiatry*, 196: 404–11

Howes, O.D. and Kapur, S. (2009) 'The dopamine hypothesis of schizophrenia: Version III—The final common pathway' *Schizophrenia Bulletin*, 35, 3: 549–62

HSE (2007) *Managing the Causes of Work-Related Stress: A step-by-step approach using the Management Standards HSG218* (second edition), London: HSE Books

Huijbregts, K.M.L., van der Feltz-Cornelis, C.M., van Marwijk, H.W.J., de Jong, F.J., van der Windt, D.A.W.M. and Beekman, A.T.F. (2010) 'Negative association of concomitant physical symptoms with course of major depressive disorder: A systematic review' *Journal of Psychosomatic Research*, 68, 6: 511–19

Hunot, V., Churchill, R., Teixeira, V. and Silva de Lima, M. (2007) 'Psychological therapies for generalised anxiety disorder' *Cochrane Database of Systematic Reviews*, Issue 1. Art. No. CD001848

Hunsley, J. and Westmacott, R. (2007) 'Interpreting the magnitude of the placebo effect: Mountain or molehill?' *Journal of Clinical Psychology*, 63, 4: 391–9

Huppert, F.A. and Whittington, J. (1995) 'Symptoms of psychological distress predict seven-year mortality' *Psychological Medicine*, 25: 1073–1086

Huppert, F.A. and Whittington, J.E (2003) 'Evidence for the independence of positive and negative wellbeing: Implications for quality of life assessment' *British Journal of Health Psychology*, 8: 107–122

Institute of Medicine (1994) *Reducing Risks for Mental Disorders: Frontiers for preventive intervention research*, Washington, DC: National Academy Press

Issa, A.M. (2006) 'The efficacy of omega-3 fatty acids on cognitive function in aging and dementia: A systematic review' *Dementia and Geriatric Cognitive Disorders*, 21: 88–96

Iversen, A.C., Fear, N.T., Ehlers, A., et al. (2008) 'Risk factors for post-traumatic stress disorder among UK Armed Forces personnel' *Psychological Medicine*, 38, 4: 511–22

Iveson, C. (2002) 'Solution-focused brief therapy' *Advances in Psychiatric Treatment*, 8: 149–56

Jablensky, A. and Sartorius, N. (2008) 'What did the WHO studies really find?' *Schizophrenia Bulletin*, 34, 2: 253–5

Jacobson, N. and Curtis, L. (2000) 'Recovery as policy in mental health services: Strategies emerging from the States' *Psycho-social Rehabilitation Journal*, 23, 4: 333–41

Jaffee, S.R., Caspi, A., Moffitt, T.E. and Taylor, A. (2004) 'Physical maltreatment victim to antisocial child: Evidence of an environmentally mediated process' *Journal of Abnormal Psychology*, 113, 1: 44–55

Jahoda, M. (1958) *Current Concepts of Positive Mental Health*, New York: Basic Books

Jahoda, M. (1979) 'The psychological meanings of unemployment' *New Society*, 6 Sept.: 492–5

Jahoda, M., Lazarsfeld, P. F. and Zeisl, H. (1933/1972) *Marienthal: The sociography of an unemployed community*. London: Tavistock.

Jamison, K.R. (1993) *Touched with Fire: Manic depressive illness and the artistic temperament*, New York: Free Press

Jamison, K.R. (1997) *An Unquiet Mind: A memoir of moods and madness*, London: Picador

Jansson, L.B. and Parnas, J. (2007) 'Competing definitions of schizophrenia: What can be learned from polydiagnostic studies?' *Schizophrenia Bulletin*, 33, 5: 1178–1200

Jaremko, M.E. (1983) 'Stress inoculation training for social anxiety, with emphasis on dating anxiety' in Meichenbaum, D. and Jaremko, M.E. (eds) *Stress Reduction and Prevention*, New York: Plenum Press

Jekeliek, S.M., Moore, K.A. and Hair, E.C. (2002) *Mentoring Programs and Youth Development: A synthesis*, Washington, DC: Child Trends

Jenkins, R., Bebbington, P., Brugha, T., et al. (2003) 'The National Psychiatric Morbidity Surveys of Great Britain—Strategy and methods' *International Review of Psychiatry*, 15: 5–13

Jessop, D.J. and Stein, R.E.K. (1991) 'Who benefits from a pediatric home care program?' *Pediatrics*, 88, 3: 497–505

Jones, K.W. (1999) *Taming the Troublesome Child: American families, child guidance, and the limits of psychiatric authority*, Cambridge, MA: Harvard University Press

Jones, P., Rodgers, B., Murray, R. and Marmot, M. (1994) 'Child development risk factors for adult schizophrenia in the British 1946 birth cohort' *The Lancet*, 344: 1398–1402

Jones, P.B., Rantakallio, P., Hartikainen, A-L., Isohanni, M. and Sipila, P. (1998) 'Schizophrenia as a long-term outcome of pregnancy, delivery, and perinatal complications: A 28-year follow-up of the 1966 North Finland general population birth cohort' *American Journal of Psychiatry*, 155: 355–64

Jordanova, V., Wickramesinghe, C., Gerada, C. and Prince, M. (2004) 'Cross validation of a general population survey diagnostic interview: A comparison of CIS-R with SCAN ICD-10 diagnostic categories' *Psychological Medicine*, 34, 6: 1013–24

Joseph, J. (2004) 'Schizophrenia and heredity: Why the emperor has no genes' in Read, J., Mosher, L.R. and Bentall, R.B. (eds) *Models of Madness*, London: Routledge

Jourard, S.M., and Landsman, T. (1980) *Healthy Personality: An approach from the viewpoint of humanistic psychology*, New York: Macmillan

Juster, H.R., Loomis, B.R., Hinman, T.M., et al. (2007) 'Declines in hospital admissions for acute myocardial infarction in New York State after implementation of a comprehensive smoking ban' *American Journal of Public Health*, 97, 11: 2035–9

Kabat-Zinn, J. (2005) 'Bringing mindfulness to medicine: An interview with Jon Kabat-Zinn, PhD. Interview by Karolyn Gazella' *Advances in Mind–Body Medicine*, 21, 2: 22–7

Kanter, J., Lamb, H.R. and Loeper, C. (1987) 'Expressed emotion in families: A critical review' *Hospital and Community Psychiatry*, 38, 4: 374–80

Kaptchuk, T.J., Kelley, J.M., Conboy, L.A., et al. (2008) 'Components of placebo effect: Randomised controlled trial in patients with irritable bowel syndrome' *British Medical Journal*, 336, 7651: 999–1003

Karasek, R.A. and Theorell, T. (1990) *Healthy Work*, New York: Basic Books

Kardiner, A. and Spiegel, H. (1947) *War, Stress and Neurotic Illness*, New York: Hoeber

Karoly, L.A. (2010) *Toward Standardization of Benefit–Cost Analyses of Early Childhood Interventions*, Working Paper 823, Santa Monica, CA: Rand

Kavanagh, D. (1992) 'Recent developments in expressed emotion and schizophrenia' *British Journal of Psychiatry*, 160: 601–20

Kelly, L., Lovett, J. and Regan, L. (2005) *A Gap or a Chasm? Attrition in reported rape cases*, London: Child and Women Abuse Studies Unit

Kelly, M., Morgan, A., Ellis, S., Younger, T., Huntley, J. and Swann, C. (2010) 'Evidence based public health: A review of the experience of the National Institute of Health and Clinical Excellence (NICE) of developing public health guidance in England' *Social Science & Medicine*, 71: 1056–62

Kendell, R. and Jablensky, A. (2003) 'Distinguishing between the validity and utility of psychiatric diagnoses' *American Journal of Psychiatry* 160, 1: 4–12

Kendler, K.S. (2004) 'Major depression and generalised anxiety disorder: Same genes, (partly) different environments-Revisited' *Focus*, 2, 3: 416–25

Kendler, K.S. (2008) 'Book review: Horwitz, A.V. and Wakefield, J,C. (2007) 'The Loss of Sadness: How psychiatry transformed normal sadness into depressive disorder' *Psychological Medicine*, 38: 148–50

Kendler, K.S., Heath, A.C., Martin, N.G. and Eaves, L.J. (1987) 'Symptoms of anxiety and symptoms of depression: Same genes, different environments?' *Archives of General Psychiatry*, 44, 5: 451–7

Kendler, K.S., Bulik, C.M., Silburg, J., Hettema, J.M., Myers, J. and Prescott, C.A. (2000) 'Childhood sexual abuse and adult psychiatric and substance use disorders in women: An epidemiological and cotwin control analysis' *Archives of General Psychiatry*, 57: 953–9

Kendler, K.S., Gardner, C.O. and Prescott, C.A. (2002) 'Toward a comprehensive developmental model for major depression in women' *American Journal of Psychiatry* 159: 1133–45

Kendler, K.S., Hettema, J.M., Butera, F., Gardner, C.O. and Prescott, C.A. (2003) 'Life event dimensions of loss, humiliation, entrapment, and danger in the prediction of onsets of major depression and generalized anxiety' *Archives of General Psychiatry*, 60: 789–796

Kessler, R.C. (1994) 'The National Comorbidity Survey of the United States' *International Review of Psychiatry*, 6, 4: 365–77

Kessler, R.C. and Walters, E.E. (1998) 'Epidemiology of DSM-III-R depression and minor depression among adolescents and young adults in the national co-morbidity survey' *Depression and Anxiety*, 7: 3–14

Kessler, R.C. and Merikangas, K.R. (2004) 'The National Comorbidity Survey Replication (NCS-R): Background and aims' *International Journal of Methods in Psychiatric Research*, 13, 2: 60–8

Kessler, R.C., Demler, O., Frank, R.G., et al. (2005) 'Prevalence and treatment of mental disorders, 1990 to 2003' *New England Journal of Medicine*, 352, 24: 2515–23

Kessler, R.C., Pecora, P.J., Williams, J., et al. (2008) 'Effects of enhanced foster care on the long-term physical and mental health of foster care alumni' *Archives of General Psychiatry*, 65, 6: 625–33

Kestenbaum, C.J. (1980) 'Children at risk from schizophrenia' *American Journal of Psychotherapy*, 34, 2: 164–77

Keyes, C.L.M. (2002) 'The mental health continuum: From languishing to flourishing in life' *Journal of Health and Social Behavior*, 43, 207–22

Kiecolt-Glaser, J.K., Page, G.G., Marucha, P.T., MacCallum, R.C. and Glaser, R. (1998) 'Psychological influences on surgical recovery: Perspectives from psychoneuroimmunology' *American Psychologist*, 53: 1209–18

Kiecolt-Glaser, J.K., McGuire, L., Robles, T.R. and Glaser, R. (2002a) 'Emotions, morbidity, and mortality: New perspectives from psychoneuroimmunology' *Annual Review of Psychology*, 53: 83–107

Kiecolt-Glaser, J.K., McGuire, L., Robles, T.R., and Glaser, R. (2002b) 'Psychoneuroimmunology: Psychological influences on immune function and health' *Journal of Consulting and Clinical Psychology*, 70, 3: 537–47

Kilcommons, A.M., Morrison, A.P., Knight, A. and Lobban, F. (2008) 'Psychotic experiences in people who have been sexually assaulted' *Social Psychiatry and Psychiatric Epidemiology*, 43: 602–611

Kim-Cohen, J., Caspi, A., Rutter, M., Tomá, M.P. and Moffitt, T.E. (2006) 'The caregiving environments provided to children by depressed mothers with or without an anti-social history' *American Journal of Psychiatry*, 163, 6: 1009–18

Kirby, A., Woodward, A., Jackson, S., Wang, Y. and Crawford, M.A. (2010) 'A double-blind, placebo-controlled study investigating the effects of omega-3 supplementation in children aged 8–10 years from a mainstream school population' *Research in Developmental Disabilities*, 31: 718–30

Kirby, D. (2007) *Emerging Answers 2007: Research findings on programs to reduce teen pregnancy and sexually transmitted diseases*, Washington, DC: National Campaign to Prevent Teen and Unplanned Pregnancy

Kirby, D. (2009) 'Editorial: Reducing pregnancy and health risk behaviours in teenagers' *British Medical Journal*, 339: b2054

Knapp, M., McDaid, D. and Parsonage, M. (2011) *Mental Health Promotion and Mental Illness Prevention: The economic case*, London: DH

Koenen, K.C., Stellman, S.D., Sommer, J.F. and Stellman, J.M. (2008) 'Persisting post-traumatic stress disorder symptoms and their relationship to functioning in Vietnam veterans: A 14-year follow-up' *Journal of Traumatic Stress*, 21, 1: 49–57

Kouvonen, A.M., Väänänen, A., Vahtera, J., et al. (2010) 'Sense of coherence and psychiatric morbidity: A 19-year register-based prospective study' *Journal of Epidemiology and Community Health*, 64: 255–261

Kuh, D., Hardy, R., Rodgers, B. and Wadsworth, M.E.J. (2002) 'Lifetime risk factors for women's psychological distress in midlife' *Social Science & Medicine*, 55: 1957–73

Kuipers, E., Onwumere, J. and Bebbington, P. (2010) 'Cognitive model of caregiving in psychosis' *British Journal of Psychiatry*, 196: 259–65

Kutchins, H. and Kirk, S.A. (1995) 'Response to Janet Williams and Robert Spitzer' *Journal of Social Work Education*, 31, 2: 153–8

Kutchins, H, and Kirk, S.A. (1997) *Making us Crazy: DSM: The psychiatric bible and the creation of mental disorders*, New York: The Free Press

Lang, T. (2006) 'Foreword to Van de Weyer, C.' *Changing Diets, Changing Minds: How food affects mental wellbeing and behaviour*, London: Sustain

Laub, J.H. and Sampson, R.J. (2003) *Shared Beginnings, Divergent Lives: Delinquent boys to age 70*, Cambridge, MA: Harvard University Press

Layard, R. (2006a) *Happiness: Lessons from a new science*, London: Penguin

Layard, R. (2006b) *The Depression Report: A new deal for depression and anxiety disorders*, London: London School of Economics

Lazarus, R.S. (1976) *Patterns of Adjustment*, New York: McGraw-Hill

Lazarus, R.S. (1993) 'Coping theory and research: Past, present and future' *Psychosomatic Medicine*, 55: 234–47

Lazarus, R.S. (2003) 'Author's response: The Lazarus Manifesto for positive psychology and psychology in general' *Psychological Inquiry*, 14, 2: 173–89

Lazarus, R.S. and Folkman, S. (1984) *Stress, Appraisal, and Coping*, New York: Springer

Ledesma, D. and Kumano, H. (2009) 'Mindfulness-based stress reduction and cancer: A meta-analysis' *Psycho-Oncology*, 18: 571–579

Leff, J. (2000) 'Expressed emotion: Measuring relationships', in Harris, T.O. (ed) *Where Inner and Outer Worlds Meet*, London: Routledge

Leff, J.P. and Vaughn, C.E. (1980) 'The influence of life events and relatives expressed emotion in schizophrenia and depressive neurosis' *British Journal of Psychiatry*, 136: 146–53

Leff, J.P. and Vaughn, C.E. (1985) *Expressed Emotion in Families: Its significance for mental illness*, London: Guilford

Leff, J.P., Kuipers, L., Berkowitz, R. and Sturgeon, D. (1985) 'A controlled trial of social intervention in the families of schizophrenia patients: Two year follow-up' *British Journal of Psychiatry*, 146: 594–600

Leighton, A. (1982) *Caring for Mentally Ill People: Psychological and social barriers in a historical context*, Cambridge: Cambridge University Press

Lenior, M.E., Dingemans, P., Schene, A.H., Hart, A.A.M. and Linszen, D.H. (2002) 'The course of parental expressed emotion and psychotic episodes after family intervention in recent-onset schizophrenia: A longitudinal study' *Schizophrenia Research*, 57: 183–90

Levine, M. (1981) *The History and Politics of Community Mental Health*, New York: Oxford University Press

Lewis, G., Pelosi, A.J., Araya, R. and Dunn, G. (1992) 'Measuring psychiatric disorder in the community: A standardized assessment for use by lay interviewers' *Psychological Medicine*, 22: 465–86

Lim, K-L., Jacobs, P. and Dewa, C. (2008) *IHE Report: How much should we spend on mental health?* Edmonton, Canada: Institute of Health Economics

Lim, W.-S., Gammack, J.K., Van Niekerk, J.K. and Dangour, A. (2006) 'Omega 3 fatty acid for the prevention of dementia' *Cochrane Database of Systematic Reviews*, 2006, Issue 1, Art. No. CD005379

Link, B.G., Cullen, F.T., Frank, J. and Wozniak, J. F. (1987) 'The social rejection of former mental patients: Understanding why labels matter' *American Journal of Sociology*, 92, 2: 1461–1500

Link, B.G. and Phelan, J.C. (2001) 'Conceptualising stigma' *Annual Review of Sociology*, 27, 363–85

Lloyd, G.G. (1985) 'Emotional aspects of physical illness' in Granville-Grossman, K. (ed) *Recent Advances in Clinical Psychiatry, vol. 5*, Edinburgh, UK: Churchill Livingstone

Lorant, V., Deliège, D., Eaton, W., Robert, A., Philippot, P. and Ansseau, M. (2003) 'Socioe-conomic inequalities in depression: A meta-analysis' *American Journal of Epidemiology*, 157: 98–112

Lovallo, W. R. (2005) *Stress and Health: Biological and psychological interactions* (2nd ed.), London: Sage

Love, J.M., Kisker, E.E., Ross, C.M., et al. (2002/2004) *Making a Difference in the Lives of Infants and Toddlers and Their Families: The impacts of Early Head Start, Vol 1*, Washington, DC: DHHS

Lundberg, O., Yngwe, M.A., Stjärne, M.K., et al. (2008) 'The role of welfare state principles and generosity in social policy programmes for public health: An international comparative study' *The Lancet*, 372: 1633–4

Luthar, S.S. (2006) 'Resilience in development: A synthesis of research across five decades' in Cicchetti, D. and Cohen, D.J. (eds) *Developmental Psychopathology: Risk, disorder, and adaptation, Volume 3 (2nd edition)*, New York: Wiley

McClusky, J. (2009) 'Letters: Predictions are overly dire' *British Medical Journal*, 338: b775

McCormick, A., Fleming, D. and Charlton, J. (1995) *Morbidity Statistics from General Practice: Fourth national study 1991–1992*, London: HMSO

McCrone, P., Dhanasiri, S., Patel, A., Knapp, M. and Lawton-Smith, S. (2008) *Paying the Price: The cost of mental health care in England to 2026*, London: Kings Fund

McGrath J.J. (2005) 'Myths and plain truths about schizophrenia epidemiology – The NAPE lecture 2004' *Acta Psychiatrica Scandinavica*, 111: 4–11

McGrath, J., Saari, K., Hakko, H., et al. (2004) 'Vitamin D supplementation during the first year of life and risk of schizophrenia: A Finnish birth cohort study' *Schizophrenia Research*, 67, 2/3: 237–46

McManus, F., Grey, N. and Shafran, R. (2008) 'Cognitive therapy for anxiety disorders: Current status and future challenges' *Behavioural and Cognitive Psychotherapy*, 36: 695–704

MacMillan, H.L., Thomas, B.H., Jamieson, E., et al. (2005) 'Effectiveness of home visitation by public-health nurses in prevention of the recurrence of child physical abuse and neglect: A randomised controlled trial' *The Lancet*, 365: 1786–93

Madge, N., Hewitt, A., Hawton, K., et al. (2008) 'Deliberate self-harm within an international community sample of young people: Comparative findings from the Child & Adolescent Self-harm in Europe (CASE) Study' *Journal of Child Psychology and Psychiatry*, 49, 6: 667–77

Mäki, P., Veijola, J., Jones, P.J., et al. (2005) 'Predictors of schizophrenia – A review' *British Medical Bulletin*, 73–74, 1: 1–15

Malaspina, D., Corcoran, C., Kleinhaus, K.R., et al. (2008) 'Acute maternal stress in pregnancy and schizophrenia in offspring: A cohort prospective study' *BMJ MC Psychiatry*, 8: 71

Malmgren K.W. and Meisel, S.M. (2004) 'Examining the link between child maltreatment and delinquency for youth with emotional and behavioural disorders' *Child Welfare*, LXXXIII: 175–88

Marmot, M. (2001) 'Economic and social determinants of disease' *Bulletin of the World Health Organization*, 79, 10: 988–9

Marmot, M. (2004) *Status Syndrome: How your standing directly affects your health and life expectancy*, London: Bloomsbury

Marmot, M. G., Rose, G., Shipley, M. and Hamilton, P. J. (1978) 'Employment grade and coronary heart disease in British civil servants' *Journal of Epidemiology and Community Health*, 32: 244–9

Marmot Review (2010) *Fair Society, Healthy Lives*, London: Marmot Review, www.ucl.ac.uk/marmotreview (accessed 25 October 2010)

Marom, S., Munitz, H., Jones, P.B., Weizman, A. and Hermesh, H. (2005) 'Expressed Emotion: Relevance to rehospitalization in schizophrenia over 7 years' *Schizophrenia Bulletin*, 31, 3: 751–8

Marshall, M., Lewis, S., Lockwood, A., Drake, R., Jones, P. and Croudace, T. (2005) 'Association between duration of untreated psychosis and outcome in cohorts of first-episode patients: A systematic review' *Archives of General Psychiatry*, 62: 975–83

Martin, P. (1998) *The Sickening Mind: Brain, behaviour, immunity and disease*, London: Flamingo

Mead, N., Lester, H., Chew-Graham, C., Gask, L. and Bower, P. (2010) 'Effects of befriending on depressive symptoms and distress: Systematic review and meta-analysis', *British Journal of Psychiatry*, 196: 96–101

Meaney, M.J. (2010) 'Epigenetics and the biological definition of gene × environment interactions' *Child Development*, 81, 1: 41–79

Mechanic, D. (1966) 'Response factors in illness: The study of illness behavior' *Social Psychiatry*, 1: 11–20

Mechanic, D. (1975) 'Socio-cultural and social psychological factors affecting personal responses to psychological disorder' *Journal of Health and Social Behaviour*, 16, 4: 393–404

Mechanic, D. (2003) 'Is the prevalence of mental disorder a good measure of the need for services?' *Health Affairs*, 22, 5: 8–20

Meichenbaum, D. and Jaremko, M.E. (1983) *Stress Reduction and Prevention*, New York: Plenum Press

Meltzer, H., Gatward, R., Goodman, R. and Ford, T. (2003) 'Mental health of children and adolescents in Great Britain' *International Review of Psychiatry*, 15: 185–7

Menezes, N.M., Arenovich, T. and Zipursky, R.B. (2006) 'A systematic review of longitudinal outcome studies of first-episode psychosis' *Psychological Medicine*, 36, 10: 1349–62

Meyer, R.J. and Haggerty, R.J. (1962) 'Streptococcal infection in families: Factors altering individual susceptibility' *Pediatrics*, 29: 539–49

Meyer, T.D. and Scott, J. (2008) 'Cognitive behavioural therapy for mood disorders' *Behavioural and Cognitive Psychotherapy*, 36: 685–93

Miller, W.R. & Rollnick, S. (1991) *Motivational Interviewing: Preparing people to change addictive behaviors*, New York: Guilford

Mills, M. (ed) (1993) *Prevention, Health and British Politics*, Aldershot, UK: Ashgate

Mills, M. and Saward, M. (1993) 'Liberalism, Democracy and Prevention' in Mills, M. (ed) *Prevention, Health and British Politics*, Aldershot, UK: Ashgate

Moffitt, T.E. and Caspi, A. (1998) 'Annotation: Implications of violence between intimate partners for child psychologists and psychiatrists' *Journal of Child Psychology and Psychiatry*, 39: 137–44

Moffitt, T.E. and the E-risk study team (2002) 'Teen-aged mothers in contemporary Britain' *Journal of Child Psychology and Psychiatry*, 43, 6: 727–42

Moore, N., McGlinchey, A. and Carr, A. (2002) 'Prevention of teenage pregnancy, STDs and HIV infection' in Carr, A. (ed) *Prevention: What works for children and adolescents*, Hove, UK: Brunner-Routledge

Morrison, A.P. (2004) 'Cognitive therapy for people with psychosis' in Read, J., Mosher, L.R. and Bentall, R.P. (eds) *Models of Madness*, Hove, UK: Routledge

Morrison, A.P., French, P., Walford, L., et al. (2004) 'A randomised controlled trial of early detection and cognitive therapy for the prevention of psychosis in people at ultra-high risk' *British Journal of Psychiatry*, 185: 291–297

Moxnes, K. (2003) 'Risk factors in divorce: Perceptions by the children involved' *Childhood*, 10, 2: 131–46

Mrazek, P. J. and Haggerty, R. J. (eds) (1994) *Reducing Risks for Mental Disorder: Frontiers for preventive intervention research*, Washinton, DC: National Academy Press

Murphy, C.M. and Maiuro, R.D. (2009) *Motivational Interviewing and Stages of Change in Intimate Partner Violence*, New York: Springer

Murray, C.J.L., and Lopez, A.D. (eds) (1996) *The Global Burden of Disease: A comprehensive assessment of mortality and disability from diseases, injuries, and risk factors in 1990 and projected to 2020*, Cambridge, MA: Harvard School of Public Health

Myers, J.K., Lindenthal, J.J. and Pepper, M.P. (1975) 'Life events, social integration and psychiatric symptomatology' *Journal of Health and Social Behavior*, 16, 4: 421–7

National Council for Mental Hygiene (1927) 'The probable causes of mental disorder', Appendix to the *Fourth Report of the National Council for Mental Hygiene 1926–7*, London

National Statistics (2003) *Census 2001: Commentaries by theme and region*, London: ONS

NCH Action for Children (1994) *The Hidden Victims: Children and domestic violence*, London: NCH

NEMO Study Group (2007) 'Effect of a 12-month micronutrient intervention on learning and memory in well-nourished and marginally nourished school-aged children: Two parallel, randomized, placebo-controlled studies in Australia and Indonesia' *American Journal of Clinical Nutrition*, 86, 4: 1082–93

Neria, Y., Nandi, A. and Galea, S. (2008) 'Post-traumatic stress disorder following disasters: A systematic review' *Psychological Medicine*, 38: 467–80

Nesse, R.M. (2008) 'Evolution: Medicine's most basic science' *The Lancet*, 372: S21–7

Newton, J. (1988) *Preventing Mental Illness*, London: Routledge

Newton, J. (1992) *Preventing Mental Illness in Practice*, London: Routledge

NHS Information Centre (2011) *Attidtudes to Mental Illness – 2011 survey report*, NHS Information Centre, www.ic.nhs.uk (accessed 31 January 2012)

NICE (2006) *Parent-Training/Education Programmes in the Management of Children with Conduct Disorders*, London: NICE

NICE (2010) *Schizophrenia: Core interventions in the treatment and management of schizophrenia in adults in primary and secondary care (update)*, London: BPS and RCPsych

NIMH Prevention Research Steering Committee (1994) *The Prevention of Mental Disorders: A national research agenda*, Washington, DC: NIMH

NSPCC (2007) *Incidence of Official Records Of Child Maltreatment in Different Countries*, www.nspcc.org.uk/Inform (accessed 31 July 2011)

O'Connor, D.B. and Shimizu, M. (2002) 'Sense of personal control, stress and coping style: A cross-cultural study' *Stress and Health*, 18: 173–83

O'Connor, W. and Nazroo, J. (eds) (2002) *Ethnic Difference in the Context and Experience of Psychiatric Illness: A qualitative study*, London: The Stationery Office

OECD (2008) *Growing Unequal? Income distribution and poverty in OECD countries*, www.oecd.org/els/social/inequality (accessed 28 October 2010)

OECD (2009b) *Doing Better for Children*. Chapter 2 Comparative Child Wellbeing across the OECD. Chapter 7 The Way Forward

OECD Family Database (2008) *SF8: Marriage and Divorce Rates*, www.oecd.org/els/social/family/database (accessed 15 May 2010)

OECD Family Database (2009) *SF2: Children in Families*, www.oecd.org/els/social/family/database (accessed 15 May 2010)

OECD Family Database (2010) *SF2.3: Mean age of mother at first childbirth.* Paris: OECD Social Policy Division, Directorate of Employment, Labour and Social Affairs

Ogden, T., Forgatch, M.S., Askeland, E., Patterson, G.R. and Bullock, B.M. (2005) 'Implementation of parent management training at the national level: The case of Norway' *Journal of Social Work Practice*, 19, 3: 317–29

Ogden, T. and Hagen, K.A. (2008) 'Treatment effectiveness of parent management training in Norway: A randomized controlled trial of children with conduct problems' *Journal of Consulting and Clinical Psychology*, 76, 4: 607–21

O'Kearney, R.T., Anstey, K. and von Sanden, C. (2006) 'Behavioural and cognitive behavioural therapy for obsessive compulsive disorder in children and adolescents' *Cochrane Database of Systematic Reviews*, Issue 4, Art. No. CD004856

Oken, E., Østerdal, M.L., Gillman, M.W., et al. (2008) 'Associations of maternal fish intake during pregnancy and breastfeeding duration with attainment of developmental milestones in early childhood: A study from the Danish National Birth Cohort' *American Journal of Clinical Nutrition*, 88, 3: 789–96

Oldehinkel, A.J., Ormel, J. and Neeleman, J. (2000) 'Predictors of time to remission from depression in primary care patients: Do some people benefit more from positive life change than others?' *Journal of Abnormal Psychology*, 109, 2: 299–307

Olds, D.L. (2002) 'Prenatal and infancy home visiting by nurses: From randomized trials to community replication' *Preventive Science*, 3: 153–72

Olds, D.L. (2008) 'Preventing child maltreatment and crime with prenatal and infancy support of parents: The nurse–family partnership' *Journal of Scandinavian Studies in Criminology and Crime Prevention*, 9: 2–24

Olds, D.L., Henderson, C.R., Chamberlin, R. and Tatelbaum, R. (1986a) 'Preventing child abuse and neglect: A randomized trial of nurse home visitation' *Pediatrics*, 78: 65–78

Olds, D.L., Henderson C.R., Tatelbaum, R. and Chamberlin, R. (1986b) 'Improving the delivery of prenatal care and outcomes of pregnancy: A randomized trial of nurse home visitation' *Pediatrics*, 77: 16–28

Olds, D.L., Robinson, J., Pettitt, L., et al. (2004) 'Effects of home visits by paraprofessionals and by nurses: Age-four follow-up of a randomized trial' *Pediatrics*, 114: 1560–8

Olds, D.L., Kitzman, H., Hanks, C., et al. (2007) 'Effects of nurse home visiting on maternal and child functioning: Age-9 follow-up of a randomized trial' *Pediatrics*, 120, 4: e832–45

ONS (Meltzer, H. and Gatward, R.) (2000) *The Mental Health of Children and Adolescents in Great Britain*, London: TSO

ONS (Meltzer, H., Gatward, R., Corbin, T., Goodman, R. and Ford, T.) (2003a) *Persistence, Onset, Risk Factors and Outcomes of Childhood Mental Disorders*, London: TSO

ONS (Meltzer, H., Gatward, R., Corbin, T., Goodman, R. and Ford, T.) (2003b) *The Mental Health of Young People Looked After by Local Authorities in England*, London: TSO

ONS (Green, H., McGinnity, A., Meltzer, H., Ford, T. and Goodman, R.) (2005) *Mental Health of Children and Young People in Great Britain*, London: Palgrave Macmillan

ONS (2009a) *National Population Projections: 2008-based*, London: ONS

ONS (2009b) (McManus, S., Meltzer, H., Brugha, T., Bebbibgton, P. and Jenkins, R.) *Adult Psychiatric Morbidity in England 2007: Results of a household survey*, Leeds: NHS Information Centre

Patterson, G.R. (1982) *A Social Learning Approach: 3.Coercive family process*, Eugene, OR: Castalia

Patterson, G.R., DeGarmo, D. and Forgatch, M.S. (2004) 'Systematic changes in families following prevention trials' *Journal of Abnormal Child Psychology*, 32, 6: 621–33

Paulson, D.S., Krippner, S. and Kirkwood, J. (2007) *Haunted by Combat: Understanding PTSD in war veterans*, Westport, CT: Greenwood

Paykel, E., Abbott, R., Jenkins, R., Brugha, T. and Meltzer, H. (2003) 'Urban–rural mental health differences in Great Britain: Findings from the National Morbidity Survey' *International Review of Psychiatry*, 15, 97–107

Pearlin L.I., Menaghan, E.G., Lieberman, M.A. and Mullen, J.R. (1981) 'The stress process' *Journal of Health and Social Behaviour*, 22: 337–56

Pecora, P.J., White, C.R., Jackson, L.J. and Wiggins, T. (2009) 'Mental health of current and former recipients of foster care: A review of recent studies in the USA' *Child and Family Social Work*, 14: 132–46

Peen, J., Dekker, J., Schoevers, R., Have, M., Graaf, R. and Beekman, A. (2007) 'Is the prevalence of psychiatric disorders associated with urbanization?' *Social Psychiatry & Psychiatric Epidemiology*, 42, 12: 984–9

Peet, M. (2004) 'International variations in the outcome of schizophrenia and the prevalence of depression in relation to national dietary practices: An ecological analysis' *British Journal of Psychiatry*, 184: 404–408

Pelosi, A. and Birchwood, M. (2003) 'Debate: Is early intervention a waste of valuable resources?' *British Journal of Psychiatry*, 182: 196–8

Perkins, D.O., Gu, H., Boteva, K. and Lieberman, J.A. (2005) 'Relationship between duration of untreated psychosis and outcome in first-episode schizophrenia: A critical review and meta-analysis' *American Journal of Psychiatry*, 162, 10: 1785–804

Persson, G. and Skoog, I. (1996) 'A prospective population study of psycho-social risk factors for late onset dementia' *International Journal of Geriatric Psychiatry*, 11: 15–22

Peters, T. and Waterman, R. (1982) *In Search of Excellence*, New York: Harper & Row

Peterson, C. and Seligman, M.E.P. (2004) *Character Strengths and Virtues: A handbook and classification*, Washington, DC: American Psychological Association

Pfeffer, J. (1998) *Human Equation: Building profit by putting people first*, Boston: Harvard Business School Press

Pharoah, F., Mari, J., Rathbone, J. and Wong, W. (2010) 'Family intervention for schizophrenia (Cochrane Review)' *The Cochrane Library*, Issue 11

Phillips, J. (2010) *Expert Patients Programme: Self-care reduces costs and improves health – The evidence*, http://www.expertpatients.co.uk (accessed 20 November 2011)

Philo, G. (1994) 'Media images and popular beliefs' *Psychiatric Bulletin*, 18: 173–4

Pini, S., de Queiroz, V., Pagnin, D., et al. (2005) 'Prevalence and burden of bipolar disorders in European countries' *European Neuropsychopharmacology*, 15, 4: 425–34

Platt, S.D. and Kreitman, N. (1984) 'Trends in para-suicide and unemployment among men in Edinburgh, 1968–82' *British Medical Journal*, 289: 1029–32

Pollett, S.L. (2009) 'A nationwide survey of programs for children of divorcing and separating parents' *Family Court Review*, 47, 3: 523–43

Porter, R. (1987) *Mind Forg'd Manacles: Madness and psychiatry in England from the Restoration to Regency*, London: Athlone

Power, A. (1996) 'Area-based poverty and resident empowerment' *Urban Studies*, 33, 9: 1535–64

Power, A. (1999) *Estates on the Edge*, London: Macmillan

Power, A. and Willmot, H. (2007) *Social Capital within the Neighbourhood*, London: LSE CASE Report 38

Price, J.S. (1968) 'The genetics of depressive behaviour' in Coppen, A. and Walk, A. (eds) *Recent Developments in Affective Disorders*, London: Royal Medico-Psychological Association, pp. 37–54

Price, J.S., Gardner, R., Wilson, D.R., Sloman, L., Rohde, P. and Erickson, M. (2007) 'Territory, rank and mental health: The history of an idea' *Evolutionary Psychology*, 5, 3: 531–54

Prochaska, J.O. and DiClemente, C.C. (1984) *The Transtheoretical Approach: Crossing traditional boundaries of change*, Homewood, IL: Dorsey Press

Prochaska, J.O., DiClemente, C.C. and Norcross, J.C. (1992) 'In search of how people change: Applications to addictive behaviors' *American Psychologist*, 47, 9: 1102–14

Prudo, R., Harris, T.O. and Brown, G.W. (1984) 'Psychiatric disorder in a rural and an urban population: 3. Social integration and the morphology of affective disorder' *Psychological Medicine*, 14: 327–45

Putnam, R.D. (2000) *Bowling Alone: The collapse and revival of American community*, New York: Simon & Schuster

Putnam, R.D. (2004) Commentary: 'Health by association: Some comments' *International Journal of Epidemiology*, 33: 667–71

QResearch (Hippisley-Cox, J. and Jumbu, G.) (2008) *Trends in Consultation Rates in General Practice 1995 to 2007: Analysis of the QRESEARCH database*, London: NHS Information Centre

Quinton, D. and Rutter, M. (1984a) 'Parents with children in care: I. Current circumstances and parenting' *Journal of Child Psychology and Psychiatry*, 25: 211–29

Quinton, D. and Rutter, M. (1984b) 'Parents with children in care: II. Intergenerational continuities' *Journal of Child Psychology and Psychiatry*, 25: 231–50

Quinton, D., Rutter, M. and Liddle, C. (1984) 'Institutional rearing, parenting difficulties and marital support' *Psychological Medicine*, 14: 107–21

Quinton, D., Pickles, A., Maugham, B. and Rutter, M. (1993) 'Partners, peers and pathways: Assertive mating and continuities in conduct disorder' *Development and Psychopathology*, 5: 763–83

Rajji, T.K., Ismail, Z., and Mulsant, B.H. (2009) 'Age at onset and cognition in schizophrenia: Meta-analysis' *British Journal of Psychiatry*, 195: 286–293

Ramel, W., Goldin, P.R., Carmona, P.E. and McQuaid, J.R. (2004) 'The effects of mindfulness meditation on cognitive processes and affect in patients with past depression' *Cognitive Therapy and Research*, 28, 4: 433–55

Rapp, C.A. (1998) *The Strengths Model: Case management for people suffering from severe and persistent mental illness*, New York: Oxford University Press.

Ravens-Sieberer, U., Erhart, M., Gosch, A., Wille, N. and the KIDSCREEN Group (2008) 'Mental health of children and adolescents in 12 European Countries – Results from the European KIDSCREEN Study' *Clinical Psychology & Psychotherapy*, 15: 154–63

RCPsych (Royal College of Psychiatrists) (2010) *No Health without Public Mental Health: The case for action. Position statement*, London: RCPsych

Read, J., Agar, K., Argyle, N. and Aderhold, V. (2003) 'Sexual and physical abuse during childhood and adulthood as predictors of hallucinations, delusions and thought disorder' *Psychology and Psychotherapy: Theory, Research and Practice*, 76, 1–22

Read, J., Goodman, L., Morrison, A.P., Ross, C.A. and Aderhold, V. (2004) 'Childhood trauma, loss and stress' in Read, J., Mosher, L.R. and Bentall, R.P. (eds) *Models of Madness*, Hove, UK: Routledge

Read, J., Seymour, F. and Mosher, L.R. (2004) 'Unhappy families' in Read, J., Mosher, L.R. and Bentall, R.P. (eds) *Models of Madness*, Hove, UK: Routledge

Read, M. (1993) 'Seat belts and freedom of the individual' in Mills, M. (ed) *Prevention, Health and British Politics*, Aldershot, UK: Ashgate

Regan, L. and Kelly, L. (2003) *Rape: Still a forgotten issue*, London: London Metropolitan University Child and Women Abuse Studies Unit, www.rcne.com/downloads/RepsPubs/Attritn.pdf (accessed 11 October 2010)

Reid, J.B. and Patterson, G.R. (1989) 'The development of anti-social behaviour problems in childhood and adolescence' *European Journal of Personality*, 3: 107–19

Reiss, D. and Price, R.H. (1996) 'National research agenda for prevention research' *American Psychologist*, 51, 11: 1109–15

Report of the Surgeon General (1999) *Mental Health: A report of the Surgeon General*, www.surgeongeneral.gov/library/mentalhealth/pdfs/c1.pdf (accessed 2 October 2011)

Rethink (2002) *Reaching People Early*, Kingston upon Thames, UK: Rethink

Richardson, A.J. (2006) 'Omega-3 fatty acids in ADHD and related neurodevelopmental disorders' *International Review of Psychiatry*, 18, 2: 155–7

Richardson, A.J. (2007) *Presentation to UK Parliamentary Food and Health Forum: Omega 3 for child behaviour and learning*, www.fhf.org.uk/inquiry (accessed 16 August 2009)

Rinaldi, M., Perkins, R., Glynn, E., Montibeller, T., Clenaghan, M. and Rutherford, J. (2008) 'Individual placement and support: From research to practice' *Advances in Psychiatric Treatment*, 13: 50–60

Rinaldi, M., Killackey, E., Smith, J., Shepherd, G., Singh, S.P. and Craig, T. (2010) 'First episode psychosis and employment: A review' *International Review of Psychiatry*, 22, 2: 148–62

Roberts, N.P., Kitchiner, N.J., Kenardy, J. and Bisson, J. (2009) 'Multiple session early psychological interventions for the prevention of post-traumatic stress disorder' *Cochrane Database of Systematic Reviews*, Issue 3, Art. No. CD006869

Robins, L.N. (1966) *Deviant Children Grown-Up: A sociological and psychiatric study of sociopathic personalities*, Baltimore, MD: Williams & Wilkins

Robins, L.N. (1978) 'Psychiatric epidemiology' *Archives of General Psychiatry*, 35, 6: 697–702

Robins, L.N., and Regier, D.A. (1991) *Psychiatric Disorders in America: The Epidemiologic Catchment Area Study*, New York: Free Press

Robins, L.N., Wing, J.K., Wittchen, H.-U., et al. (1988) 'The composite international diagnostic interview: An epidemiologic instrument for use in conjunction with different diagnostic systems and in different cultures' *Archives of General Psychiatry*, 45: 1069–77

Robitschek, C. and Keyes, C.L.M. (2009) 'Keyes's model of mental health with personal growth initiative as a parsimonious predictor' *Journal of Counseling Psychology*, 56, 2: 321–9

Rose, D. (1995) *Official Social Classifications in the UK: Social research update, University of Surrey, Issue 9*, http://sru.soc.surrey.ac.uk/SRU9.html (accessed 3 August 2010)

Rose, G. (1981) 'Strategy of prevention: Lessons from cardiovascular disease' *British Medical Journal*, 282: 1847–51

Rose, G. (1985) 'Sick individuals and sick populations' *International Journal of Epidemiology*, 14: 32–8

Rose, G. (1992) *The Strategy of Preventive Medicine*, Oxford: Oxford University Press

Rose, G. and Day, S. (1990) 'For debate: The population mean predicts the number of deviant individuals' *British Medical Journal*, 301: 1031–4

Rowe, D. (2003) *Depression: The way out of your prison (third edition)*, London: Routledge

Royal College of Psychiatrists (2009) *Cognitive Behavioural Therapy Information Leaflet*, London: RCP

Rushton, A., Monck, E., Leese, M., McCrone, P. and Sharac, J. (2010) 'Enhancing adoptive parenting: A randomized controlled trial' *Clinical Child Psychology and Psychiatry*, 15, 4: 529–542

Russell, D.E.H. (1986) *The Secret Trauma*, New York: Basic Books

Russell, L.B. (2009) 'Preventing chronic disease: An important investment, but don't count on cost savings' *Health Affairs*, 28, 1: 42–5

Rutter, M. (1981) *Maternal Deprivation Reassessed (2nd edition)*, Harmondsworth, UK: Penguin

Rutter, M. (2006) 'Is Sure Start an effective preventive intervention?' *Child and Adolescent Mental Health* 11, 3: 135–41

Rutter, M., Cox, A., Tupling, C., Berger, M. and Yule, W. (1975a) 'Attainment and adjustment in two geographical areas: I. The prevalence of psychiatric disorder' *British Journal of Psychiatry*, 126: 493–509

Rutter, M., Yule, B., Quinton, D., Rowlands, O., Yule, W. and Berger, M. (1975b) 'Adjustment in two geographical areas: III. Some factors accounting for area differences' *British Journal of Psychiatry*, 126: 520–33

Rutter, M., Maughan, B., Mortimer, P. and Ousten, J. (1979) *Fifteen Thousand Hours: Secondary schools and their effects on children*, London: Open Books

Saha, S., Welham, J., Chant, D. and McGrath, J. (2006) 'Incidence of schizophrenia does not vary with economic status of the country: Evidence from a systematic review' *Social Psychiatry and Psychiatric Epidemiology*, 41: 338–40

Saint-Paul, G. (2008) 'Alternative strategies for fighting unemployment: Lessons from the European experience' *World Economics Journal*, 9, 1: 35–55

Salmon, A. (1985) *The Haunted Heroes*, film, London: BBC

Sampson, O.C. (1980) *Child Guidance: Its History, provenance and future*, London: British Psychological Society

Sampson, R.J., Morenoff, J.D. and Earls, F. (1999) 'Beyond social capital: Spatial dynamics of collective efficacy for children' *American Sociological Review*, 64, 5: 633–60

Sanders, M. R. (1999) 'Triple P-Positive Parenting Program: Towards an empirically validated multilevel parenting and family support strategy for the prevention of behavioural and emotional problems in children' *Clinical Child and Family Psychology Review*, 2, 71–90

Sastry, J. and Ross, C.E. (1998) 'Asian ethnicity and the sense of personal control' *Social Psychology Quarterly*, 61: 101–20

Sayce, L. (1998) 'Stigma, discrimination and social exclusion, what's in a word?' *Journal of Mental Health*, 7, 4: 331–44

Sayce, L. (2000) *From Psychiatric Patient to Citizen: Overcoming discrimination and social exclusion*, Basingstoke, UK: Macmillan

Scarpetta, S., Sonnet, A. and Manfredi, T. (2010) 'Rising youth unemployment during the crisis: How to prevent negative long-term consequences on a generation?' *OECD Social, Employment and Migrations Working Papers No. 106*, Paris: OECD

Scheff, T. (1966) *Being Mentally Ill: A sociological theory*, Chicago: Aldine

Schilling, E., Aseltine, R. and Gore, S. (2007) 'Young women's social and occupational development and mental health in the aftermath of child sexual abuse' *American Journal of Community Psychology*, 40, 1/2: 109–24

SCMH (Sainsbury Centre for Mental Health) (2007) *Mental Health and Employment. Briefing No. 33*, London: Centre for Mental Health

Scott, J. (2008) 'Cognitive behavioural therapy for severe mental disorders: Back to the future?' *British Journal of Psychiatry*, 192: 401–3

Scott, K.M., Von Korff, M., Alonso, J., et al. (2009) 'Mental–physical co-morbidity and its relationship with disability: Results from the world mental health surveys' *Psychological Medicine*, 39, 33–43

Scott, S. and Dadds, M.R. (2009) 'Practitioner review: When parent training doesn't work: Theory-driven clinical strategies' *Journal of Child Psychology and Psychiatry*, 50, 12: 1441–50

Scott, S., Knapp, M., Henderson, J. and Maughan, B. (2001a) 'Financial cost of social exclusion: Follow up study of antisocial children into adulthood' *British Medical Journal*, 323: 1–5

Scott, S., Spender, Q., Doolan, M., Jacobs, B. and Aspland, H. (2001b) 'Multicentre controlled trial of parenting groups for childhood antisocial behaviour in clinical practice' *British Medical Journal*, 323: 1–6

Secker, J., Grove, B. and Seebohm, P. (2001) 'Challenging barriers to employment, training and education for mental health service users: The service user's perspective' *Journal of Mental Health*, 10, 4: 395–404

Segerstrom, S.C. (2006) *Breaking Murphy's Law: How optimists get what they want from life – and pessimists can too*, New York: Guilford Press

Seligman, M.E.P. (1975) *Helplessness: On depression, development and death*, San Francisco: W.H. Freeman

Seligman, M.E.P., Steen, T.A., Park, N. and Peterson, C. (2005) 'Positive psychology progress: Empirical validation of interventions' *American Psychologist*, 60, 5: 410–21

Seligman, M.E.P., Rashid, T. and Parks, A.C. (2006) 'Positive psychotherapy' *American Psychologist*, 61: 774–88

Selten, J.P., Veen, N.D., Hoek, H.W., et al. (2007) 'Early course of schizophrenia in a representative Dutch incidence cohort' *Schizophrenia Research*, 97, 1–3: 79–87

Seymour, L. and Grove, B. (2005) *Workplace Interventions for People with Common Mental Health Problems: Evidence review and recommendations*. London: BOHRF

Shay, J. (1994) *Achilles in Vietnam: Combat trauma and the undoing of character*, New York: Atheneum

Shay, J. (2002) *Odysseus in America: Combat trauma and the trial of homecoming*, New York: Scribner

Shen, Y., Zhang, M., Huang, Y., et al. (2006) 'Twelve-month prevalence, severity, and unmet need for treatment of mental disorders in metropolitan China' *Psychological Medicine*, 36, 2: 257–67

Shepherd, M. (1978) 'Epidemiology and clinical psychiatry' *British Journal of Psychiatry*, 133: 289–98

Shinman, S. (1981) *A Chance for Every Child: Access and response to pre-school provision*, London: Tavistock

Shorter, E. (1997) *A History of Psychiatry: From the era of the asylum to the age of Prozac*, Chichester, UK: Wiley

Siegel, M., Albers, A., Chenq, D., Hamilton, W. and Biener, L. (2008) 'Local restaurant smoking regulations and the adolescent smoking initiation process' *Archives of Pediatric and Adolescent Medicine*, 162, 5: 477–83

Siegrist, J. and Theorell, T. (2006) 'Socio-economic position and health: The role of work and employment' in Siegrist, J. and Marmot, M. (eds) *Social Inequalities in Health*, Oxford: Oxford University Press

Silver, E., Mulvey, E.P. and Swanson, J.W. (2002) 'Neighborhood structural characteristics and mental disorder: Faris and Dunham revisited' *Social Science & Medicine*, 55, 8: 1457–70

Simkiss, D.E., Snooks, H.A., Stallard, N., et al. (2010) 'Measuring the impact of a universal group based parenting programme: Protocol and implementation of a trial' *BMC Public Health*, 10: 364

Simon, G.E., Goldberg, D.P., Von Korff, M. and Ustun, T.B. (2002) 'Understanding cross-national differences in depression prevalence' *Psychological Medicine*, 32: 585–594

Sin, N.L. and Lyubomirsky, S. (2009) 'Enhancing wellbeing and alleviating depressive symptoms with positive psychology interventions: A practice-friendly meta-analysis' *Journal of Clinical Psychology: In Session*, 65, 5: 467–87

Singer, M.T. and Wynne, L.C. (1966) 'Communication styles in parents of normals, neurotics and schizophrenics' *Psychiatric Research Report*, 20: 25–38

Singh, S.P. and Burns, T. (2006) 'Race and mental health: There is more to race than racism' *British Medical Journal*, 333: 648–51

Singleton, N., Bumpstead, R., O'Brien, M., Lee, A. and Meltzer, H. (2001) *Psychiatric Morbidity among Adults Living in Private Households, 2000*, London: The Stationery Office

Smith, R. (1985) '"I'm just not right": The physical health of the unemployed' *British Medical Journal*, 291: 1626–9

Social Exclusion Unit (1999) *Teenage Pregnancy*, London: SEU

Sofi, F., Cesari, F., Abbate, R., Gensini, G.F. and Casini, A. (2008) 'Adherence to Mediterranean diet and health status: Meta-analysis' *British Medical Journal*, 337, 7671: 673–5

Solomon, A. (2001) *The Noonday Demon*, New York: Simon & Schuster

Sorgaard, K.L., Sandanger, I., Sorensen, T., Ingebrigtsen, G. and Dalgard, O.S. (1999) 'Mental disorders and referrals to mental health specialists by general practitioners' *Social Psychiatry and Psychiatric Epidemiology*, 34: 128–135

Spataro, J., Mullen, P.E., Burgess, P.M., Wells, D.L. and Moss, S.A. (2004) 'Impact of child sexual abuse on mental health: Prospective study in males and females' *British Journal of Psychiatry*, 184: 416–21

Spijker, J., de Graaf, R., Ormel, J., Nolen, W.A., Grobbee, D.E. and Burger, H. (2006) 'The persistence of depression score' *Acta Psychiatrica Scandinavica*, 114: 411–16

Sproston, K. and Nazroo, J. (2002) *Ethnic Minority Psychiatric Illness Rates in the Community (EMPIRIC): Quantitative report*, London: The Stationery Office

Stansfeld, S.A., Head, J., Fuhrer, R., Wardle, J. and Cattell, V. (2003) 'Social inequalities in depressive symptoms and physical functioning in the Whitehall II study: Exploring a common cause explanation' *Journal of Epidemiology & Community Health*, 57: 361–7

Stegmann, M.E., Ormel, J., de Graaf, R., et al. (2010) 'Functional disability as an explanation of the associations between chronic physical conditions and 12-month major depressive episode' *Journal of Affective Disorders*, 124, 1/2: 38–44

Stein, M. (2006) 'Research review: Young people leaving care' *Child and Family Social Work*, 11, 3: 273–9

Stein, M. and Wade, J. (2000) *Helping Care Leavers: Problems and strategic responses*, London: Department of Health

Stephenson, J.M., Strange, V., Forrest, S., et al. (2004) 'Pupil-led sex education in England (RIPPLE study): Cluster-randomised intervention trial' *The Lancet*, 364: 338–46

Stephenson, J.M., Strange, V., Allen, E., et al. (2008) 'The long-term effects of a peer-led sex education programme (RIPPLE): A cluster randomised trial in schools in England' *PLoS Medicine*, 5: 1579–90

Stewart, J. (2006) 'An "enigma to their parents": The founding and aims of the Notre Dame Child Guidance Clinic, Glasgow' *The Innes Review*, 57, 1: 54–76

Stone, M.H. (1998) *Healing the Mind: A history of psychiatry from antiquity to the present*, London: Pimlico

Straub, R.E. and Weinberger, D.R. (2006) 'Schizophrenia genes – Famine to feast' *Biological Psychiatry*, 60: 81–3

Stroud, C.B., Davila, J. and Moyer, A. (2008) 'The relationship between stress and depression in first onsets versus recurrences: A meta-analytic review' *Journal of Abnormal Psychology*, 117, 1: 206–13

Surtees, P., Wainwright, N., Luben, R., Khaw, K. and Day, N. (2003) 'Sense of coherence and mortality in men and women in the EPIC-Norfolk United Kingdom prospective cohort study' *American Journal of Epidemiology*, 158: 1202–9

Sutherland, S. (1976) *Breakdown*, London: Palladin

Szreter, S. and Woolcock, M. (2004) 'Health by association? Social capital, social theory, and the political economy of public health' *International Journal of Epidemiology*, 33: 1–18

Teasdale, J.D., Scott, J., Moore, R.G., Hayhurst, H., Pope, M. and Paykel, E.S. (2001) 'How does cognitive therapy prevent relapse in residual depression? Evidence from a controlled trial' *Journal of Consulting and Clinical Psychology*, 69, 3: 347–57

Teng, Y.M. (2007) *Living Arrangements among the Elderly in Southeast Asia*, Paper for UN seminar, www.unescap.org (accessed 24 January 2012)

Thomas, R. and Zimmer-Gembeck, M.J. (2007) 'Behavioral outcomes of parent–child interaction therapy and Triple P – Positive Parenting Program: A review and meta-analysis' *Journal of Abnormal Child Psychology*, 35: 475–95

Thompson, M.J.J., Coll, X., Wilkinson, S., Uitenbroek, D. and Tobias, A. (2003) 'Evaluation of a mental health service for young children: Development, outcome and satisfaction' *Child and Adolescent Mental Health*, 8, 2: 68–77

Tierney, J.P., Grossman, J.B. and Resch, N.L. (2000) *Making a Difference: An impact study of Big Brothers/Big Sisters*, Philadelphia: Public/Private Ventures

Time to Change, www.time-to-change.org.uk (accessed 2 October 2011)

Time to Change (2008) *Stigma Shout: Service user and carer experiences of stigma and discrimination*, London: Time to Change

Titmuss, R. (1970) *The Gift Relationship: From human blood to social policy*, London: Allen & Unwin

Toshiyuki, K., Motoichiro, K., Reverger, R., Gusti Rai, T. and Kashima, H. (2005) 'Never-treated patients with schizophrenia in the developing country of Bali' *Schizophrenia Research*, 79, 2/3: 307–13

Tremblay, R.E. (2010) 'Developmental origins of disruptive behaviour problems: The "original sin" hypothesis, epigenetics and their consequences for prevention' *Journal of Child Psychology and Psychiatry*, 51, 4: 341–67

Tuke, S. (1813) *Description of the Retreat, an Institution near York, for Insane Persons of the Society of Friends*, Reprinted by Process Press, London, 1996

UNICEF (2003) 'A league table of child maltreatment deaths in rich nations' *Innocenti Report Card No. 5*, Florence, Italy: UNICEF Innocenti Research Centre

UNICEF (2007) 'Child poverty in perspective: An overview of child wellbeing in rich countries' *Innocenti Report Card No. 7*, Florence: UNICEF Innocenti Research Centre

US Department of Health and Human Services, Administration on Children, Youth and Families (2009) *Child Maltreatment 2007*, Washington, DC: US Government Printing Office

Van de Weyer, C. (2011) *Changing Diets, Changing Minds: How food affects mental wellbeing and behaviour*, London: Sustain

Van Straten, A., Geraedts, A., Verdock-de Leeuw, I., Andersson, G. and Cuijpers, P. (2010) 'Psychological treatment of depressive symptoms in patients with medical disorders: A meta-analysis' *Journal of Psychosomatic Research*, 69: 23–32

Vaughn, C.E. and Leff, J.P. (1976) 'The influence of family and social factors on the course of psychiatric illness: A comparison of schizophrenic and depressed neurotic patients' *British Journal of Psychiatry*, 129: 125–37

Veen, N.D., Selten, J.-P., van der Tweel, I., Feller, W.G., Hoek, H.W. and Kahn, R.S. (2004) 'Cannabis use and age at onset of schizophrenia' *American Journal of Psychiatry*, 161, 3: 501–6

Velayudhan, L., Poppe, M., Archer, N., Proitsi, P., Brown, R.G. and Lovestone, S. (2010) 'Risk of developing dementia in people with diabetes and mild cognitive impairment' *British Journal of Psychiatry*, 196: 36–40

Vickerman, K.A. and Margolin, G. (2009) 'Rape treatment outcome research: Empirical findings and state of the literature' *Clinical Psychology Review*, 29: 431–48

Von Korff, M.R., Scott, K.M. and Gureje, O. (eds) (2009) *Global Perspectives on Mental–Physical Comorbidity in the WHO World Mental Health Surveys*, New York: Cambridge University Press

Waddell, G. and Burton, K. (2006) *Is Work Good for Your Health and Wellbeing?* London: TSO

Wade, J. (2008) 'The ties that bind: Support from birth families and substitute families for young people leaving care' *British Journal of Social Work*, 38: 39–54

Wade, J. and Dixon, J. (2006) 'Making a home, finding a job: Investigating early housing and employment outcomes for young people leaving care' *Child & Family Social Work*, 11, 3: 199–208

Walker, G. (2007) *Mentoring, Policy and Politics*, Philadelphia: Public/Private Ventures

Warner, R. (1994/2004) (2nd & 3rd editions) *Recovery from Schizophrenia: Psychiatry and political economy*, Hove, UK: Brunner-Routledge

Warner, R. (2000) *The Environment of Schizophrenia: Innovations in practice, policy and communications*, London: Brunner-Routledge

Warner, R. (2003) 'Fact versus fantasy: A reply to Bentall & Morrison' *Journal of Mental Health*, 12, 4: 351–57

Warner, R. and Mandiberg, J. (2003) 'Changing the environment of schizophrenia at the community level' *Australasian Psychiatry*, 11, Supp.: S58–64

Webster-Stratton, C. and Hancock, L. (1998) 'Training for parents of young children with conduct problems: Content, methods, and therapeutic processes' in Briesmeister, J.M. and Schaefer, C.E. (eds) *Handbook of Parent Training*, 2nd ed., New York: Wiley

Weder, N. and Kaufman, J. (2011) 'Critical periods revisited: Implications for intervention with traumatized children' *Journal of the American Academy of Child and Adolescent Psychiatry* 50, 11: 1087–9

Weiss, R.S. (1982) 'Relationship of social support and psychological wellbeing' in Schulberg, H.C. and Killilea, M. (eds) *The Modern Practice of Community Mental Health*, San Francisco: Jossey-Bass

Weissberg, R.P. and Greenberg, M.Y. (1998) 'Prevention science and collaborative community action research: Combining the best from both perspectives' *Journal of Mental Health*, 7, 5: 479–492

Weissman, A., Gotlieb, L., Ward, S., Greenblatt, E. and Casper, R.F. (2000) 'Use of the Internet by infertile couples' *Fertility and Sterility*, 73: 1179–82

Weissman, M.M., Bland, R.C., Canino, G.J., et al. (1996) 'Cross-national epidemiology of major depression and bipolar disorder' *Journal of the American Medical Association*, 276: 293–9

Welham, J., Isohanni, M., Jones, P. and McGrath, J. (2009) 'The antecedents of schizophrenia: A review of birth cohort studies' *Schizophrenia Bulletin*, 35, 3: 603–23

Werner, E.E. (1995) 'Resilience in development' *Current Directions in Psychological Science*, 4, 3: 81–5

West, R. (2005) 'Editorial – Time for a change: Putting the transtheoretical (stages of change) to rest' *Addictions*, 100: 1036–9

WHO (1992) *International Statistical Classification of Diseases and Related Health Problems – Tenth Revision (ICD-10)*, Geneva, Switzerland: World Health Organization

WHO (1999) *Report of the Consultation on Child Abuse Prevention, 29–31 March 1999*, Geneva, Switzerland: World Health Organization

WHO (2001) *Strengthening Mental Health Promotion*, Geneva, Switzerland: World Health Organization (Fact sheet No. 220)

WHO (2002) Chapter 3: 'Child abuse and neglect by parents and other caregivers' in *World Report on Violence and Health*, Geneva, Switzerland: World Health Organization

WHO (2004) *Promoting Mental Health*, Geneva, Switzerland: World Health Organization

Wiggins, M., Bonell, C., Sawtell, M., et al. (2009) 'Health outcomes of youth development programme in England: Prospective matched comparison study' *British Medical Journal*, 339: b2534

Wilkinson, R.G (1996) *Unhealthy Societies: The afflictions of inequality*, London: Routledge

Williams, Stern & Associates (2005) *Healthy Families Florida Evaluation Report: January 1, 1999 – December 31, 2003*, Miami, FL: WSA, www.healthyfamiliesfla.org/pdfs/Final_Evaluation_1999-2003.pdf (accessed 9 March 2010)

Wing, J.K., Babor, T., Brugha, T., et al. (1990). 'SCAN: Schedules for Clinical Assessment in Neuropsychiatry' *Archives of General Psychiatry*, 47: 589–593

Wipfli, B.M., Rethorst, C.D. and Landers, D.M. (2008) 'The anxiolytic effects of exercise: A meta-analysis of randomized trials and dose–response analysis' *Journal of Sport & Exercise Psychology*, 30, 4: 392–410

Wolchik, S.A., Sandler, I.N., Winslow, E. and Smith-Daniels, V. (2005) 'Programs for promoting parenting of residential parents: Moving from efficacy to effectiveness' *Family Court Review*, 43, 1: 65–80

Wolfe, D.A. (2006) 'Preventing violence in relationships: Psychological science addressing complex social issues' *Canadian Psychology*, 47, 1: 44–50

Wolfe, D.A., Wekerle, C., Scott, K., Straatman, A.-L., Grasley, C. and Reitzel-Jaffe, D. (2003) 'Dating violence prevention with at-risk youth: A controlled outcome' *Evaluation Journal of Consulting and Clinical Psychology*, 71, 2: 279–91

Wolfensberger, W. (1983) 'Social role valorization: A proposed new term for the principle of normalization' *Mental Retardation*, 21, 6: 234–239

Wolpert, L. (2001) *Malignant Sadness: The anatomy of depression*, London: Faber & Faber

World Bank (2000) *World Development Report 1999–2000*, Washington, DC: World Bank

Wyatt, R.J., Green, M.F. and Tuma, A.H. (1997) 'Long term morbidity associated with delayed treatment of first admission schizophrenic patients' *Psychological Medicine*, 27, 261–268

Young, M. and Willmott, P. (1962) *Family and Kinship in East London*, London: Pelican

Zeilinski, D.S. and David, S. (2009) 'Child maltreatment and adult socio-economic well-being' *Child Abuse & Neglect*, 33, 10: 666–78

Index

Page references in *italic* indicate Figures and Tables.

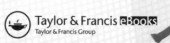